MODERN PERSPECTIVES IN PSYCHIATRY

Edited by John G. Howells

5

MODERN PERSPECTIVES
IN
PSYCHO-OBSTETRICS

MODERN PERSPECTIVES IN PSYCHIATRY
Edited by John G. Howells

MODERN PERSPECTIVES IN PSYCHO-OBSTETRICS

Edited by

JOHN G. HOWELLS

M.D., F.R.C.Psych., D.P.M.

Director, The Institute of Family Psychiatry
The Ipswich Hospital
England

BRUNNER/MAZEL *Publishers* · New York

Published by
BRUNNER/MAZEL, INC.
64 University Place, New York, N. Y. 10003

Originally published in United Kingdom by Oliver & Boyd, Edinburgh

Library of Congress Catalog Card No. 72-79142
SBN 87630-056-5

MANUFACTURED IN THE UNITED STATES OF AMERICA

EDITOR'S PREFACE

This fifth volume in the Modern Perspectives in Psychiatry Series aspires to the same goals as its predecessors. It aims to bring the facts from the growing points in a particular field of psychiatry to the clinician at as early a stage as possible. Thus, a single volume in this series is not a textbook; a psychiatric textbook has the double disadvantage of rapidly becoming out of date and of restricting to one, or at best to a few, authors the coverage of a field as large as psychiatry. However, the eventual scope of the volumes in the whole series is such as to constitute a complete international system in the theory and practice of psychiatry.

Contributions likely to be significant in the development of international psychiatry are selected from all over the world. It is hoped that the series will be a factor in effecting integration of world psychiatry and that it will supply a forum for the expression of creative opinion wherever it may arise. In the present volume will be found original contributions of authorities from Canada, France, Sweden, the United Kingdom, the United States of America and the Union of Soviet Socialist Republics.

Each chapter is written by an acknowledged expert, often the leading authority in his field. He was entrusted with the task of selecting, appraising and explaining his special subject for the benefit of colleagues who may be less well acquainted with it. Each chapter is not an exhaustive review of the literature on the subject, but contains what the contributor regards as relevant to clinical practice in that field. This volume will be valuable to both obstetrician and psychiatrist, the general medical practitioner, and allied professions.

Volumes in the Modern Perspectives in Psychiatry Series are complementary. Readers of this volume will find of especial interest the already published Volume 1, *Modern Perspectives in Child Psychiatry*, and Volume 3, *Modern Perspectives in International Child Psychiatry*. In Volume 1 the relevant chapters are: The genetical aspects of child psychiatry; Normal child development and handicapped children; The psychiatric aspects of adoption; The aetiology of mental subnormality; The neuropsychiatry of childhood; and in Volume 3: The child's hazards in utero; Genesis of behaviour disorders; Mother-infant relations at birth; Fathering. The list of contents of the volumes already published will be found at the back of this volume.

The place of the series as a major work of reference is assured by the appearance of cumulative indices in each volume. As in the previous volumes, the cumulative indices of this volume have again been prepared by my Editorial Assistant, Mrs. M. Livia Osborn. My grateful thanks are due to her for her valuable work and for her indefatigable help with many matters of preparation, presentation and editing.

Grateful acknowledgement is also made to the following publishers and editors of journals, and to the Authors concerned for kind permission to reproduce the material mentioned: Dr. Myre Sim and Dr. Alun Jones for the cases in Ch. IV on pages 79 and 79–80, respectively: Fig. 1 of Ch. IV was reproduced as Plate 134 in *Chinese Art* by S. W. Bushell (Victoria and Albert Museum: Board of Education 1909) and in *The Philosophy of the Bed* by M. Eden and R. Carrington (Hutchinson, 1961); Dr. George J. Train for the quotation from "Psychodynamics in obstetrics and gynecology", *Psychosomatics*, 1965, **6**, in Ch. VII; the Association for the Aid of Crippled Children for portions of "Pregnancy, childbirth and the outcome: a review of patterns of culture and future research needs" by Niles Newton from the chapter by Margaret Mead and Niles Newton in *Childbearing—its social and psychological aspects*, edited by Stephen A. Richardson and A. F. Guttmacher, Williams and Wilkins, 1967 and *Journal of the American Medical Association*, 1964, **188** for portions of "Some aspects of primitive childbirth" by Niles Newton in Ch. VIII; Syntex Information Service, Ch. IX, Figs. 1, 2 and 3; Dr. J. Stallworthy and *The Practitioner*, 1970, **204**, Ch. X, Figs. 1 and 2; *Canadian Medical Association Journal*, 1961, **84**: 647, and 1961, **84**: 1064. Ch. XIV, Tables II, IV, and V; Tavistock Publications Ltd. for material from *Key concepts in community psychiatry* used in Ch. XV; *New England Journal of Medicine*, 1967 for Drs. N. and M. Newton's paper on "Psychological aspects of lactation", and *Clinical Obstetrics and Gynecology*, 1962, for portions of their paper on "The normal course and management of lactation", in Ch. XXI; *American Journal of Psychiatry*, 1969, 1970, **126**, for significant portions of Ch. XXII.

CONTENTS

PART TWO

CLINICAL

PRE-NATAL

PERI-NATAL

PART ONE

GENERAL

I

BIRTH PROCESSES AND MATERNAL BEHAVIOR IN SOME FAMILIAR LABORATORY MAMMALS*

HOWARD MOLTZ

PH.D.

and

MICHAEL LEON

M.A.

The University of Chicago
Chicago, Illinois, U.S.A.

1

Introduction

For any mammalian species to survive, it must not only reproduce, it must also care for its young. Why mammals exhibit this care, why they come to nurse and otherwise nurture their offspring, is the subject of the present chapter.

Before approaching that subject, however, it must first be emphasized that maternal behavior is not expressed uniformly throughout the mammalian series; rather, it is expressed in a diversity of ways, a diversity which seems limited only by the requirements of litter survival. Some mammals build nests prior to parturition, such as rat and mouse, for example; others, such as the rabbit, build nests either before or during parturition, depending on the species (Ross et al.[84]); and still others, dogs and cats, do not build at any time. Placentophagy is widespread among mammals but there are several families which do not exhibit this behavior—Camilidae is one such family (Pitters[69]) and Phocidae is another (Bartholomew[6]). The rat and mouse retrieve young when the young wander from the nest, but under the same circumstances the rabbit remains indifferent. And finally, while all mammals of course nurse their young, the time they actually spend in this activity shows wide variation. At one extreme is the tree shrew (family Tupaiidae) which nurses only at 48-hour intervals and then for only five or ten minutes per session (Martin[55]); at the other extreme perhaps is the

* This chapter was written while the senior author was in receipt of Research Grant 5R01HD03651 from the National Institutes of Health of the Public Health Service.

laboratory rat which, at least during the first three or four days following parturition, spends some 20 hours a day in contact with young (Holland[39]).

To the extent that the interspecific divergences we have just mentioned reflect fundamental differences in physiological organization and psychological complexity, to that extent no single explanation of maternal behavior is likely to obtain across the entire class of mammals; and of course there is no reason to expect it should. The mammalian series, after all, includes an enormous diversity of species, each representing in some degree a distinct level of biological and behavioral integration (Schneirla[90]). For each, then, to nurture its young in exactly the same way and, in particular, for each to have that behavior governed by the same causal determinants, would be most improbable indeed.

The natural history of mammals, as Lehrman[52] has pointed out, has not inspired as widespread or as intense an interest as that of birds. As a result, we simply do not have, except for a few familiar mammals, any really precise and complete descriptions of maternal behavior. Rather, the bulk of our information consists of scattered and fragmentary facts about the way in which one species nurses and the other retrieves. Such facts, while sufficient to highlight interspecific differences in maternal behavior, are not sufficient to provide the kind of descriptive data needed to begin the search for causal determinants. For this, we must know, for example, whether the female characteristically builds a nest, and, if so, just how it is constructed. We must know also the behavioral details of the birth process and just when, in relation to the time the young emerge, the various items of the maternal complex appear. Finally, since the litter situation does not remain static, there must also be included in every maternal profile a detailed description of the way in which the mother-young interaction changes to reflect changes in both the physiological condition of the mother and the stimulus characteristics of the young.

There is still another point that must be emphasized. Before attempting to explain the maternal behavior of any species, we must have available for that species not only the kinds of observational details just mentioned, but some knowledge as well of the intraorganic mechanisms underlying gestation and birth. Unfortunately, it is only for the rat, and to a much more limited extent for the rabbit, that we have both sufficient behavioral data and sufficient physiological evidence to support an integrated analysis. Of necessity, then, it is upon the rat and rabbit that the present chapter must focus. However, it is hoped that detailed consideration of these two species will at least raise experimental questions relevant to the development and subsequent expression of maternal behavior in other mammalian forms.

2

Characteristics of Maternal Behavior in the Rat

Gestation in the rat is characteristically 22–23 days in duration. Beginning about 24 hours before term, the female begins to construct a nest. The material employed—usually paper, hay or excelsior—which heretofore was used to build a flat, mat-like structure, is now used to construct what can be designated as the "preparturient nest". To build such a nest, the female pushes and plies the available material, usually with her mouth but often with her paws, until a circular or semi-circular mound is formed. Although distinctly different from the mat-like structure referred to above, the preparturient nest is only loosely constituted, having sides rarely exceeding one or two inches in height. Beginning almost immediately after parturition, however, the nest material is reworked to form a mound that is at once higher (four to six inches) and more compact. This the female accomplishes usually by reaching out with her mouth and pulling the material at first toward and then over her. When completed, the postparturient nest often hides from view both mother and pups. In the laboratory, the pre- and post-parturient nests are almost always constructed in that corner of the cage which the female had previously selected for sleeping (Eibl-Eibesfeldt[20]).

The birth of the young takes place in the preparturient nest and is heralded by peristaltic-like waves passing posteriorly along the flank musculature. For a period of some 10 hours prior to parturition the female lies quietly, usually with the ventral surface of her body against the floor and with her legs stretched backwards. As the uterine contractions become more vigorous, however, and as the interval between contractions shortens, she begins to arch her back, pressing her abdomen hard against the floor. Suddenly her posture changes, as a result, presumably, of the first fetus entering the lower birth canal; at this time she adopts what Sturman-Hulbe and Stone[101] appropriately enough, called "the head between heels position". When in such a position, she vigorously licks the vaginal orifice, often biting and tearing the surrounding tissue as well. As the first fetus begins to emerge, it also is licked, and within a short time passes clear of the birth canal. When the placenta is expelled, the female takes the pup between her forepaws and devours the fetal membranes; the placenta and umbilicus are eaten thereafter in rapid order. As soon as the pup is free of fetal tissue, the mother begins to lick its body surface, coming gradually to concentrate on its anogenital area.

The second and subsequent deliveries occur in essentially the same way as the first, except that during these deliveries the female is less likely to adopt the "head-between-heels position". The interval between deliveries is variable and, in the case of a large litter, the delivery process may take several hours. Once the young are born and each has been cleaned, the female proceeds to rebuild the nest, transforming it from the low and loosely structured preparturient nest to the high and compact postparturient nest.

Nursing begins almost immediately after parturition, with the mother crouching over the young in such a way as to expose her mammary region. As the thermotactic pups begin to nuzzle in her fur, she adjusts her posture, allowing attachment first to one nipple then to another. After the pups are attached and suckling has begun, the mother usually either remains entirely passive or engages in no activity other than that of readjusting her position to sustain attachment.

Although simple in appearance, nursing is in fact a complex response. The mother must not only inhibit her own motor activity while adopting a posture that permits sucking, but at the same time must crouch in such a way as to maintain the body temperature of the young at approximately 100°F. Both these functions invariably demand subtle positional changes in response to movement of the pups. Just how subtle these adjustments actually are is exemplified occasionally by the female, which to all appearances seems to be nursing but whose pups are discovered to be cold and either dead or moribund.

Retrieving, the last maternal response item to be discussed, can be observed beginning at parturition. The mother grasps the pup, usually with the incisors and usually at the mid-dorsal region, although seizing a pup by its head or paw is not uncommon. Once seized, that pup is rapidly transported back to the nest.

In the laboratory, retrieving can most easily be elicited by removing the young from the nest and depositing them along the floor of the cage. Once aware that they are thus deployed, the female will grasp each in turn and transport them back to the nest. The fact that the pups are brought to the nest and not simply deposited at random, distinguishes retrieving from what might be called "carrying". Retrieving is directed, and serves to collect the young at a specific location; carrying is apparently aimless, and ends by leaving the young scattered. Occasionally, a puerperal female that has failed to establish a stable nest site will be seen to carry rather than retrieve. Such a female responds quickly enough to scattered young, but in transporting these young, she will drop some in one and some in another quadrant of the cage. Thus dispersed, a few will invariably die of neglect. (The reader is urged to consult also the excellent descriptions of maternal behavior in the rat provided by Rosenblatt & Lehrman,[81] and Wiesner and Sheard.[108])

3

Immediate Display of Maternal Behavior in the Puerperal Rat

An important fact in understanding the ontogeny of maternal behavior is that a nulliparous female, if kept continuously in the presence of young, will begin eventually to display interest in these young (Rosenblatt;[80] see

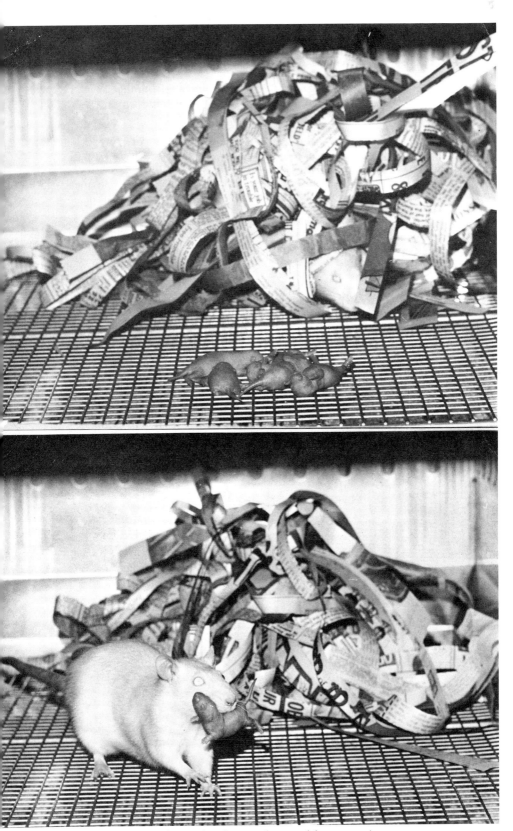

Mother rat retrieving her pups and returning them to the nest. (also see over)

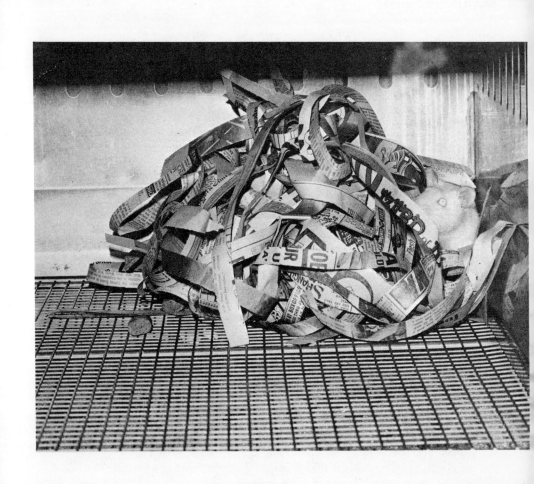

also Cosnier[13] and Wiesner and Sheard[108]). She will begin, in other words, to build a nest, lick, retrieve, and finally crouch in a nursing posture, indistinguishable from the puerperal female. That these responses are not instigated by hormonal changes resulting from enforced association with pups is evidenced by the fact that they occur with the same reliability in similarly confined nulliparae that have been either ovariectomized or hypophysectomized (Rosenblatt[80]).

But whereas the nulliparous female requires, on the average, some six or seven days of continuous exposure to pups before she will begin attending to them, her puerperal counterpart responds immediately upon their emergence from the birth canal. What accounts for this alacrity on the part of the puerperal female? Or, to put it another way, why is it that in such a female maternal behavior occurs in almost precise synchrony with the birth of the young? The need for this synchrony is of course obvious and it is to the events responsible that we now turn our attention. The correlative question of why the nulliparous female responds to young at all, will be considered in a later section.

The Experience of Parturition

Perhaps the difference in response latency between the puerperal and the nulliparous female can be explained by reference to an event as obvious as the occurrence of parturition. As is well known, parturition in the rat, as in most other mammalian forms, is characterized by a complex of responses that includes self-licking—particularly of the vaginal area—the ingestion of birth fluids, and the consumption of fetal and placental membranes. These events, paralleled by such endogenous phenomena as oxytocin release, uterine contractions, and the emergence of the fetuses, might by their very nature be instrumental in orienting the puerperal female toward the young and consequently in instigating immediate responsiveness.

This view of parturition as providing experiences important, and perhaps even essential, for the characteristic behavior of the puerperal female has been advanced previously by several investigators. Schneirla,[91] for example, speaks of "parturitive behavior" as "facilitating initiation of nursing and other stimulative relations of mother and new-born" (p. 421). Similarly, Rosenblatt and Lehrman,[81] in discussing the immediate responsiveness of the puerperal female, suggest that it might be occasioned, in part at least, by the experience gained during the parturitive process itself.

In an effort to determine whether parturition can be invoked to explain the difference in latency between puerperal and nulliparous rats, Moltz, Robbins, and Parks[64] undertook to deliver near-term females (21 days, 6 hours *post coitum*) by caesarean section. These females, half of whom were breeding for the first time (primiparous), and half of whom had reared two previous litters (multiparous), had fetuses and placentas removed surgically and then, after a period of time sufficient to permit mammary parenchyma to reach a secretory level comparable to that found in normal puerperae, were presented with normally-delivered foster pups. The data left no doubt about the answer to the question. Each caesarean-sectioned female, multiparous as well as primiparous, responded to foster young with an alacrity indistinguishable from that of the normally-delivered female. That the behavior thereafter was also indistinguishable was revealed by systematic observations of the mother, as well as by the weight of each litter at the time of weaning. Obviously enough, whatever role the experience of parturition plays in the induction of maternal behavior, it is not of sufficient importance to account for the difference in latency between the puerperal and the nulliparous female.

Relief from Uterine Distension

It is possible that it is not the experience of parturition as such, but simply the relief from uterine distension, that is the critical event underlying puerperal responsivity. If such were in fact the case, then of course whether the near-term conceptus was removed surgically or delivered vaginally would be irrelevant, because in each case the female would be expected to show immediate maternal behavior.

Klein[42] undertook to investigate this possibility by ligating the lower end of each uterine cornu in the mid-pregnant rat. At the expected time of parturition, but of course while still retaining their own fetuses, such females were offered new-born foster young. Despite the continuance of uterine distension, each quickly showed what the experimenter referred to as "quite normal nestling and maternal behavior" (p. 86).

In a second study, Klein extraverted each fetus into the peritoneal cavity, leaving only the placentas inserted in the uterine wall. These females were at mid-pregnancy at the time of the operation; and, although the operation afforded virtually complete relief from uterine distension, they showed no maternal behavior when offered foster young.

It is possible of course that the stimulative events related to the evacuation of the conceptus do play a role in instigating nurtural responsivity in the puerperal female. But, like the experience of parturition, this role appears to be in no way critical.

Mammary Engorgement

It is well known that in the rat, and of course in other mammals as well, the onset of lactation occurs at about the time of parturition, so that when the young emerge the mammae are already distended with milk (Kuhn,[45, 46] Kuhn and Lowenstein,[47] Shinde et al.[97]). In this condition, the puerperal female promptly begins to nurse, and, as we have already mentioned, begins with equal promptness to exhibit other maternal responses. Perhaps it is mammary engorgement or, more precisely, the peripheral stimulation accompanying that engorgement, that can explain the latency difference between puerperal and nulliparous females. Already present in the puerperal female during parturition, such stimulation may induce nursing as soon as pups to be nursed become available—and nursing in turn may induce retrieving and nest-building in rapid sequence. The nulliparous female, of course, experiences no intramammary stimulation, and thus, in contrast to her puerperal counterpart, may lack a stimulative dimension critical for inducing immediate attention to young.

One way of determining the criticality of mammary engorgement in the behavior of the puerperal female is to determine whether such a female will display nursing, nest-building, and retrieving with characteristic alacrity, even when deprived of all mammary tissue and hence of all mammary stimulation.

Moltz, Geller, and Levin[59] subjected weanling rats to a total mammectomy and, incidentally, to a total thelectomy (surgical removal of the nipples) as well. When these animals matured and were then impregnated and allowed to give birth normally, they behaved in a manner indistinguishable from intact puerperae. Obviously, intramammary tension is not a critical event in the initiation of maternal behavior, nor, of course, can it be enlisted to explain puerperal-nulliparous differences in maternal latency.

Self-licking

The nulliparous rat spends a significant amount of time in grooming or self-licking, focusing this activity primarily on the head and forepaws and on the shoulders and upper back (Roth & Rosenblatt[87]). Although she licks other areas of her body as well, they receive scant attention as compared with the areas just mentioned. With the advent of pregnancy, however, this pattern of self-licking changes. Now the female focuses most of her attention on those parts of her body which before she had largely ignored— vagina, pelvis, and nipples (Roth and Rosenblatt;[87] see also Steinberg and Bindra[98]).

Undoubtedly, there are many events underlying this shift in licking. One such class of events, as Roth and Rosenblatt themselves point out, probably arises from pregnancy-induced changes, which come to be localized largely in what has been called the "critical body regions". For example, the nipples enlarge during pregnancy with the base of each nipple becoming bare of fur, the abdomen increases in girth, and the vagina partially evaginates and discharges fluid. In addition to these peripheral changes, however, self-licking during pregnancy may be regulated as well by an increased need for salt, a need which, as Lehrman[51] and Bindra[9] have suggested, could be met by the ingestion of the presumably "salty" vaginal exudate. In support of this suggestion, Steinberg and Bindra[98] found that the addition of sodium chloride to the diet of the pregnant rat significantly reduced genital-licking, while leaving unaffected the licking of nipples and pelvic region.

Irrespective, however, of just what it is that induces so marked a change in licking focus, the important question for our purposes is what role, if any, this change plays in the induction of maternal behavior? Having had, in other words, the kind of licking experience that pregnancy alone brings, is the puerperal female thereby "prepared" for the appearance of the young in ways that the nulliparous female is not?

Birch[10] raised female rats with rubber collars around their necks, thereby preventing licking of any body area posterior to the collar. Removing the collars some two to three hours prior to parturition, he found his experimental subjects markedly deficient in maternal behavior. More specifically, the majority either cannibalized at the time of birth or simply remained indifferent; and even in those cases in which some attention was paid to young, the latencies were, in Birch's words, "abnormally long". On the basis of these data, Birch, and other investigators following him (e.g., Lehrman[51]), hypothesized that ventral and, in particular, vaginal licking during pregnancy is transferred to the pup, as the pup, in emerging from the birth canal, becomes an extension of the mother's body.

This is a simple and attractive hypothesis, one that has been repeatedly invoked to account for the behavioral difference between puerperal and nulliparous females. Unfortunately, however, the data on which it is based have not been confirmed. Coomans (cited in Eibl-Eibesfeldt[19]), Friedlich,[29] and Kirby and Horvath[41] have each repeated Birch's study but without obtaining Birch's results. Christopherson and Wagman[11] have also tried to replicate these results, even depriving their rats of self-licking at as early an age as eleven days. They too, however, failed to affect in any way the characteristic behavior of the puerperal female. Although it is difficult to account for Birch's original data, what seems clear is that the unique pattern of self-licking displayed by the pregnant female does not underlie the immediate interest in young she subsequently shows at the time of parturition.

The Hormones of Parturition

Thus far, neither the experience of parturition, mammary engorgement, relief from uterine distension, nor self-licking during pregnancy has provided a clue to the maternal behavior of the puerperal female. But of course there is still another dimension along which she differs from her nulliparous counterpart.

As long ago as 1925, Stone[99] advanced the hypothesis that the endocrine changes accompanying the termination of pregnancy might underlie the onset of maternal behavior also. This is an obvious idea of course, readily suggested by the observation that such maternal actions as nursing, nest-building, and retrieving are each initiated in the puerperal female in close temporal association with the birth process. But just what are the hormonal events which characteristically precipitate parturition and perhaps also maternal behavior? A complete answer, unfortunately, cannot be given, since even now there are too many gaps in our understanding of the mammalian birth process. Nonetheless, many investigators of maternal behavior have attempted to manipulate the blood concentrations of the gonadal steroids and the pituitary gonadotrophins. The aim, of course, was to induce immediate or near-immediate maternal behavior in the nulliparous female.

Stone[99] joined pairs of females in parabiotic union by means of a small abdominal junction. One of the twins of each pair was then impregnated and allowed to give birth. This female, despite her enforced union, gave birth normally and displayed maternal behavior immediately upon the emergence of the young; her nulliparous twin, in contrast, remained indifferent to foster pups offered her. But there is serious question here as to just which hormones, if any, passed from the parturient female to the nulliparous twin. Estrogen evidently did not, as evidenced by the condition of the vaginal epithelium; neither did prolactin apparently, since none of the nulliparae showed signs of mammary change.

Using direct injections of plasma rather than hoping for diffusion across a parabiotic union, Terkel and Rosenblatt,[104] recently accomplished what Stone had set out to do—they demonstrated that substances present in the blood at the time of parturition can induce maternal behavior. Specifically, they compared nulliparous females given plasma taken from puerperal females with those given plasma taken from proestrus and diestrus females, respectively. Only those nulliparous subjects given the "maternal plasma" showed a significant reduction in the onset of maternal behavior, responding to foster young, on the average, 48 hours after they were proffered (with a good deal of variability, however). Each of the remaining groups did not differ significantly from untreated nulliparae, taking, as is characteristic of such females, some six or seven days to respond.

Terkel[103] has recently developed a method for effecting a continuous cross-transfusion of blood between two freely-moving rats. Using this technique to transfuse "maternal blood", he was able to reduce not only the latency with which his nulliparae responded to foster young but the high variability they had previously exhibited following discrete injections.

This reduction in latency is impressive, although it is counted in hours rather than in minutes. Perhaps the endocrine agents actually involved require time to condition or excite the neuronal substrate mediating the several response items of the maternal complex. In any event, there can be no doubt that substances in the blood of puerperal females can "increase the readiness of virgins to respond maternally to pups" (Terkel and Rosenblatt,[104] p. 481). Of course, as the experimenters themselves point out, their studies do not offer any clues as to precisely which hormone or hormones were in fact responsible for the results obtained. The studies now to be reviewed have each been addressed to this more specific question.

Wiesner and Sheard[108] used a battery of hormones—or more precisely a battery of crude hormone extracts—prepared, respectively, from mare and human pregnancy urine, bovine corpora lutea, minced human placenta, and bovine anterior pituitary tissue. Both intact and ovariectomized nulliparae were injected with one or another of these extracts and tested daily for retrieving. In some of the experiments reported, the foster young were housed with the experimental females; in others they were available only during the retrieving test. Neither the luteal, urinary, nor placental products induced either retrieving or any other response item in the maternal complex. Anterior pituitary extracts, on the other hand, were somewhat more effective, although even here only about 33% of the nulliparae tested responded maternally. A frequency of 33% is of course not an impressive finding and, in the present case, is particularly difficult to interpret because of the crude nature of the pituitary extracts employed. Interestingly enough, of all the agents that must have been contained in these pituitary extracts, prolactin was specifically dismissed as responsible for inducing the limited retrieving that was observed. The grounds for this dismissal, simply enough, was that it seemed "exceedingly unlikely that the same factor [would be] responsible for both mammary secretion and maternal behavior, quite apart from the mutual independence of the two phenomena" (p. 234).

Riddle and his associates reported a series of studies that have been widely cited in the literature and as widely misinterpreted. Having previously found that broodiness in fowl "seems to be induced only or chiefly by prolactin", they attempted to determine whether prolactin—and a variety of other hormones and chemical agents as well—would induce maternal behavior in the rat (Riddle,[75] Riddle et al.,[76, 77, 78, 79]). Nulliparous females of between 60 and 70 days were used, some of which remained intact, while others were ovariectomized. After eliminating what Riddle et al. called "normal reactors", i.e., females which spontaneously showed interest in young during a series of 10-minute tests prior to treatment, each animal was injected daily for 10 days and then tested each day for 10 minutes with a single pup. If the pup was retrieved, the female was considered to have acted maternally.

Riddle et al. found prolactin, intermedin, and luteinizing hormone to induce retrieving in some 50 to 80% of both their intact and ovariectomized females. In contrast, whole anterior pituitary extract was effective in only the intact females, while follicle stimulating hormone (with thyrotrophin), pregnant mare's serum, "adrenotropin", and "Prolan" were each largely without effect. Among the steroid hormones used, progesterone, testosterone, and pellet implants (but not injections) of desoxycorticosterone were followed by retrieving in at least 65% of the animals tested. Phenol and thyroxine were also effective in inducing retrieving, but only in ovariectomized females. Estrone proved to have special properties—it terminated retrieving in animals that had begun to respond after injection of one or another of the above-mentioned substances.

Needless to say, the present results are difficult to interpret. In the first place, one would have wished Riddle et al. to have observed items in addition to retrieving and under conditions that involved more than a single foster pup presented for only 10 minutes. Maternal behavior, obviously enough, includes a complex of responses patterned over time and focused typically on an entire litter. These responses—retrieving, nursing, nestbuilding, and licking—are each essential for litter survival, and t~ this end must each be integrated by the female into an effective temporal sequence. To study retrieving alone, then, is not to study "maternal behavior"—it is to study retrieving. And under stimulation from just a single pup, it is doubtful whether even retrieving can be tested meaningfully.

In the second place, Riddle *et al.* used a bewildering variety of compounds, some of which seemed effective in one type of experimental female and some in another. It is instructive that the experimenters themselves do not suggest that each of these agents function also to induce retrieving in the puerperal female. On the contrary, in such females they suggest the action of a single hormone that (a) is released in increased amounts at the time of parturition, (b) exerts an antigonadal effect, and (c) excites either directly or indirectly the "sensorimotor mechanism" mediating maternal behavior. Prolactin, according to Riddle *et al.* "best fits these requirements." As to progesterone, desoxycorticosterone, and the several other agents claimed effective in inducing retrieving in nulliparae, the experimenters have little to say, except that these agents might have induced retrieving through their release of prolactin.

There have been several attempts to confirm the findings of Riddle *et al.* but each has been without success. Lott,[53] for example, injected ·25 mg of progesterone into nulliparous females every day for a period of ten days. On Day 11, 24 hours after the last injection, each experimental and each control (oil-injected) female was tested with a single foster pup for ten minutes daily for three days. There was no significant difference between groups and in fact little evidence of retrieving. Lott and Fuchs[54] administered 40 IU prolactin daily for ten days and once again found little evidence of retrieving. Finally, Beach and Wilson[7] injected 400 IU of prolactin daily for five days, following which not one but six foster pups were proffered each day for three consecutive days. In a second experiment, they administered estrogen for twenty-one consecutive days followed, concurrently, by injections of prolactin and progesterone. Neither of these regimens induced retrieving with any appreciable frequency.

Contradictory results are always difficult to explain. Lott, Lott and Fuchs, and Beach and Wilson used strains of rats different from the strain employed by Riddle *et al.*; they also used pituitary hormones of greater chemical purity. What is certain is that under the conditions of these experiments, neither prolactin, progesterone, nor even prolactin in combination with progesterone was found effective in inducing retrieving.

Convinced that further attempts to replicate the findings of Riddle *et al.* would be futile, other experimenters adopted a different approach to the problem of hormonal induction. Taylor[102] and Denenberg *et al.*,[16] for example, imposed a hormone regimen previously found effective in evoking maternal nest-building in ovariectomized nulliparous rabbits (Zarrow *et al.*[114]). This regimen involved injection of both estrogen and progesterone, with the subsequent withdrawal of progesterone prior to the termination of estrogen treatment. For use with the ovariectomized nulliparous rat estradiol (either ·2 μg or 1 μg) was administered from Day 1 to Day 19 and pro-gesterone (2 mg) from Day 2 to Day 15. In a second study, the progesterone treatment was extended to 19 days, and the estradiol treatment (now at a dose level of either 2 or 4 μg) to 27 days. The only index of maternal behavior employed was dowel-shredding which, like nest-building, has been found to exhibit a peak at, or just prior to, the time of parturition.[102] Contrary to expectation, there was no increase in the amount of material shredded following either the withdrawal of progesterone (Day 15 or Day 19) or the termination of estradiol (Day 19 or Day 27). If, as the experi-menters claim, an increase in dowel-shredding is "representative of maternal nest-building" (Denenberg et al.,[16] p. 14), then in the rat maternal nest-building cannot be evoked by an estrogen-progesterone regimen found effective in the rabbit.

Over the past several years a series of studies has been carried out in the authors' laboratory addressed also to the problem of hormonal induction. The approach adopted initially involved not the nulliparous but the pre-parturient female and the question asked was whether, in such females, selective disruption of the endocrine events accompanying parturition would subsequently interfere with the display of maternal behavior. If it did—if an imposed hormonal imbalance were in fact to render the puerperal female indistinguishable from her nulliparous counterpart—, then perhaps some insight would be gained into the problem of maternal latency.

In our first study,[65] we drew attention to the fact that associated with the birth process, and in some part responsible for the occurrence of that pro-cess, is a dramatic change in ovarian output, one that reverses the prevailing gestational ratio of estrogen to progesterone (Eto et al.,[23] Zarrow[112]). Simply enough, the question posed was whether or not manipulation of this appar-ently focal event would affect the onset of maternal behavior and, if it did, whether the influence thus exerted would be manifested differentially in primiparous and multiparous puerperae.

To this end, we ovariectomized (and of necessity delivered by caesarean section) each of our animals shortly before term. In response to the steroid imbalance imposed by our ovariectomy, only 50% of our primiparous females accepted immediately the foster litters offered them; the remaining 50% delayed acting maternally until, after three days, the young died of neglect. In contrast, virtually all of the multiparous animals behaved in characteristic puerperal fashion.

The ovariectomy just referred to resulted, of course, in the reduction of circulating levels of estrogen and, in view of the positive feedback effect of this steroid on prolactin discharge (Deis,[15] Everett,[24] Meites and Nicoll,[56] Nicoll and Meites,[66] Ramirez and McCann,[72] Ratner et al.,[73] Rothchild and Schwartz,[89] Welch et al.[105]) probably in the reduction of circulating prolactin as well. In addition, removing the ovaries also resulted in a decrease in plasma progesterone.

It seemed to us unlikely that the reduced concentration of progesterone effected through ovariectomy was responsible for the observed delay of maternal behavior among our primiparous females. As already mentioned, associated with the birth process in the rat is a shift in ovarian output, resulting, *inter alia*, in a *decrease* in progesterone titer. Both from the time course of this decrease (Fajer and Barraclough,[25] Grota and Eik-Nes,[36] Hashimoto *et al.*[38]) and from the fact that maternal behavior is initiated typically at a point of low progesterone concentration, we did not think our ovariectomy could have produced the observed behavioral effect merely as a result of having realized a still further reduction in progesterone titer. Indeed, not only did we consider this particular consequence of the operation to be irrelevant for the results obtained, but, on the contrary, we hypothesized that if the characteristic near-term decrease in blood progesterone were to be prevented from occurring, then the initiation of maternal behavior in turn would effectively be delayed (*cf.* Richards,[74] Rothchild[88]). Accordingly, we attempted to determine whether such manipulation of progesterone would in fact delay the appearance of maternal behavior and, if so, whether the effect thus exerted would once again be manifested differentially in the primiparous and multiparous female (Moltz, Levin and Leon[60, 61]).

Once again, both primiparous and multiparous females were used. Each, beginning on Day 19 of pregnancy, was injected with 2 mg of progesterone. On Day 21, caesarean sections were performed, necessitated by the failure of our rats to give birth normally under the progesterone dosage administered.

The results obtained paralleled those of our ovariectomy study. There, as here, a significant proportion of the primiparous females delayed responding to young until the young died of neglect. At the same time, virtually all the multiparous females responded immediately.

There is no doubt that selected hormonal manipulation can affect the latency to maternal behavior. However, before proceeding to discuss just which endocrine mechanisms are actually involved in governing the onset of maternal behavior in the puerperal female, it might be well at this point to ask how the observed influence of breeding history was mediated, of how, in other words, our multiparous females came to respond in a manner different from our primiparous females.

We can assume that selected hormonal agents function to increase the excitability of all or some of the neuronal mechanisms mediating maternal behavior, with the result that the puerperal female becomes immediately responsive to the sight, sound, and perhaps odor, of the young. We can also assume that these same neuronal mechanisms are modified by previous breeding experience in such a way as to increase their responsiveness to endocrine activation.

A plausible model for conceptualizing the effects such an increase might exert would involve the idea of threshold. Specifically, the very fact that the normal primiparous mother is as maternally proficient as the normal multiparous mother (Moltz and Robbins[63]) indicates that the substrate mediating maternal behavior is already differentiated and organized by the time the first birth is completed. Since a substrate of this kind must surely have threshold characteristics unique, in part at least, to each female, individual differences in tissue excitability would be expected to exist among primiparous animals—some primiparous animals, of course, having much lower arousal thresholds than others. Previous parity might increase the level of tissue excitability, so that, although individual differences persist, the average level of tissue excitability among multiparous animals would be higher than the average level that already prevails among primiparous animals. The threshold distribution of a multiparous group would then have a lower mean value than that of a primiparous group, but the distributions of these two groups would overlap because of individual differences in tissue excitability, which are unrelated to the occurrence of parity.

Clearly enough, a primiparous-multiparous difference of this kind, assuming it does typically exist, would not be manifested in behavior under conditions in which stimulating hormones prevail at blood concentrations above that demanded for arousal by even the most elevated tissue thresholds. Presumably, these are the concentrations that characteristically obtain following normal delivery and apparently following caesarean delivery as well. However, if only residual titers of key hormones are made to prevail, or if neuronal responsiveness to these key hormones is made to decrease, then only tissue mediators having low thresholds of arousal might respond. As a consequence, immediate maternal behavior would be seen only in animals possessing these particular thresholds.

In brief, we are suggesting that low thresholds to hormonal stimulation prevail among multiparous females but that, because of individual differences in tissue excitability, some primiparous animals have thresholds which fall within the lowered threshold distribution of the multiparous population. This suggestion could explain (a) why a significantly smaller incidence of immediate acceptance was found among the primiparous than among the multiparous females of both our ovariectomy and progesterone studies, and (b) why as many as half these primiparae nonetheless behaved without delay.

But of course the major problem still remains, namely the identity of the inductor hormones. Included in the report of our progesterone study was the hypothesis that these hormones are estrogen and prolactin, or more precisely the synergy of estrogen and prolactin. We now believe that progesterone is also essential. Consider first the titers of these endocrine agents in the normal pregnant female.

Progesterone, as assayed in both peripheral plasma (Grota and Eik-Nes,[36] Wiest et al.[110]) and ovarian venous plasma (Eto et al.,[23] Fajer and Barraclough,[25] Hashimoto et al.,[38] begins to increase on Day 4 of pregnancy, reaching maximal concentrations on Day 14. Thereafter the output of the steroid starts to fall slowly until, on Day 20, the decline becomes abrupt.

(This apparently is due to the sharp increase of 20 alpha-hydroxysteroid dehydrogenase, the enzyme largely responsible for the conversion of progesterone to 20 alpha-hydroxypregn-4-en-3-one (Kuhn,[46] Wiest,[109] Wiest et al.[110]).

That progesterone is taken up in rat brain during most of pregnancy can reasonably be inferred from studies showing the ready accumulation of the tritiated preparation in the non-pregnant female (Hamburg,[37] Laumas and Farooq,[50] Raisinghani et al.[70]). In such an animal, it has been found to elevate activation thresholds in cortical (Arai et al.,[2] Beyer et al.,[8] Komisaruk et al.,[44] Ramirez et al.[71]), diencephalic (Barraclough and Cross[4]), and hippocampal (Kobayashi et al.[43]) neurons. Probably many other neurons are similarly affected, since—unlike estrogen—progesterone shows no evidence of selective uptake in the central nervous system (Seiki et al.,[95, 96]).

Virtually coincident with the onset of progesterone withdrawal is a characteristic increase in plasma estrogen (Yoshinaga et al.[111]). Prevailing evidently at low concentrations prior to the time of mid-pregnancy, the secretory rate of estrogen begins increasing about Day 15. At first slowly, and then more rapidly, estrogen rises to peak value on or shortly before the day of parturition. It is selectively bound in specific brain regions, at least in the nonpregnant female, as the studies of Eisenfeld and Axelrod,[21, 22] Pfaff,[67, 68] and Stumpf[100] show.

Prolactin, the third hormone conceived essential for the immediate induction of maternal behavior, is released at the time of coition (Dilley and Adler[18]) but thereafter is maintained at low plasma concentrations until about Day 20 of pregnancy (Grindeland et al.,[35] Kwa and Verhofstad[49]). On Day 22, the day of parturition, it is seen to increase sharply (Amenomori et al.[1]). To the authors' knowledge, there is no evidence concerning prolactin uptake in the central nervous system; nor, in turn, is there evidence concerning the effect of prolactin on the uptake of other hormones.

At this point it might be well to ask why, of all the endocrine changes occurring at or near the time of parturition, progesterone, estrogen, and prolactin were selected as critical? What of the role of other hormones, particularly other hypophyseal and ovarian hormones?

The pituitary content of follicle stimulating hormone (FSH) increases dramatically between Days 12 and 16 of pregnancy, remaining at "remarkably high levels" until the day of delivery (Greenwald[34]). These high levels, however, reflect merely increased storage rather than increased synthesis and release as evidenced by the fact that the number of vesicular follicles remains constant throughout pregnancy.

There is a three-fold increase in the pituitary content of luteinizing hormone (LH) between Day 1 and Day 8 of pregnancy, but thereafter the content remains at a fairly steady level (Greenwald[34]). Apparently it is only following delivery—and several hours after maternal behavior has been established—that a surge of LH occurs. It is this surge that triggers the postpartum ovulation exhibited characteristically by the female rat.

Oxytocin, a polypeptide hormone synthesized in the hypothalamus and stored in the posterior pituitary (e.g. Cross[14]) has long been suspected of being one of the endocrine agents responsible for the initiation of labor. This suspicion has been strengthened recently by the detection of oxytocin during parturition in the jugular blood of sheep, cows, horses, and goats (cf. Fitzpatrick[28]). In the rat, however, assays of oxytocin have not been carried out, and consequently for this species we simply do not know whether concentrations of the peptide in peripheral blood change in any systematic way during labor and prior to the onset of maternal behavior.

Finally, there is the question of 20^α-hydroxypregn-4-en-3-one (20^α-OH) and its possible effect on the behavior of the puerperal female. As we have already mentioned, 20^α-OH is a metabolite of progesterone, synthesized within the ovary by the enzyme 20^α-hydroxysteroid dehydrogenase. Assays of peripheral blood have revealed a sharp increase in the concentration of 20^α-OH between Days 19 and 21 of gestation (Wiest et al.[110]). In itself, however, this near-term increase is probably without functional significance, 20^α-OH representing merely a byproduct of the "enzymatic process by which progesterone levels in the peripheral plasma and uterus are lowered" (Wiest,[109] p. 1183). But thus far 20^α-OH has been studied only in relation to the initiation of labor (Wiest[109]); its possible effect on the initiation of maternal behavior has not been investigated directly.

As is evident, we cannot decisively reject the possibility that oxytocin, or 20^α-OH, or even FSH is involved in the induction of maternal behavior. Nonetheless, these hormones were not manipulated by the present authors in the attempt to identify the endocrine mechanisms underlying the responsivity of the puerperal female. It was simply that, for purposes of experimentation, a choice had to be made, and progesterone, estrogen, and prolactin seemed functionally more relevant to the induction of maternal behavior than other ovarian and hypophyseal hormones. Moreover, it was possible to picture just how they might operate to evoke immediate attention to young.

We conceive of the maternal mediating system as being essentially insensitive to both estrogen and prolactin arousal so that at even relatively high titers these critical hormones characteristically fail to exert an activational effect. Probably before such an effect can occur, the mediating system must be primed, or, in other words, must be made to sustain lower-than-normal thresholds to estrogen and prolactin. It is here that progesterone, or rather that progesterone withdrawal, is believed to function.

Existing at high concentrations during the larger part of pregnancy, progesterone probably acts at first to maintain or even to increase activation thresholds within the mediating system. Beginning, however, on Day 15, blood levels of progesterone, as we have already mentioned, typically start to decline. It is conceivable that this decline, occurring from the high progesterone titers of pregnancy brings about within the mediating system an effect functionally akin to what Kawakami and Sawyer[40] called the "rebound from progesterone dominance". As pictured here, such a rebound would not only decrease selected thresholds within the mediating system but would carry these thresholds to levels lower than normal. It would, in other words, have the effect—at a time more or less coincident with the birth process—of rendering the mediating system sensitive to endocrine influence, particularly to the influence of estrogen and prolactin. It is only then, presumably, that estrogen and prolactin, themselves conditioned by near-term secretory rates, are able to excite the mediating substrate to a point that makes it acutely responsive to the sight, sound and odor of the young. Thus affected, the puerperal female can respond not in six or seven days but as soon as the young emerge from the birth canal.

With this picture in mind, we began to manipulate progesterone, estrogen and prolactin in the attempt to reduce the latency to maternal behavior in the nulliparous female. The experimental regimen that we finally adopted can be described briefly (Moltz, Lubin, Leon, and Numan[62]).

At between 90 and 110 days of age, nulliparous females were ovariectomized and three weeks later administered estradiol, progesterone and prolactin. The estradiol was injected once daily from Day 1 through Day 11 at a dosage level of 12 μg per injection; the progesterone twice daily on Days 6 through 9 at a dosage level of 3 mg per injection; and the prolactin on the evening of Day 9 and the morning of Day 10 each at a dosage of 50 IU. On the afternoon of Day 10—approximately 20 hours after the progesterone had been withdrawn—six foster pups, 10–15 hours old, were given each female. The pups remained until the following morning, at which time a fresh litter was substituted. This procedure continued until maternal behavior was displayed or, failing maternal behavior, until seven days had elapsed. To be scored as maternal, a female was required not only to retrieve, but to build a nest, assume a nursing posture, lick the young, and keep them warm. She was, in other words, obliged to exhibit the full spectrum of nurtural attachment.

Of the ten nulliparous females subjected to our hormone schedule, each, without exception, showed full maternal behavior at between 35 and 40 hours from the time the pups were first proffered. Not only does this represent a significant reduction in latency from the average of six to seven days characteristic of untreated nulliparae, but it also represents a uniformity in time of onset closely approaching that exhibited by the puerperal female. In contrast, control females, given, respectively, only two of the three "inductor hormones" (the vehicle in each case having been substituted for the hormone omitted) or simply injected with all three vehicles, showed marked variability in onset and, of course, a significantly higher median latency. Fig. 1 represents the data graphically.

The picture that we now have of maternal behavior places in perspective the roles played by both pup-related stimuli and endogenously-produced hormones. Clearly, the presence of young, quite apart from any endocrine intervention, can activate the neuronal system mediating the expression of nursing, nest-building, retrieving and licking. But activation by pups alone takes some six or seven days, an interval altogether too long for the survival of a neonatal litter. In the puerperal female, then, endocrine intervention becomes necessary to insure immediate responsiveness. Here our data enable us to conceive of the action of a triad of hormones. Beginning with

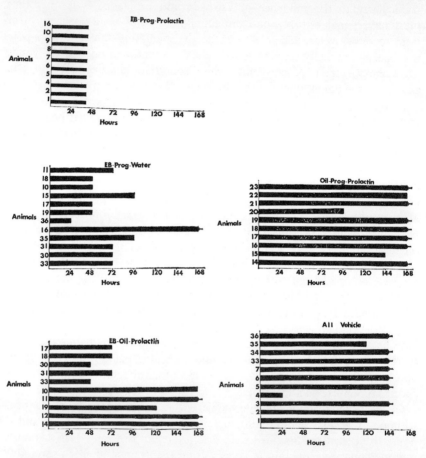

Fig. 1.   The latency and variability in time of onset for the display of maternal behavior in experimental and control females. Broken bar indicates animal had failed to act maternally at the conclusion of the observation period (From Moltz, Lubin, Leon & Numan, 1970).

progesterone, or rather with progesterone withdrawal, the mediating system becomes primed or sensitized to the activational effects of estrogen and prolactin. Estrogen and prolactin, in turn, are then pictured as bringing the system to a point that renders it acutely responsive to the sight, sound and odor of young.

Although the nulliparous females subjected to our triad of hormones showed a significant reduction in latency as well as a marked uniformity in the time of onset of maternal behavior, the question still remains as to why they took as long as 35 to 40 hours to respond. This may indicate that the dosage level of one or another of the hormones administered was too low, or perhaps too high. Or it may indicate that progesterone, estrogen, and prolactin are in themselves sufficient to effect only a limited reduction in latency, and that to induce immediate maternal behavior additional hormones must be administered. Or finally, it may simply mean that the time elapsing between the injection of one or another of our inductor agents was not optimal. As regards this last possibility, we already know that when progesterone is injected on Days 4 through 7, rather than as in our present schedule on Days 6 through 9, only 20% of our ovariectomized nulliparous females respond within the 40 hours found to obtain previously. Correlatively, when progesterone is extended to the morning of Day 10, rather than terminated on the evening of Day 9, 60%, instead of 100%, display full maternal behavior. It is at least conceivable that a different scheduling of the present regimen would reduce our obtained latency of 35 to 40 hours to one of perhaps 15 to 20 hours (cf. Terkel[103]). However, whether with discrete injections one can ever duplicate the effects of endogenous release—and thereby induce immediate attention to young— has yet to be determined.

Maternal Behavior in the Adult Male Rat

Like the nulliparous female, the adult male also responds to young. Given the same six or seven days of exposure to foster pups, he too begins to act maternally, building a nest, licking, retrieving, and finally hovering in a nursing posture (Rosenblatt,[80] Wiesner and Sheard[108]). That the male can exhibit these nurtural responses and in the appropriate temporal sequence, indicates that he also possesses a fully developed mediating system which, like that of the female, is capable of responding to pup-related stimuli alone. The question that arose is whether this system is also capable of activation by our triad of inductor hormones (Moltz, Lubin, Leon and Numan[62]).

Male rats were castrated and subjected to the same endocrine regimen as experimental nulliparous females, namely, estrogen and prolactin imposed on progesterone withdrawal. In contrast to their female counterparts, these males did not respond at 35 to 40 hours, but instead responded, as did control animals, taking six to seven days.

These data lead us to suspect that the mediating system of the male is refractory to endocrine excitation; that, while it can respond to pup-related stimuli, it cannot be sensitized to these same stimuli through hormone injection. However, it may simply be that males require a higher dosage level of one or another of our inductor agents. Thus far we have not attempted to vary dosage level systematically, although to some gonadectomized males we did administer twice the amount of estrogen and progesterone found effective in our nulliparous females. It is instructive that these males still failed to show any significant reduction in latency.

But whether the mediating system of the male is susceptible to hormonal facilitation or not, it evidently differs in sensitivity from that of the female. It becomes of interest to determine how this difference might have arisen.

During the past decade, there has been much research on the role of androgen in the neonatal male, revealing, among other effects, its influence in suppressing the reactivity of the neuronal system mediating lordotic behavior. (Barraclough,[3] Barraclough and Gorski,[5] Feder, Phoenix and Young,[26] Feder and Whalen,[27] Gerall and Ward,[33] Whalen and Edwards,[106, 107]). Neonatal androgen may well have a parallel effect on the neuronal system mediating maternal behavior. This system, more specifically, might begin to develop in both the male and the female rat at, or perhaps even before, the time of birth. In the male, however, androgen may come early in ontogeny to exert an effect on threshold, making his maternal mediating system subsequently insensitive to hormonal excitation. If this is correct, the result might well be that of a system which, although capable of supporting full maternal behavior in response to young, remains refractory to endocrine facilitation.

In contrast to the male, the female of course is not exposed to androgen during neonatal life and in fact is only first exposed to endogenous estrogen at about Day 14 postpartum (Cierciorowska and Russfield[12]). As a consequence, her maternal control system may escape the kind of "desensitization" to which the male is subjected.

<h1 style="text-align:center">4</h1>

Birth and Maternal Behavior in the Rabbit

For the rabbit, as for the rat, the main source of progesterone during pregnancy is the ovary, and in both species removal of the ovary leads to abortion. Like the rat, the rabbit also evidences a marked change in progesterone output during the course of gestation. As measured in ovarian vein blood (Mikhail et al.[57]), progesterone in the rabbit begins to increase on the second day after mating, reaching maximal values on Day 16 of her 31- to 32-day gestation period. From there the concentration decreases gradually until a few days before parturition, at which time it begins to decline abruptly. By Day 4 postpartum, progesterone can no longer be detected. Unfortunately, neither estrogen nor prolactin levels have been measured in the pregnant rabbit.

Parturition in the rabbit differs significantly from that in the rat. In the rat, strong uterine motility can often be observed beginning as early as three days prior to delivery, with delivery itself frequently taking as long as two hours. In the rabbit, however, intra-uterine pressure waves (as measured both by radio-telemetry and balloon insertion) show a sudden onset, followed almost immediately by the rapid expulsion of the fetuses (Fuchs,[30, 31, 32] Kuriyama and Csapo,[48] Schofield[92, 93, 94]). This difference in the time of occurrence of uterine contractions and in the duration of labor may reflect, as several investigators have suggested, a difference in the role played by oxytocin. In the rabbit, oxytocin release probably occurs suddenly and, along with progesterone withdrawal, is likely instrumental in initiating delivery; in the rat, delivery is probably initiated by progesterone withdrawal alone, with oxytocin entering only during the second or final stage of the delivery process.

Maternal behavior in the rabbit is in some respects similar to, and in other respects different from, that in the rat. Depending on the strain, the rabbit begins to build a nest either a few days before parturition or on the day of parturition itself (Ross et al.[84]). In the laboratory, the nest is usually built of hay, straw, or other materials of a similar nature, while in the wild, first a burrow is dug and then the nest is constructed of natural compost (Deutsch,[17] Ross et al.[85]). In either case, the female lines the site with hair plucked from her own body, hair that had already started to loosen a few days before parturition. Whether or not the quality of the nest improves with successive breeding experiences has been debated. The rat clearly shows no improvement, the primiparous female being as proficient in nest building as her multiparous counterpart (Moltz and Robbins[63]). For the laboratory rabbit, however, Ross et al.[83] have presented evidence of a linear increase in nest quality from the first to the fourth parturition. Deutsch,[17] however, questions the generality of this evidence, maintaining that under natural conditions—when presumably opportunities for nest construction are optimal—the primiparous doe builds a nest that in no way differs from that built by the multiparous doe.

Delivery, of course, whether in the wild or in the laboratory, takes place in the nest. As soon as the young emerge, the female becomes attentive; she quickly licks and cleans her pups and within only a few minutes begins to nurse (Ross et al.[86]). Unlike the rat, however, the portparturient doe nurses only once a day and then for only two or three minutes at a time (Deutsch,[17] Zarrow et al.[113]). Also retrieving, one of the most interesting components of rodent maternal behavior, has never been observed reliably either in wild or in laboratory-reared rabbits (Ross et al.[82]).

Unfortunately, there has been no attempt to determine whether the nulliparous doe, if simply kept in continuous association with young, will come to respond maternally. However, there have been a number of attempts to induce through hormone injection maternal behavior, or more precisely maternal nest-building, in the nulliparous doe. Taking ovariectomized females, Zarrow et al.[114, 115, 116] administered both estradiol and progesterone for some four weeks in one experiment and for about two weeks in another. When injection of both steroids were terminated simultaneously, maternal nest-building failed to occur. However, when progesterone was terminated two or three days before the cessation of estradiol, nest-building was observed in all experimental animals. Evidently, progesterone withdrawal is as critical for the induction of maternal behavior (or at least for the induction of maternal nest-building) in the nulliparous rabbit as it is in the nulliparous rat. Moreover, it is significant that in both species maternal behavior did occur, not immediately after progesterone withdrawal, but only after some period of time: in the rabbit about two to three days, and in the rat, as we have already mentioned, about 40 hours. Unfortunately, Zarrow *et al.* did not proffer foster young; so we do not know whether the induction of nest-building in the nulliparous doe would have been followed also by the induction of licking and nursing.

Endocrine manipulation in the pregnant rabbit has also provided some interesting parallels with the rat. In both species, sustained injections of progesterone beginning near term will delay the onset of parturition and, at dosages of 4 mg, will, in many females, also inhibit the appearance of maternal behavior (Zarrow *et al.*[115]). However, once again our information is incomplete; we do not know whether the does used by Zarrow *et al.* were primiparous or multiparous, and consequently whether the behavioral inhibition observed following the sustained progesterone injections can be modified in the pregnant rabbit by previous breeding experience. It will be recalled that in the pregnant rat such modification was found to occur readily.

Thus far we have not mentioned specifically the role of prolactin in the induction of maternal behavior in the rabbit. That the nulliparous rat fails to respond only to estrogen- and progesterone-withdrawal is clear, that superimposed on these steroids must be exogenous prolactin. In contrast, it would seem that the nulliparous rabbit does not require exogenous prolactin, but will respond in most cases simply to the steroids alone. However, as Zarrow *et al.* point out, the role of prolactin in the induction of nest-building in the doe cannot be assessed properly until hypophysectomized animals are tested. In other words, it is possible that the extended estrogen injections found necessary to induce nest-building in the rabbit functioned to discharge sufficient prolactin from the female's own pituitary (e.g. Welch *et al.*[105]) to make injection of the gonadotrophin superfluous. Perhaps, had a more abbreviated schedule been employed, approaching, for example, that used with the rat, then exogenous prolactin may have been found critical.

One final comparison between the rabbit and the rat remains to be discussed, namely, that relating to maternal behavior in the male. It will be recalled that in the rat, we were unsuccessful in reducing the latency to maternal behavior in the male, that even when estrogen and progesterone dosages were doubled, the male still took six or seven days to respond to young. Zarrow *et al.* report essentially the same observation in the rabbit. More specifically, castrated male rabbits were administered 10 μg, rather than 5 μg, of estradiol and 8 mg, rather than 4 mg., of progesterone under the same schedule found effective in inducing nest-building in the nulliparous female. Despite these dosages, the male failed to show any signs of nest-building following progesterone-withdrawal.

Perhaps in the rabbit, as well as in the rat, the presence of androgen early in ontogeny is critical in affecting thresholds to endocrine activation within the maternal mediating system. If this were the case, then for the rabbit also we would expect neonatal (or perhaps prenatal) castration—in freeing the male from the "desensitizing" effects exerted by endogenous androgen during a critical period in ontogeny—to increase subsequently his reactivity to inductor hormones. Correlatively, androgen injection during a critical period in the ontogeny of the genetic female might raise her hormone-sensitivity to a threshold level characteristic of the normal male.

From what has already been said, it is obvious that maternal behavior in the rat and rabbit defies dichotomization into categories such as "innate" and "acquired". It is of course neither "innate" in the sense of being encoded isomorphically in the genome nor "acquired" in the sense of being learned or conditioned (cf. Moltz[58]). Rather, it can be understood only by reference to a complex of intraorganic events and extrinsic stimulative conditions interacting to excite a mediating substrate whose reactivity thresholds in turn have been affected by neonatal steroid levels and by previous breeding experience. This is the picture that now emerges for the rat and rabbit. It is obvious that much additional research, carried out systematically on a variety of mammalian forms, will be needed before the full spectrum of interspecific differences and similarities in the mechanisms underlying maternal behavior become apparent. Such an endeavor, although difficult, should prove richly rewarding for both physiology and psychology alike.

REFERENCES

1. AMENOMORI, Y., CHEN, C. L. and MEITES, J. 1970. Serum prolactin levels in rats during different reproductive states. *Endocrinology*, **86**, 506–510.
2. ARAI, Y., HIROL, M., MITRA, J. and GORSKI, R. A. 1967. Influence of intravenous progesterone administration on the cortical electroencephalogram of the female rat. *Neuroendocrinology*, **2**, 275–282.
3. BARRACLOUGH, C. A. 1965. Mating behavior in the androgen-sterilized female rat and its relation to the hypothalamic regulation of sexual behavior. In L. Martini and A. Pecile (eds.). *Hormonal steroids*. New York: Academic Press.
4. BARRACLOUGH, C. A. and CROSS, B. A. 1963. Unit activity in the hypothalamus of the cyclic female rat: Effect of genital stimuli and progesterone. *J. Endocr.*, **26**, 339–359.
5. BARRACLOUGH, C. A. and GORSKI, R. A. 1962. Studies on mating behavior in the androgen-sterilized female rat in relation to the hypothalamic regulation of sexual behavior. *J. Endocr.* **25**, 175–182.
6. BARTHOLOMEW, G. A. 1959. Mother-young relations and the maturation of pup behaviour in the Alaska fur seal. *Anim. Behav.*, **7**, 163–171.
7. BEACH, F. A. and WILSON, J. R. 1963. Effects of prolactin, progesterone, and estrogen on reactions of non-pregnant rats to foster young. *Psychol. Rep.*, **13**, 231–239.
8. BEYER, C., RAMIREZ, V. D., WHITMOYER, D. I. and SAWYER, C. H. 1967. Effects of hormones on the electrical activity of the brain in the rat and rabbit. *Exp. Neurol.*, **18**, 313–326.
9. BINDRA, D. 1959. *Motivation: a systematic reinterpretation*. New York: Ronald Press.

10. BIRCH, D. 1956. Sources of order in the maternal behavior of animals. *Amer. J. Orthopsychiat.*, **26**, 279–284.

11. CHRISTOPHERSEN, E. R. and WAGMAN, W. 1965. Maternal behavior in the albino rat as a function of self-licking deprivation. *J. comp. physiol. Psychol.*, **60**, 142–144.

12. CIERCIOROWSKA, A. and RUSSFIELD, A. 1968. Determination of estrogenic activity of the immature rat ovary. *Archs Path.*, **85**, 658–662.

13. COSNIER, J. 1963. Quelques problemes poses par le "comportement maternel provoque" chez la ratte. *C. R. Soc. Biol.* (Paris), **157**, 1611–1613.

14. CROSS, P. A. 1966. Neural control of oxytocin secretion. In *Neuroendocrinology.* Vol. 1. (L. Martini and W. F. Ganog, eds.). New York: Academic Press.

15. DEIS, R. P. 1967. Mammary gland development by hypothalamic and hypophyseal estrogen implants in male rats. *Acta physiol. lat.-amer.*, **17**, 115–117.

16. DENENBERG, V. H., TAYLOR, R. E. and ZARROW, M. X. 1969. Maternal behavior in the rat: an investigation and quantification of nest building. *Behaviour*, **34**, 1–16.

17. DEUTSCH, J. A. 1957. Nest building behaviour of domestic rabbits under semi-natural conditions. *Brit. J. anim. Behav.*, **2**, 53–54.

18. DILLEY, W. G. and ADLER, N. T. 1968. Postcopulatory mammary gland secretion in rats. *Proc. Soc. exp. Biol. Med.*, **129**, 964–967.

19. EIBL-EIBESFELDT, I. 1958. Das Verhalten der Nagetiere. In *Handbuch der Zoologie* (J. Helmecke, H. V. Lengerken, and D. Starck, eds.). Berlin: Walter de Gruyter.

20. EIBL-EIBESFELDT, I. 1961. The interactions of unlearned behaviour patterns and learning in mammals. In *Brain mechanisms and learning* (J. F. Delafresnaye, ed.). Oxford: Blackwell Scientific Publications.

21. EISENFELD, A. J. and AXELROD, J. 1965. Selectivity of estrogen distributions in tissues. *J. Pharmacol. exp. Ther.*, **150**, 469–475.

22. EISENFELD, A. J. and AXELROD, J. 1966. Effect of steroid hormones, ovariectomy, estrogen pretreatment, sex and immaturity on the distribution of ^{3}H-estradiol. *Endocrinology*, **79**, 38–42.

23. ETO, T., HSOI, T., MUSUDO, H. and SUZUKI, Y. 1962. Progesterone and pregn-4-ene 20$^\alpha$-ol-3-one in rat ovarian venous blood at different stages in the reproductive cycle. *Japan. J. anim. Reprod.*, **8**, 34–40. (Title translated).

24. EVERETT, J. W. 1966. The control and secretion of prolactin. In *The pituitary gland*, Vol. II (G. Harris and B. Donovan, eds.). Berkeley: Univer. Calif. Press.

25. FAJER, A. B. and BARRACLOUGH, C. A. 1967. Ovarian secretion of progesterone and 20$^\alpha$-hydroxypregn-4-en-3-one during pseudopregnancy and pregnancy in rats. *Endocrinology*, **81**, 617–622.

26. FEDER, H. H., PHOENIX, C. H. and YOUNG, W. C. 1966. Suppression of feminine behaviour by administration of testosterone propionate to neonatal rats. *J. Endocr.*, **34**, 131–132.

27. FEDER, H. H. and WHALEN, R. E. 1965. Feminine behavior in neonatally castrated and estrogen-treated male rats. *Science*, **147**, 306–307.

28. FITZPATRICK, R. J. 1966. The posterior pituitary gland and the female reproductive tract. In *The pituitary gland*, Vol. 3 (G. W. Harris and B. T. Donovan, eds.). Berkeley: Univer. Calif. Press.

29. FRIEDLICH, O. B. 1962. A study of maternal behavior of the albino rat as a function of self-licking deprivation. Unpublished Master's Thesis, Southern Illinois University.

30. FUCHS, A. R. 1964. Oxytocin and the onset of labour in rabbits. *J. Endocr.*, **30**, 217–224b.

31. FUCHS, A. R. 1964. The role of oxytocin in the initiation of labour. *Proc. 2nd. Int. Congr. Endocr.*, 753–758a.

32. FUCHS, A. R. 1966. Studies on the control of oxytocin release at parturition in rabbits and rats. *J. Reprod. Fertil.*, **12**, 418.

33. GERALL, A. A. and WARD, J. L. 1966. Effects of prenatal exogenous androgen on the sexual behavior of the female albino rat. *J. comp. physiol. Psychol.*, **62**, 370–375.

34. GREENWALD, G. S. 1966. Ovarian follicular development and pituitary FSH and LH content in the pregnant rat. *Endocrinology*, **79**, 572–578.

35. GRINDELAND, R. E., McCULLOCH, W. A. and ELLIS, S. 1969. Radio-immuno-assay of rat prolactin. Paper presented at the 51st Meeting of the Endocrine Society.

36. GROTA, L. J. and EIK-NES, K. B. 1967. Plasma progesterone concentrations during pregnancy and lactation in the rat. *J. Reprod. Fertil.*, **13**, 83–91.

37. HAMBURG, D. 1966. Effects of progesterone on behavior. In *Endocrines and the central nervous system* (R. Levine, Ed.). Baltimore: Williams and Wilkins.

38. HASHIMOTO, I., HENRICKS, D. M., ANDERSON, L. L. and MELAMPY, R. M. 1968. Progesterone and pregn-4-en-20$^\alpha$-ol-one in ovarian venous blood during various reproductive states in the rat. *Endocrinology*, **82**, 333–341.

39. HOLLAND, H. C. 1965. An apparatus note on A.M.B.A. (Automatic Maternal Behavior Apparatus). *Anim. Behav.*, **13**, 201–202.

40. KAWAKAMI, M., and SAWYER, C. H. 1959. Neuroendocrine correlates of changes in brain activity thresholds by sex steroids and pituitary hormones. *Endocrinology*, **65**, 652–668.

41. KIRBY, H. W. and HORVATH, T. 1968. Self-licking deprivation and maternal behavior in the primiparous rat. *Canadian J. Psychol.*, **22**, 369–376.

42. KLEIN, M. 1952. Uterine distension, ovarian hormones and maternal behaviour in rodents. *Ciba Colloq. Endocrinol.*, Vol. 3. New York: Blakeston.

43. KOBAYASHI, T., KOBAYASHI, T., TAKEZAWA, S., OSHIMA, K. and KAWAMURA, H. 1962. Electrophysiological studies on the feedback mechanism of progesterone. *Endocr. jap.*, **9**, 302–320.

44. KOMISARUK, B. R. McDONALD, P. G. WHITMOYER, D. I. and SAWYER, C. H. 1967. Effects of progesterone and sensory stimulation on EEG and neuronal activity in the rat. *Exp. Neurol.*, **19**, 494–507.

45. KUHN, N. J. 1968. Lactogenesis in the rat. Metabolism of uridine diphosphate galactose by mammary gland. *Biochem. J.*, **106**, 743–748.

46. KUHN, N. J. 1969. Progesterone withdrawal as the lactogenic trigger in the rat. *J. Endocr.*, **44**, 39–54.

47. KUHN, N. J. and LOWENSTEIN, J. M. 1967. Lactogenesis in the rat. Changes in metabolic parameters at parturition. *Biochem. J.*, **105**, 995–1002.

48. KURIYAMA, H. and CSAPO, A. 1961. Placenta and myometrial block. *Amer. J. Obstet. Gynec.*, **82**, 592.

49. KWA, H. G. and VERHOFSTAD, F. 1967. Prolactin levels in the plasma of female rats. *J. Endocr.* **39**, 455–456.

50. LAUMUS, K. R. and FAROOQ, A. 1966. The uptake *in vivo* of (1, 2-^{3}H) progesterone by the brain and genital tract of the rat. *J. Endocr.*, **36**, 95–96.

51. LEHRMAN, D. S. 1956. On the organization of maternal behavior and the problem of instinct. In *L'Instinct dans le Comportement des Animaux et de l'Homme* (P. P. Grassé, ed.). Paris: Masson et Cie.

52. LEHRMAN, D. S. 1961. Hormonal regulation of parental behavior in birds and infrahuman mammals. In *Sex and internal secretions* (W. C. Young, Ed.). Baltimore: Williams & Wilkins.

53. LOTT, D. F. 1962. The role of progesterone in the maternal behavior of rodents. *J. comp. physiol. Psychol.*, **55**, 610–613.

54. LOTT, D. F. and FUCHS, S. S. 1962. Failure to induce retrieving by sensitization or the injection of prolactin. *J. comp. physiol. Psychol.*, **55**, 1111–1113.

55. MARTIN, R. D. 1966. Tree shrews: Unique reproductive mechanism of systematic importance. *Science*, 152, 1402–1404.
56. MEITES, J. and NICOLL, C. S. 1965. *In vivo* and *in vitro* effects of steroids on pituitary prolactin secretion. In *Hormonal steroids* (L. Martini and A. Pecile, eds.). New York: Academic Press.
57. MIKHAIL, G., NOALL, W. W. and ALLEN, W. M. 1961. Progesterone levels in the rabbit ovarian vein blood throughout pregnancy. *Endocrinology*, 69, 504–509.
58. MOLTZ, H. 1965. Contemporary instinct theory and the fixed action pattern. *Psychol. Rev.*, 72, 27–47.
59. MOLTZ, H., GELLER, D. and LEVIN, R. 1967. Maternal behavior in the totally mammectomized rat. *J. comp. physiol. Psychol.*, 64, 225–229.
60. MOLTZ, H., LEVIN, R., and LEON, M. 1969. Differential effects of progesterone on the maternal behavior of primiparous and multiparous rats. *J. comp. physiol. Psychol.*, 67, 36–40.
61. MOLTZ, H. LEVIN, R. and LEON, M. 1969. Prolactin in the post-partum rat: Synthesis and release in the absence of suckling stimulation. *Science*, 163, 1083–1084.
62. MOLTZ, H., LUBIN, M., LEON, M. and NUMAN, M. 1970. Hormonal induction of maternal behavior in the ovariectomized nulliparous rat. *Physiol. Behav.* 5, *1370–1377.*
63. MOLTZ, H. and ROBBINS, D. 1965. Maternal behavior of primiparous and multiparous rats. *J. comp. physiol. Psychol.*, 60, 417–421.
64. MOLTZ, H., ROBBINS, D. and PARKS, M. 1966. Caesarean delivery and the maternal behavior of primiparous and multiparous rats. *J. comp. physiol. Psychol.*, 61, 455–460.
65. MOLTZ, H. and WIENER, E. 1966. Effects of ovariectomy on maternal behavior of primiparous and multiparous rats. *J. comp. physiol. Psychol.*, 62, 382–387.
66. NICOLL, C. S. and MEITES, J. 1962. Estrogen stimulation of prolactin production by rat adenohypophysis *in vitro*. *Endocrinology*, 70, 272–277.
67. PFAFF, D. W. 1965. Cerebral implantation and autoradiographic studies of sex hormones. In *Sex research: new developments*. (J. Money, ed.). New York: Holt, Rinehart, & Winston.
68. PFAFF, D. W. 1968. Uptake of ^{3}H-estradiol by the female rat brain: An autoradiographic study. *Endocrinology*, 82, 1149–1155.
69. PITTERS, H. 1954. Untersuchungen über angeborene Verhaltensweisen bei Tylopoden, unter besonderer Berucksichtigung der neuweltlichen Formen. *Z. Tierpsychol.*, 11, 213–303.
70. RAISINGHANI K. H., DORFMAN, R. I., FORCHELLI, E., GYERMEK, L. and GENTHER, G. 1968. Uptake of intravenously administered progesterone, pregnanedione and pregnanolone by the rat brain. *Acta Endocrinologica*, 57, 395–404.
71. RAMIREZ, V. D., KOMISARUK, B. R., WHITMOYER, D. I. and SAWYER, C. H. 1967. Effects of hormones and vaginal stimulation on the EEG and hypothalamic units in rats. *Amer. J. Physiol.*, 212, 1376–1384.
72. RAMIREZ, V. D. and MCCANN, S. M. 1964. Induction of prolactin secretion by implants of estrogen into the hypothalamo-hypophyseal region of female rats. *Endocrinology*, 75, 206–214.
73. RATNER, A., TALWALKER, P. K. and MEITES, J. 1963. Effect of estrogen administration *in vivo* on prolactin release by rat pituitary *in vitro*. *Proc. Soc. exp. Biol. Med.*, 112, 12–15.
74. RICHARDS, M. P. M. 1967. Maternal behavior in rodents and lagomorphs: a review. In *Advances in reproductive physiology* (A. McLaren, ed.). New York: Academic Press. Vol. II (in press).
75. RIDDLE, O. 1937. Physiological responses to prolactin. *Cold Spr. Harb. Symp. quant. Biol.*, 5, 218–228.

76. RIDDLE, O., HOLLANDER, W. F., MILLER, R. A., LAHR, E. L., SMITH, G. C. and MARVIN, H. N. 1942. Endocrine studies. *Yearb. Carneg. Instn.*, **41**, 203–211a.
77. RIDDLE, O., LAHR, E. L. and BATES, R. W. 1935. Effectiveness and specificity of prolactin in the induction of the maternal instinct in virgin rats. *Amer. J. Physiol.*, **113**, 109a.
78. RIDDLE, O., LAHR, E. L. and BATES, R. W. 1935. Maternal behavior induced in virgin rats by prolactin. *Proc. Soc. exp. Biol. Med.*, **32**, 730–734b.
79. RIDDLE, O., LAHR, E. L. and BATES, R. W. 1942. The role of hormones in the initiation of maternal behavior in rats. *Amer. J. Psychol.*, **137**, 299–317b.
80. ROSENBLATT, J. S. 1967. Nonhormonal basis of maternal behavior in the rat. *Science*, **156**, 1512–1513.
81. ROSENBLATT, J. S. and LEHRMAN, D. S. 1963. Maternal behavior of the laboratory rat. In *Maternal behavior in mammals* (H. L. Rheingold, ed.). New York: Wiley.
82. ROSS, S., DENENBERG, V. H., FROMMER, G. P., and SAWIN, P. B. 1959. Genetic, physiological and behavioral background in the rabbit. V. Nonretrieving of neonates. *J. Mammal.*, **40**, 91–96.
83. ROSS, S., DENENBERG, V. H., SAWIN, P. and MEYER, P. 1956. Changes in nest building behaviour in multiparous rabbits. *Brit. J. Anim. Behav.*, **4**, 69–74.
84. ROSS, S., SAWIN, P. B., DENENBERG, V. H. and ZARROW, M. X. 1961. Maternal behavior in the rabbit: yearly and seasonal variation in nest building. *Behaviour*, **18**, 154.
85. ROSS, S., SAWIN, P., ZARROW, M. X. and DENENBERG, V. H. 1963. Maternal behavior in the rabbit. In *Maternal behavior in mammals* (H. L. Rheingold, ed.). New York: Wiley.
86. ROSS, S., ZARROW, M. X., SAWIN, P. B., DENENBERG, V. H. and BLUMENFIELD, M. 1963. Maternal behaviour in the rabbit under semi-natural conditions. *Anim. Behav.*, **11**, 283–285a.
87. ROTH, L. L. and ROSENBLATT,, J. S. 1967. Changes in self-licking during pregnancy in the rat. *J. comp. physiol. Psychol.*, **63**, 397–400.
88. ROTHCHILD, I. 1965. Interrelations between progesterone and the ovary, pituitary and the central nervous system in the control of ovulation and the regulation of progesterone secretion. In *Vitamins and hormones*, Vol. 23 (R. Harris, I. Wool and J. Loraine, eds.). New York: Academic Press.
89. ROTHCHILD, I. and SCHWARTZ, N. B. 1965. The corpus-luteum hypophysis relationship: The effects of progesterone and oestrogen on the secretion of luteotrophin and luteinizing hormone in the rat. *Acta Endocrinologica*, **49**, 120–137.
90. SCHNEIRLA, T. C. 1950. Levels in the psychological capacities of animals. In *Philosophy for the future* (R. W. Sellars, *et. al.*, eds.). New York: Macmillan.
91. SCHNEIRLA, T. C. 1956. Interrelationships of the "innate" and the "acquired" in instinctive behaviour. In *L'instinct dans le Comportement des Animaux et de L'Homme*. Paris: Masson et Cie.
92. SCHOFIELD, B. M. 1957. The hormonal control of myometrial function during pregnancy. *J. Physiol.*, **138**, 1.
93. SCHOFIELD, B. M. 1968. Parturition. In *Advances in reproductive physiology*, Vol. 3 (A. McLaren, ed.). New York: Academic Press.
94. SCHOFIELD, B. M. 1969. Parturition in the rabbit. *J. Endocr.*, **43**, 673–674.
95. SEIKI, K., HIGASHIDA, M., IMANISHI, Y., MIYAMOTO, M., KITAGAWA, T., and KOTANI, M. 1968. Radioactivity in the rat hypothalamus and pituitary after injection of labelled progesterone. *J. Endocr.*, **41**, 109–110.
96. SEIKI, K., MIYAMOTO, M., YAMASHITA, A. and KOTANI, M. 1969. Further studies on the uptake of labelled progesterone by the hypothalamus and pituitary of rats. *J. Endocr.* **43**, 129–130.
97. SHINDE, Y., OTA, K. and YOKOYAMA, A. 1964. Lactose content of mammary glands

of pregnant rats near term: Effect of removal of ovary, placenta and foetus. *J. Endocr.*, **31**, 105–114.

98. STEINBERG, J. and BINDRA, D. 1962. Effects of pregnancy and salt-intake on genital licking. *J. comp. physiol. Psychol.*, **55**, 103–106.

99. STONE, C. P. 1925. Preliminary note on maternal behavior of rats living in parabiosis. *Endocrinology*, **9**, 505–512.

100. STUMPF, W. E. 1968. Estradiol-concentrating neurons: typography in the hypothalamus by dry-mount autoradiography. *Science*, **162**, 1001–1003.

101. STURMAN-HULBE, M. and STONE, C. P. 1929. Maternal behavior in the albino rat. *J. comp. Psychol.*, **9**, 203–237.

102. TAYLOR, R. E. 1965. Hormones and maternal behavior in the rat. Unpublished doctoral dissertation, University of Michigan.

103. TERKEL, J. 1970. Unpublished doctoral dissertation, Rutgers University.

104. TERKEL, J. and ROSENBLATT, J. S. 1968. Maternal behavior induced by maternal blood plasma injected into virgin rats. *J. comp. physiol. Psychol.*, **65**, 479–482.

105. WELCH, C. W., SAR, M., CLEMENS, J. A. and MEITES, J. 1968. Effect of estrogen on pituitary prolactin levels of female rats bearing median eminence implants of prolactin. *Proc. Soc. exp. Biol. Med.*, **12**, 817–821.

106. WHALEN, R. E., and EDWARDS, D. A. 1966. Sexual reversibility in neonatally castrated male rats. *J. comp. physiol. Psychol.*, **62**, 307–310.

107. WHALEN, R. E. and EDWARDS, D. A. 1967. Hormonal determinants of the development of masculine and feminine behavior in male and female rats. *Anat. Rec.*, **157**, 173–180.

108. WIESNER, B. P. and SHEARD, N. M. 1933. *Maternal behaviour in the rat*. Edinburgh: Oliver & Boyd.

109. WIEST, W. G. 1968. On the function of 20^α-hydroxypregn-4-en-one during parturition in the rat. *Endocrinology*, **83**, 1181–1184.

110. WIEST, W. G.; KIDWELL, W. R. and BALOGH, K. 1968. Progesterone catabolism in the rat ovary: a regulatory mechanism for progestational potency during pregnancy. *Endocrinology*, **82**, 844–860.

111. YOSHINAGA, K., HAWKINS, R. A. and STOCKER, J. F. 1969. Estrogen secretion by the rat ovary *in vivo* during the estrous cycle and pregnancy. *Endocrinology*, **85**, 103–112.

112. ZARROW, M. X. 1961. Gestation. In *Sex and internal secretions*, Vol. II. (W. C. Young, ed.). Baltimore: Williams and Wilkins.

113. ZARROW, M. X., DENENBERG, V. H. and ANDERSON, C. O., 1965. Rabbit: frequency of suckling in the pup. *Science* **150**, 1835–1836.

114. ZARROW, M. X., DENENBERG, V. H. and KALBERER, W. D. 1965. Strain differences in the endocrine basis of maternal nest-building in the rabbit. *J. Reprod. Fertil.*, **10**, 397–401.

115. ZARROW, M. X., FAROOQ, A., DENENBERG, V. H., SAWIN, P. B. and ROSS, S. 1963. Maternal behaviour in the rabbit: Endocrine control of maternal nest-building. *J. Reprod. Fertil.*, **6**, 375.

116. ZARROW, M. X., SAWIN, P. B., ROSS, S. and DENENBERG, V. H. 1962. Maternal behavior and its endocrine basis in the rabbit. In *Roots of behavior* (E. L. Bliss. ed.). New York: Harper.

II

PSYCHOSOMATIC INFERTILITY IN THE MALE AND FEMALE

DAVID ROTHMAN

B.S., M.D.

Director, Department of Obstetrics and Gynecology
The Jewish Hospital of St. Louis
Assistant Professor of Clinical Obstetrics and Gynecology
Washington University School of Medicine
Obstetrician-in-Chief, Booth Memorial Hospital of St. Louis
U.S.A.

ALEX H. KAPLAN

B.S., M.D.

Associate Professor of Clinical Psychiatry
Washington University School of Medicine
Medical Director of the Psychoanalytic Foundation of St. Louis
U.S.A.
Past Psychiatrist-in-Chief, The Jewish Hospial of St. Louis

PSYCHOLOGICAL FACTORS PRODUCING INFERTILITY IN THE FEMALE

1

Introduction

Some women do not achieve motherhood because of psychological factors which may either prevent pregnancy or produce a spontaneous abortion. It is not always clear in every case how emotional factors produce physiological changes which prevent conception, but there is evidence to indicate that tubal spasm, the failure of ovulation, a subtle avoidance of coitus during the fertile period, the rapid expulsion of the spermatic fluid from the vagina, vaginismus and hostile cervical secretion, either alone or in combination, may be responsible. It is typical for patients whose infertility is on a psychosomatic basis to express an intense conscious desire for pregnancy and, indeed, many will go from doctor to doctor subjecting themselves to repetitive testing and treatment in an effort to conceive, and yet not until they are in psychotherapy do they become aware of the fact that pregnancy, childbirth, and motherhood are really intolerable for them. The concern with pregnancy is that it will make them unattractive and drive their husbands away. The fear of childbirth is usually that they will die in labor and/or have an abnormal child, and the anxiety about motherhood is that they will be unable to assume the responsibility of caring for a child's life. There is also the fear that the child will become a competitor for their husband's love.

These patients also present a similar belief that the reason for their inability to conceive is a form of punishment for something of which they feel guilty. Usually this is related to a conscious feeling of guilt about premarital sexual relations or induced abortion. However, it has not been found that this is a factor in the infertility: but rather, that the guilt stems from the unconscious harboring of intense hostility particularly towards the mother, along with greedy, sexual, competitive, jealous or dependent feelings or her unexpressed desire to be like the opposite sex.

The material of several investigators, including our own,[21] would seem to show that the fear of dying in childbirth is frequently related to the unresolved hostility towards the patient's mother. Since the unconscious desire is to be freed of the mother (death wish), then retribution demands that they in turn die in becoming a mother. This fear alone is enough for some women to develop a defence against conception.

Spasm of the Fallopian Tubes

Many observations[7] have been reported to suggest that stimulation from the autonomic nervous system may produce tubal spasm sufficient to prevent their visualization on salpingography. In some instances, the administration of antispasmotics has been successful in showing a release of the spasm, and in other cases pregnancy has occurred even though no other treatment was directed at remedying the blocked tubes.

To illustrate a case of infertility on the basis of tubal spasm, the following material is of interest. This 22-year-old patient had a problem of primary infertility for three-and-a-half years and her X-rays showed tubal occlusion at the isthmus. Only because of her marked depression and desperation for not achieving motherhood was she asked to talk about her feelings. One session led to another, until it became apparent to the patient that, unconsciously, becoming a mother was too great a threat for her. As a child, this patient felt rejected by her parents unless she could please them by doing a perfect job. For example, her father taught her how to drive the car, but if she made one mistake, he would take over the wheel. In the same manner her mother, in teaching her how to sew, would relieve her of the job if she did not do it properly. She felt forced to make perfect grades in school, where she became known as the "brain". Her mother found fault with all her friends, feeling that none of them was good enough to associate with her daughter. The birth of her brother was associated with intense feeling of rejection. She felt so pressured by her parents that she had daydreams of running away from home and of dying. The deep hurt she felt as a child resulted in repressed hostility, with overconcern for her family and marked dependency.

In the early sessions, these attitudes were shown in her anxiety about her mother's health, which necessitated a phone call every morning to assure herself that her mother was not ill. As the therapy progressed, she became consciously aware of her hostility and wanted her mother "out of her hair". As she became more comfortable with her hostile feelings, she was able to recall dreams of her mother's death which were associated with a great deal of anxiety, as were thoughts of her brother dying when he was in the army. Her feelings of guilt were intensified by the mother, who denied herself and smothered the patient with material gifts all under the guise of love. If the patient then attempted to show anger, the mother's comment was, "Look at all I do for you; how can you make me so unhappy," or "You'll be sorry after I'm gone." As a result of this guilt, the patient's need for punishment, which seemed to relate itself to the inability to get pregnant, was expressed in the following material.

After talking about the hate that she felt for her mother, the patient made the statement, "Maybe I'm better off not being pregnant now, because I would not be a good mother." On recalling a dream of the death of her mother, she became panicky and stated that she felt guilty because "it is wrong to hate your mother. If I get pregnant, something will happen to me or the child." Several times in referring to her inability to get pregnant, the patient stated, "Nothing goes right for me; God is punishing me." Much time was spent by the patient talking of her marked feelings of inadequacy as well as her dependency, with the realization that the responsibility of motherhood was frightening to her. She often cried on being separated from her husband; and with older friends she felt like a child among adults.

It was with great effort that the patient finally admitted that she really didn't want a baby, because there would be competition for her husband's love. Only with considerable difficulty did she admit that this had been a conscious thought of hers at the time she was married. This patient did conceive after sixteen sessions and had an uneventful delivery of a full-term child.

Failure to Ovulate

It is a fairly well-established fact that the failure to ovulate can be on a psychogenic basis. Three patients in our series demonstrated this as the only recognizable factor in the causation of their infertility. It was interesting that two of them had first names that could be those of a boy. All three of them described themselves more like boys than girls. They were always their father's little boy in earlier years. However, despite the masculine identification, these women still remained overly dependent, giving evidence of being over-protected by their parents.

Such a patient was first seen after she had been married for two-and-a-half years without sexual relations being successfully consummated. No physical abnormalities were noted on examination and she was referred to a psychiatrist, with whose help she resolved the problem. A few years later, she reported with a problem of infertility. A routine infertility work-up on both husband and wife revealed that the patient was subject to anovulatory menstrual cycles. A trial of hormone therapy was not effective and psychotherapy was then suggested.

The patient was the youngest of three daughters. A sister three years older was the mother's favorite, and the patient was constantly being compared unfavorably with this older sister; which resulted in intense feelings of rejection and inadequacy. Because her mother was so critical, she found it impossible to make decisions on her own and became markedly dependent upon her mother. The patient also found it impossible to express her anger towards her mother, as the mother would then withdraw and intensify the patient's feeling of rejection. The patient, however, was her father's favorite and, as she expressed it, "she was her father's boy". She behaved as a tomboy when she was a child and can remember that in her teens she wouldn't kiss a boy because her father had expressed disapproval. She compared her husband to her father and stated that her husband was aware of the fact that he was father figure to her.

Her failure to become pregnant was disturbing to her for two reasons: first, she had to prove that she was an adequate woman; and second, it was important that she give her husband a child, because otherwise he might not love her. It occurred to her, however, that she had recently sat on her father's lap and then had the disturbing fantasy of her own child in this position. Her thought was, "I still want to be a child to my father for the few years he has remaining. Maybe I don't want a child of my own." It was her father who waited up for her when she returned from dates, and he was not very enthusiastic when she did marry. As a matter of fact, her father still calls her every day.

In therapy, the patient became aware of the intense anger which she felt towards her over-protective and rejecting parents; and along with it, she felt marked feelings of guilt. She felt that she was the cause of their unhappiness. The usual response of the parents to her anger was, "You don't love us." The mother also responded that her blood pressure would go up and she would die. The patient remembered that as a child she frequently wanted to run away from home. She often dreamt of the death of her parents. Eventually she realized that this was her unconscious wish—her one way of getting even with her parents. Finally, she accepted the fact that her mother's unhappiness was not her responsibility. The patient conceived two months after the final visit, in which period there were a total of seventeen sessions over a period of eight months.

This patient was helped by being able to resolve some of the intensity of her hostility towards her parents and the guilt that went along with it. She had an intense need to please and be loved by her father to the point of being her father's boy, and earlier she denied the feminine role. Therapy helped work through her marked dependency and ambivalent reaction to her parents; so too did the fact that she sought to solve her rejection by developing more acceptable tomboy attitudes. As a result of therapy, she apparently was able to give up the desire to sit on her father's knee, to be a baby herself, and consequently could ovulate as a mature woman and had a child of her own.

The Subtle Avoidance of Coitus

In spite of the intense conscious desire for pregnancy, when the fear of conception is great the patient may avoid the fertile period without consciously recognizing it. This was demonstrated by a patient who usually could tell the time of ovulation because of the presence of mittelschmerz, and yet without conscious appreciation, she did not have coitus during this time. The turning point in her therapy came when she recognized this and stated, "Instead of my looking forward to the time of ovulation, I find that I am disturbed and anxious and have a sense of relief after I feel that this time has passed." The work of Benedek and Rubenstein[3] on the sexual cycle in women, in which the relationship between hormones and emotion show that the analyst was not only able to tell when ovulation occurred, but could also predict the phase of the menstrual cycle from the content of the patient's material in the analytic sessions. The woman's unconscious would, therefore, be sensitive to the chemical changes occurring at ovulation, and the patient could unconsciously avoid sexual contact.

Rapid Expulsion of Spermatic Fluid and Vaginismus

An interesting experience occurred with one of our patients, which demonstrated that the muscular activity of the vagina may rapidly expel the spermatic fluid. The husband of this young lady was sent to a psychiatrist because of a problem of ejaculatory impotence, and the wife was being seen by a gynecologist who was using the husband's sperm obtained through masturbation to inseminate his wife artificially. Because all tests in the standard infertility investigation were negative; and because artificial insemination was not proving successful, the patient was seen in psychotherapy. Her case will be discussed again later. However, at about the time she was involved with feelings about an unresolved Oedipal erotic attachment to her father, she had a dream which dealt with insemination (having sexual relations) by her gynecologist (father). Consciously, at this time, she had expressed uncomfortable feelings about the insemination and was not sure she wanted them continued. Her gynecologist, of course, was not aware of the patient's feelings as being expressed in the psychotherapeutic sessions, but also at this time he had written a note in the patient's chart that usually the method for the insemination was to place the ejaculatory fluid in a cup placed against the cervix, except on this one occasion when he merely placed the specimen in the posterior fornix of the vagina and noticed its immediate expulsion.

This case has many interesting facets, as it reveals a method by which a woman can unconsciously produce infertility, why some cases of artificial insemination are not successful, and also illustrates infertility due to an unresolved Oedipal attachment to the father. Therese Benedek et al.[2] have reported a similar case.

In our patient, the inseminations eventually did result in pregnancy, but only after she had spent considerable time in talking about her intense (incestuous) feelings towards her father. He had given her nightgowns as a gift at the time of her marriage which were to be used on her honeymoon and he would not speak to her husband for two weeks after the marriage, which the patient felt at the time was a peculiar reaction. She recalled that her father belittled her when she was a girl, but he had also impressed her with the fact that he expected her to look after him in his later years. Also, it occurred to her that her father seemed to be jealous of her dating other boys and warned her against sex play. She, in turn, had tried to run away from her mother. Even today she recognized a feeling of discomfort if her father put his arm around a younger girl. The patient was not sure that she believed in a God any more, but she stated, "If I did, I would feel that I was being punished."

In addition to the mechanism of rapidly expelling the spermatic fluid, the muscular action about the vagina may prevent pregnancy by producing vaginismus to the degree that coitus is not possible. When no organic factors are present to produce this discomfort, it is usually a symptom of a marked disturbance in the patient's psychosexual development and requires psychotherapy.

One-child Infertility

M. Heiman[11] has reported on a psychoanalytical evaluation of the problem of one-child sterility or secondary infertility on a psychosomatic basis in which he found that these women have a greater need for being mothered than for motherhood. The first child becomes the only child because unconsciously it represents a re-establisment of the child-mother relationship between the woman and her own mother. The twosomeness of this mother-child relationship does not permit the intrusion of a third person, be it either a second child or the patient's husband. This explains the observation in such cases of the husband being relegated to a secondary role. We have seen patients with secondary infertility who seem to fall into the pattern described by Dr. Heiman.

Such a case was one who had had a child three years before and had been unable to conceive since. During this three-year period, she had received the accepted infertility work-up by another gynecologist, and our tests as well as his revealed no pathologic condition to explain the infertility. The patient was the youngest of three children born during the depression. She was told by her mother that she was an unwanted child. This feeling was reinforced in many ways, so that as a child the patient felt deeply rejected. For example, the patient was punished for being a poor eater by being left at home when the family took a trip. This was recalled in therapy with deep feelings of depression over being abandoned. As a reaction to these feelings, she felt compelled to make good grades at school in order to keep up with her older sister, who was the mother's favorite. Her feeling was one of not being good enough to be loved. Any expression of anger would cause her mother to cry and withdraw, or would lead to the admonition, "God will punish you for being a bad girl."

The patient was, therefore, convinced that she was the cause of her mother's unhappiness. This led to both repressed hostility and marked dependence on her mother. The intense feeling of rejection and deep hostility towards her mother was expressed in dreams of her mother's dying and in anxiety about her mother's health. A considerable period of time was spent by the patient in therapy becoming conscious of this anger with the associated feeling of guilt. She felt that, since she wished for the death of her mother, God was punishing her and therefore she would not become a mother, but that, if she did get pregnant, either she or the baby would die. When the patient finally appreciated that her anger towards her mother was unconditionally accepted by her doctor, a great deal of anxiety was relieved and she felt as though a heavy weight had been lifted from her. It was following this period in therapy that she was able to establish a better relationship with her four-year-old son and to separate from him. Up to this point, he was not allowed out of her sight. Subsequently, he was sent to nursery school and his behavior improved.

The raising of this child had been a heavy burden to her, for it revived her own ambivalence towards her mother, causing her unconsciously to reject her own child and over-protect him. She was finally able to acknowledge that having another child would markedly increase her burdens and she also became aware that the responsibilities of motherhood were very threatening to her in another way; as she expressed it, "A child under two months is helpless and alone. If I make a mistake, I might harm him", emphasizing her unconscious hostility to her first child because of her own wish to be a child. A major turning-point in the therapy occurred when the patient became consciously aware of the fact that she really did not want to become pregnant because of all the emotional threats involved. Her expression was, "Instead of my looking forward to the time of ovulation, I find that I am disturbed and anxious and have a sense of relief after I feel that this time has passed".

This is the patient who was previously referred to—the case in which there had been a subtle avoidance of coitus during the fertile period. Having another child was too great a burden for her, since it symbolized her own older unresolved mother-child relationship, as well as its counterpart in her overprotective attitude toward her child. In this case, as in the series of Dr. Heiman, the husband was relegated to a secondary role. After working through her feelings towards her mother and child, she was free to talk about her repressed sexual feelings which repression had been intensified by her mother's attitudes. The onset of menstruation frightened her; she thought she was bleeding to death. During her first pregnancy she had some bleeding after sex relations and lost her sexual desires. Feeling that a pregnant woman may be injured persisted until after she had discussed these feelings in therapy. Pregnancy occurred within two months after her last session and she was delivered of a normal male infant without difficulty. There had been twenty-two sessions of therapy over a period of a year.

2

Psychological Testing

Rubenstein[22] was impressed in his psychological treatment of six cases of infertility, in which five did conceive that the central conflict was related to an identification with a hostile mother and therefore suggested that besides the usual sterility studies, preliminary psychological tests be made on all patients, and when an intensely hostile mother is inferred to exist, psychotherapy be recommended. From 1960 to 1964, sixty-six of our patients who were seen with the problem of infertility were given the Family Problems Scale (Loevinger and Sweet) and the Sentence Completion Test (Elizabeth Nettles) as part of their investigation. Then after a period of a couple of years, these tests were evaluated by two psychologists independently to see whether they could select the patients whose infertility problem was, indeed, on a non-organic basis. However, unfortunately, they were unable to select these cases with any degree of accuracy.

We then had the test material analyzed in detail by two other psychologists, Rodney M. Coe and Anita Artstein, with the following results. Of the 66 cases, only 51 were considered for the study as in 6 instances the infertility problem was due to the husband and 9 women were lost to follow-up. The Family Problems scale has 210 questions which measure items divided into five clusters: (1) authoritarian family ideology, (2) acceptance of conventional social role for women, (3) harmony and discord in the home, (4) fear of intrusion and distrust of others, and (5) impulse control, aggression and disorder. Because only 8 patients had a definitely proven organic etiology to their infertility, the customary statistical procedures could not be used to compare the scores on the various clusters with the 43 patients in the non-organic infertile group. However, a comparison of percentages does lead to some tentative conclusions in that in clusters 1 and 2 (Authoritarian Family Ideology and Acceptance of Convenional Role of Women), the organic infertility case scored low—25·0% in cluster 1 and 37·5% in cluster 2, compared with 67·5% in cluster 1 and 72·5% in cluster 2 in the non-organic group. This means essentially that non-organically infertile females more often come from homes which might be characterized as overly permissive.

An inference may also be made that social roles of family members in permissive environs are less clearly articulated, that is there may be more overlapping among the role tasks associated with each complementary role. If so, it could be expected that non-organically infertile females would exhibit less acceptance of the conventional social role of women (cluster 2). One might also believe that the more authoritarian a family is in ideology and practice, the clearer are the wives on what they are expected to do and be in the family.

The Sentence Completion test did not reveal any significant differences in the two groups.

It would seem to indicate that the psychological tests used were not sensitive enough to differentiate this problem or, more likely, that the psychodynamics in the cases of infertility are not unique. They are also found in many neurotic women seen in therapy for other problems besides infertility.

Four patients had been studied with an extensive battery of psychological tests including the Rorschach, Thematic Apperception Test, Bender-Gestalt, Draw-A-Person, Sentence Completion and the Family Problems Scale. Testing was done subsequent to their psychotherapy and after delivery of their children. The women gave evidence of anxiety and feelings of inadequacy and weakness. Since this was after a successful pregnancy, it throws light on the question that is often raised about the anxiety and feelings of inferiority in the feminine role that may stem specifically from the inability to have a child. The tests would suggest that these women are chronically anxious and plagued by doubts about their ability to measure up to adult roles.

The basic conflicts over dependency and hostility were apparent in all four cases, with variable insight and conscious appreciation of conflict areas. Hysterical features with emphasis on repression and naïve denial were common, and the hysterical component probably accounts in part for the effectiveness of the type of therapy given. For the most part, the tests substantiated the material obtained in the psychotherapeutic sessions. In no case did the disturbance seem to be psychotic-like, but there was considerable range in the degree of clinical pathology that one would expect to observe. They have considerable strength to deal with their discomfort and make a reasonable adjustment to motherhood in spite of general neurotic patterns and specific sexual complexes.

It would certainly simplify the treatment of the infertile couple if psychological tests could be developed which would single out the cases of psychosomatic infertility.

3

Summary

An evaluation of the week by week therapy notes on these patients indicates that the early hours were filled with much self-criticism, involving the feeling that the lack of conception was a punishment for earlier wrong-doings or bad feelings and thoughts. There was much protestation about the eagerness to become pregnant and the almost universal presentation of ideal family experiences. However, as time went on, the women began to recognize their own disinclination for pregnancy and were able to admit a fear of pregnancy, feeling they might be destroyed in the process. Often there were feelings indicating a marked jealousy of mother figures as well as the unborn child. Patients soon became aware of their marked ambivalent feelings towards their mothers. This was intense and universal in all the patients. The patients were either overcome with guilt when they felt hostility or spoke with a fear that their parents, especially the mother, would die if anger were expressed. With the therapist encouraging the expression of the previous blocked hostile feelings, the patients were able to be critical of parental figures without guilt and to recognize the many ways in which their over-protective upbringing was, in effect, a rejection by the parents of them as individuals.

To protect themselves against such an unacceptable early situation, the patients developed a markedly dependent identification with their hostile mothers or an over-identification with their fathers. This resulted in the women's developing insecure and immature attitudes about their femininity or development of tomboyish attitudes. The ability to express their blocked angry feelings without guilt also facilitated the expression of warm, affectionate womanly feelings to the therapist. This development of a positive transference was nearly always followed by an increased feminine attitude on the part of the patient as well as an increased appetite for sexual relations with their husbands. The development of the warm, positive emotional relationship between the patient and the therapist nearly always preceded the occurrence of conception. Very frequently the patients, through dreams or expressed feelings, could accurately predict their pregnancy.

PSYCHOLOGICAL FACTORS PRODUCING INFERTILITY IN THE MALE

1

Introduction

While some women do not achieve motherhood because of psycho-pathological factors within themselves which prevent pregnancy or produce a spontaneous abortion, it is also obvious that psychological and organic factors may play a role as regards the male function and the propagative act. While there has been no meaningful evidence as yet that emotional factors in the male may produce biophysiological changes resulting in reduced sperm count or defective sperm, there has been an occasional impressionistic report of a reduced emission as a result of anxiety surrounding the collection and examination of the ejaculate.[9] There is considerable evidence that emotional factors are responsible for certain types of impotence in the male which effectively negate the possibility of conception in the female. Besides erectile impotence (*impotentia coeundi*) and ejaculatory impotence (*ejaculatio retardata*, or retarded ejaculation), the male may phobically avoid coitus. All of these conditions may be responsible for the lack of conception.

Despite the large number of articles on the problem of male potency disorders, there has been no prevalence study except that carried out by Kinsey.[16] However, there have been two important studies of the natural history of male potency disorders,[6, 12] and one interesting statistical study attempting to delineate the psychological factors causally related to impotence.[24] Even the definition of the syndrome is unclear, so it is not always certain that the authors are talking about the same problem.

Definition of Impotence

In many of the articles on male potency disorders, specific definitions of male impotence are not used; and when they are given, they do not correspond to other definitions of the syndrome. In Webster's *Third New International Dictionary*, the term "impotent" is simply defined as "the inability to copulate". As clinically used, while related to the inability to copulate, impotence is often used to refer not only to the man's own sexual satisfaction, but to his inability to bring the woman to orgasm. This fact distorts the definition to a point where it becomes meaningless, since the woman's gratification is not exclusively dependent on the male. As used in this paper, impotence will refer only to the man's own sexual satisfaction.

Male potency disorders can be subdivided into the following three major types: (1) erectile impotence (*impotentia coeundi*), (2) ejaculatory impotence (*ejaculatio retardata*), and (3) premature ejaculation (*ejaculatio praecox*).

Erectile impotence is described as that condition where the male cannot obtain or maintain a penile erection satisfactory to him for purposes of heterosexual coitus. Ejaculatory impotence refers to the inability to ejaculate during sex relations. Sometimes this inability relates also to masturbation. However, all males with ejaculatory impotence do have nocturnal emissions.

Premature ejaculation is defined as that condition where the male reaches orgasm and ejaculation before he wishes to do so. Since this generally occurs *intra vaginam* and may be a problem as regards orgastic gratification in the female and pleasurable gratification for the male, it will not be considered at any length at this time because, regardless of the lack of orgastic gratification, conception may take place.

In addition, male impotence is also described as primary (having always been present) or secondary (occurring after having been potent). The question of specificity is also of significance, since impotence may be absolute (under no circumstances), or selective (occurring with certain individuals and not with others).

Incidence and Prevalence of Impotence

As with the definition of impotence, there are also problems concerning the incidence or prevalence of male impotence. There has been little work done on the problem of individual differences, and apart from Kinsey's,[16] no significant prevalence studies have been carried out. This leaves the whole question of incidence or prevalence very much in doubt, since different authors have committed themselves to a wide range of statistics. For example, it had been popularly stated, without statistical evidence, that men are 50% impotent during the wedding night and that men become increasingly more impotent as they get older.[25] In 1963, Lyman Stewart, a urologist, claimed without statistical evidence, that 10% of all males are impotent; from the age of 50 to 65, he said, the incidence rises to 38% and after the age of 65, 52% are impotent.[26]

Kinsey[16] in his studies found that ejaculatory impotence was present in six men and "more or less permanent erectile impotence" in 66 men out of 4108 males studied. These statistics do not include "instances of temporary incapacity in younger individuals. . . At ages under 36, erectile or ejaculatory impotence accounts for no more than a few stray cases of low-rates of outlet. Only 0·4% of males under 25 were troubled with erectile impotence, 1% of males under 35, 25% at 65 and 75% at 80." These statistics in older men were the result of only a small number of subjects.

We are in general agreement with Kinsey's prevalence studies regarding ejaculatory and erectile impotence and his general remarks concerning the psychological etiology. "Impotence in a male under 55 years of age is almost always the product of psychologic conflict, except in those exceedingly few cases where there has been mechanical injury of the genitalia or of the portion of the central nervous system which control erections, or in those similarly few cases where venereal or other disease has interfered with nervous function. There is even some evidence that much of the impotence which is seen in old age is psychologic in origin."[16] Many other authors have postulated that 90% or more of male potency disorders are psychogenic in nature.[24]

2

Ejaculatory Impotence as a Factor in Female Infertility: Case Reports

In line with the experience of other investigators, very few males suffering from impotence come voluntarily for help.

A patient, age 21, was married for nine months when referred for symptoms of primary ejaculatory impotence. His wife had earlier seen her obstetrician (Rothman) complaining of infertility due to her husband's inability to ejaculate during sex relations. There was also an inability to ejaculate during masturbation. However, nocturnal emissions were present.[15]

While at first the patient felt he had no emotional problems, he soon came to recognize his marked dependency and emotional immaturity, his inability to accept responsibility, his need to look to parental figures for guidance and direction, his inability to be competitive or aggressive, and his need to rigidly conform to cultural standards. An early feeding problem, he was frequently sick during his childhood. The youngest of three children, he had an older sister who was reasonably well adjusted and more aggressive. The second sister had many episodes of depression and was diagnosed as a manic-depressive with suicidal tendencies. Mother, overly seductive, was also over-protective and over-controlling. Until he was fourteen years of age, she frequently lay down with him when he went to sleep. The mother often engaged in much kissing and hugging. Father, busy and highly successful in business, was only occasionally available to his son. Oral traits were markedly exaggerated. Still sucking his thumb at the age of twenty-one, he had trouble with dieting, tended to be heavy. In appearance he was baby-faced, an attractive but dependent-looking male. Patient was over six feet tall, chubby but not obese. His striking personality characteristics were his passivity, his need to be cared for, and his inability to accept responsibility for decisions.

Patient's early pathological relationship with his mother and subsequent lack of identification with father, plus rivalry with his sisters, led to marked characterological changes with the focus on his need to cling to adults for support and nourishment (oral regression), latent passive homosexual tendencies, fear of his own aggression, guilt over sexuality, and a need to be like his sister. There was a marked accentuation of all oral activity; eating, kissing, talking, thumbsucking with refusal to give of himself to others. Symbolically, his penis seemed equated with breasts, semen with milk, so that he could not part with his ejaculate. There was underlying competitiveness, defended against by much pseudo-aggressive behavior projecting onto others the reason for his lack of competitiveness (paranoid tendencies?). His sexual experiences were on one hand the continuation of his pseudo-masculine role and on the other, a refusal to give something of himself to his wife. He always felt that the ejaculate was dangerous, not only to his wife, but to himself.

All his behavior was designed to bring on failure through pseudo-aggression, oral dependency, pseudo-masculinity, and ejaculatory impotence. In psychoanalytic psychotherapy, working through the emotional relationship with the therapist, first demonstrating his dependency as he originally related to his mother and then later competition and ambivalence to male figures, he learned to compete, to be more normally aggressive with his father and to identify with him. His attitudes towards women and his mother became more realistic and he developed normal masculine attitudes. This led successively to the ability to masturbate with ejaculation, followed by sex relations actively carried out by his wife and subsequently normal sex relationships with several pregnancies. In work, he accepted more responsibility, became more autonomous and self-dependent, and developed into a highly successful business executive. Improvement has been maintained for over fifteen years.

The psychodynamics of this case of ejaculatory impotence is similar in many ways to the studies of Noy. Wollstein, Kaplan-De-Nour,[19] Bergler,[4, 5] and Ovesey and Meyers.[20] Bergler was the original investigator of this syndrome. He referred to the syndrome as "oral asperma" and indicated that the symptoms are secondary manifestations cloaking a deep and masochistic attachment to the mother. The symptoms of ejaculatory impotence act as revenge against women who are considered to be symbols of the mother. What the male really wants is to be refused, so that he can enjoy the refusal masochistically.[4] Ovesey and Meyers found a strong association between the symptoms of retarded ejaculation and mild paranoid tendencies. The men were highly ambitious and competitive, but these drives were inhibited because early childish intimidation caused them to perceive all competition in terms of murderous violence, with each adversary out to kill the other. Sexual relations were considered to be a symbolic extension of a competitive struggle with men, but successful completion of the act meant not only validating the masculine role but simultaneously destroying the competitiveness. By sustaining an erection but inhibiting orgasm, the man can ward off the phantasy of retaliation while maintaining his illusion of hyper-masculinity. Detumesence is equated with castration and loss of semen with depletion of vitality.[20]

Patient with Avoidance Problem as well as Erectile Impotence

Patient, a 23-year-old male, was seen one year after he was married, with complaints of fear of approaching his wife sexually. In addition, he had a mild-to-moderate speech defect present since early childhood.

Prior to his marriage he engaged in necking and petting, with some genital contact with normal erections. Sex relations with his fiancée were delayed until after marriage. On the honeymoon, becoming sexually aroused, he "suddenly discovered that he did not know anything about the appropriate positions that might be used". After reading a book and attempting sex relations again, symptoms of erectile impotence developed. However, after additional sexual failures, patient began to feel extremely anxious when he approached his wife sexually and, in reaction, began to avoid sex; which symptoms continued for a number of years. He described periods of sexual arousal with corresponding periods of acute anxiousness, queasy feelings in his stomach, and marked fearfulness about approaching his wife. Occasionally, however, they resorted to mutual masturbation.

A frightened and fearful boy in younger years, he was afraid to fight and was anxious when his parents went out. While he had a speech problem, from the very earliest years for reasons which are unclear to him, his parents never mentioned this problem, and he finally insisted on getting some help when he was seventeen and eighteen years of age. While his older brother was wild and aggressive as a child, athletic and more self-reliant, the patient was closer to the younger sister, with whom he felt more comfortable. He remembers that, while his father and brother were impulsive and aggressive, he was more like his mother, fearful, compulsive and constricted. Outwardly markedly religious, as was the family, he often had sadistic fantasies of beating naked women with sticks. Markedly attracted to big-breasted women and married to a very attractive woman, he cannot think of his wife as a sex partner, only as the mother of his children. When he thinks of having sex relations, he is afraid that something will happen to his penis and he becomes anxious and withdraws from his wife. Sometimes when he is lying next to his wife, he becomes anxious and phantasies that some unknown man might come into the room. In some way this is related to his sexual incapacity, as if the man will have the sexual relations with his wife which he was unable to carry out.

Patient was enuretic until the age of ten. In his adolescence he was more attracted to older women on whom he could be dependent. From what he recalls, there was a considerable amount of nakedness in the home and much sexual seduction on the part of his mother. While in latency period, he thought of himself as "a hood" and frequently cheated in class, as well as truanted. Subsequently, as a reaction, he developed compulsive personality characteristics and became indecisive and ritualistic in his behavior. While his feelings were isolated, he thought of himself as being markedly omnipotent. However, he had great difficulty in expressing his feelings and giving of himself to his wife, his family and his friends. In adolescence, he enjoyed sexual arousal through voyeuristic activities, observing prostitutes and dancing girls, but was unable to allow himself any heterosexual experiences.

A psychological examination indicated that structurally all of his affects were repressed, and this added to the inner turmoil and anxiety. His control was maintained at the cost of considerable suffering and loss of self-esteem. Being highly conforming, all of his energies were channeled to the inhibitory and masking defences. He showed evidence of repression and depression. Conflict was acute, with excessive concern about morality. Sexual activity was described as not only bad but dangerous. Sex relations, in his mind, were equated with the fear of loss of love, fear of injury and the fear of his own sexual power and excitement.

Patient was essentially an overly serious, tense, rigid, frequently depressed, overly conforming and ruminative individual. While only twenty-three years of age, he gave the impression of being at least ten or fifteen years older. Bright and with good motivation, he made a real effort in psychotherapy to overcome years of chronic frustration and feelings of inadequacy associated with his symptoms of speech defect and impotence. His formal diagnosis was that of an obsessive personality trait disorder with symptoms of chronic stuttering and erectile impotence.

In psychoanalytically oriented psychotherapy, patient found it extremely difficult to express his inner affects. Resistance to therapy was very marked. Patient was frequently silent, obviously angry but unable to admit such feelings. Highly competitive, he was markedly anxious because of these feelings, and set up situations in which someone else had to assume responsibility in work, whereas the real truth lay in his own fear of committing himself to any type of business decisions.

Following a period of greater insight into his earlier ambivalent and incestuous feelings toward his mother and subsequently his wife, he was first able to have sexual relations with his wife by encouraging her to wear underwear similar to that which had stimulated him voyeuristically during adolescence. Phantasizing his wife as a depreciated love object, he was able to complete the sex act. Following another period of resistance and no further sex for some weeks, he was able to re-live and carry out those adolescent phases of sexual development which in earlier years were impossible for him.

His ability to show warm, affectionate feelings increased, but he still had difficulty competing with men and tended to maintain many compulsive defences. Now the father of three children, while still suffering from some of his earlier psychological difficulties, there are no longer any problems of erectile impotence and sexual avoidance.

Discussion of Psychodynamic Factors

The patients represented by the aforementioned clinical studies illustrate the small number of younger males suffering from primary impotence disorders which affect the fertility of the woman. These patients are not similar to those younger males who may be occasionally impotent early in marriage due to anxiety concerning sexual performance, or where the impotence reflects marital conflict or some intercurrent psychic trauma which temporarily disturbs sexual adequacy.[17] These illustrated cases are also not representative of the older males who begin to have more difficulty with potency problems at a time when problems of infertility are not pertinent. Such patients with transitory potency problems, often referred to as secondary impotence, do not have the typical psychodynamic patterns of those males with primary impotence. Their psychological problems are less deeply ingrained in personality defects and therefore can be modified more easily by muscular relaxation techniques, educative techniques, supportive emotional measures or briefer forms of psychotherapy. In fact, it is common for all males in psychotherapy and psychoanalysis to report occasional episodes of impotence at points of significant emotional stress, related most frequently to the concern over masculine adequacy. Transitory impotence may also occur in the life of any normal male, especially when coital attempts are more the result of intellectual rather than emotional decisions.

Most of the patients with symptoms of primary erectile and ejaculatory impotence seen in our clinical practice as represented by the aforementioned patients, do come from middle and upper socio-economic groups. While this situation is somewhat atypical for a clinic population, even there the impotent males are generally in the higher-class groups. Nearly all of the patients in our private practice with impotence disorders were college graduates or the equivalent thereof. They all came from intact families and all were highly successful outside of the marriage in their work. All of the patients had evidence of early psychic trauma with evidence of frequent feeding problems and physical illnesses. These patients were subjected to marked over-protection, over-indulgence and sexual seduction by their mothers. In general, nearly all of the patients were mild-mannered and self-contained. They obviously tried to please everyone and they seemed to have considerable difficulty with over-aggression, although in therapy it was learned that unconsciously they were all markedly competitive, with much repressed hostility manifesting itself in pseudo-aggressive and pseudo-masculine activities.

As a group, they were little interested in sports, especially contact sports, but were involved in impressing others by their intellectual activities. Indeed, all of them were markedly concerned and fearful about women towards whom they generally had a marked infantile dependent relationship or pseudo-aggressive relationship. In a certain sense, these men felt unable to carry out the sexual act, which they viewed as a burden placed upon them by the woman with the feeling that they had to prove themselves in sex.

Attracted more to the female breast than the genital, most of the impotent males were less interested in sex relations than the average male. There was a marked fear of the female genital, and a fear of self-destruction as a result of sex relations. They were profoundly dependent on their wives, as they had been in earlier years on their own mothers. Their attitude to males was one of marked inferiority, feeling less aggressive than other males, with prominent latent homosexual feelings towards these males. Relationships to their fathers were markedly ambivalent. Their fathers were generally distant, involved in their own competitive needs, generally successful. Most of the fathers were over-indulgent in their behavior towards their sons, and they were treated by their wives very much as their sons learned to react to other women.

In classifying the personality characteristics of such individuals, they can be described as having mixed compulsive and hysterical personalities with strong oral and phallic aspects. Their sexual behavior has a strong oral character to it designed to fail on a genital level but succeed on an infantile oral level. Sexual success was feared and equated as aggression, hostility and murderous impulses towards women, with the fear of resultant punishment by castration. This is most striking in patients with ejaculatory impotence, but is also true of men with erectile impotence. The person with erectile impotence often has premature ejaculation, and he presents his weakness by depositing the semen *ante portas* thus demonstrating the weakness, denying the wish to be assertive, potent, aggressive, and by the same token frustrating the female about whom he is so ambivalent.

The psychodynamic features described above are similar not only to earlier studies by Ferenczi,[8] Freud[10] and Stekel[25] but correspond to the statistical study by Senoussi *et al.*[24] This latter study showed that "psychogenic impotence, like organic impotence, can be attributed to more than one source . . . (a) violation of a persistent frame of reference concerning sexual acceptance; (b) heightened sensitivity because of expectations of humiliation and rejection; and (c) persistent feelings of insecurity as an individual and as a provider."

But similar genetic and psychodynamic factors may also be present in the homosexual, and even in the compulsive, hysterical and anxiety neurotics. Patients suffering from impotence problems are not psychotic, but more like neurotics. Their personality development and the character of their symptoms are closely related to the hysterical and compulsive symptomatology and personality. However, the symptoms themselves are better explained as a psychophysiologic manifestation (hypersensitivity of penis or other sexual dysfunction leading to ejaculatory impotence or erectile impotence, symptoms resulting from autonomic dysfunction).

All of the patients who entered treatment presumably for their potency disorder had many other characterological difficulties and neurotic symptoms, similar to the sexual difficulty. However, these personality characteristics were present prior to the onset of sexual maturity, and the potency disorder followed the emotional difficulties. On the other hand, few of the patients had overt anxiety. Most of the patients can be described as passive-aggressive personality trait disturbances with obsessive and hysterical features and a psychophysiological, genito-urinary disorder, impotence.

However, despite the similarity of the psychodynamic factors as described above, for the impotent male can one say that these specific psychological constellations are crucial for the development of a male potency disorder? Even Sigmund Freud in 1912[10] stated, "There is one principal objection to raise against this doctrine (specific constellation); it does too much; it explains why certain persons suffer from psychical impotence but it makes it seem puzzling that others can escape the affliction." At this point, we feel one cannot state that there are specific genetic and psychodynamic factors responsible for the development of the male potency disorders. Such psychodynamic constellations may also be present in individuals who develop hysterical neuroses, sexual perversions or have other personality trait disturbances. It is also impossible to correlate male potency disorders with any of the aforementioned early family difficulties, such as the degree of maternal seduction and over-protection or the character of paternal identification. In several male patients with symptoms of homosexuality, anxiety attacks, and serious phobias, the family backgrounds are very much the same as those males suffering from impotence.

The problem of male sexual potency is a complex one. It is also related to changing cultural attitudes. There is the strong impression that at present most men are generally concerned with whether or not they have sufficient staying power to satisfy the woman with whom they have sex relations. The cultural pressure for erective potency, more frequently in men with a college education, was demonstrated by Masters and Johnson[18] in their study of 261 subjects of college matriculation, of whom 214 expressed such a concern. However, only 7 of 51 subjects who did not reach the level of college were at all concerned about their wives' reactions in sex relations. In addition, almost every male over forty in Masters and Johnson's patients expressed a fear of secondary potency with ageing. Of course, the concern about erective potency is in line with the cultural pressure on the part of man to be successful throughout his life in all areas of endeavor. Concern about success and work and sex are, therefore, well correlated. The use of the contraceptive pill by the woman in addition to her feeling that orgasm is now her just due must also have adversely modified the cultural pressures for erective potency.

Potency problems were said to be common in the psychiatric and psychoanalytic practices of the early 1900s.[10] However, despite the apparent present cultural pressure, we still have no meaningful statistical studies of how changing cultural factors affect the incidence and prevalence of male potency disorders. In a recent unpublished study by the author, an attempt was made by questionnaire to determine the incidence of potency disorders during 1968 in all of the male patients in psychotherapy or psychoanalysis seen by the practicing psychoanalysts in St. Louis. Of the 15 psychoanalysts, 13 responded to the questionnaire. Of the 51 males in psychoanalysis, there were 9 cases of primary impotence (18%) and 13 cases of secondary impotence, of whom 6 were transitory (25%), making a total incidence of impotence of 43%. Of the 79 males in psychotherapy, there was one case of primary impotence (1·2%) and 20 cases of secondary impotence, of whom 4 were transitory (25%).[14] Certainly these statistics corroborate the earlier impression that potency problems are most common in the private practice of psychoanalytic psychiatry.

3

Therapy and Prognosis

The two illustrated cases of primary impotence were both treated by psycho-analytically oriented psychotherapy. In addition to potency problems, these men both had moderately serious personality difficulties which affected their work and social relations. Essentially, one might describe them as having impotent personality characteristics similar to their sexual difficulties. However, with psychoanalysis or psychoanalytically oriented psychotherapy, the treatment (moderate or much improved) of the 22 primary and secondary cases of impotence being treated by psychoanalysis in 1968 in St. Louis varied between 77% and 80%. Of the 21 cases of impotence (only one was a primary type) being treated by psychoanalytically oriented psychotherapy, only 52% were moderately or much improved.[14]

The statistics cited above are indicative only of selected middle and upper class patients seen in a private psychoanalytic practice. The results are only impressionistic, since the study was inadequately controlled and lacked objective criteria as to the description of symptoms, personality difficulties as well as therapy results. Urologists in private practice also routinely see many patients with symptoms of potency disorder. These symptoms are generally of transitory character, secondary in type, and the bulk of patients are over 50 years of age. Treatment by the urologists is frequently educative, emotionally supportive with the use of tranquilizing drugs and prostatic massage. The results are said to be highly satisfactory.[1]

Recently with selective patients, Semans,[23] Tuthill,[28] Johnson and Masters,[13] Wolpe,[29] and others have used re-educative techniques, muscular relaxation techniques, emotional support, provision from the sexual partner for maximum co-operation and stimulation, sex education and reconditioning techniques with apparent success (66% to 100%). Involvement of the marital couple as a unit is an important aspect of treatment, as is the encouragement of the male to be more passive while the woman at first assumes a more active role.

However, studies of clinic populations by Alan J. Cooper[6] and J. Johnson[12] of the natural history of male potency disorders and the effect of therapy, indicate a rate of improvement of between 33.3% and 37%. According to Cooper,[6] other scientists' impressive results occurred either because they treated carefully selected patients or because the criteria for improvement were apparently lax. J. Johnson[12] pointed out that the improvement rate of impotence if it is largely psychogenic in character, with or without therapy, was far below the spontaneous rate of improvement in the neurosis (65%). He therefore assumed there may be constitutional factors which limit therapeutic effectiveness. Constitutional factors may also be "the eradicable effects of early experience".[27]

While Cooper's results were similar to those of Johnson, and while he also predicates the importance of unknown constitutional factors, his studies suggest that psychogenic impotence occurs with any frequency only in young males, and then only represents a fraction (15%) of the bulk of potency disorders seen in the general psychiatric clinic. However, the higher success rate of treatment in this young group (7 cures out of 8 patients) supports the validity made about the psychogenic ideology. But the corollary of this fact, that predominantly "biological disorders of potency" could not be expected to respond to any extent to psychological treatment, was also demonstrated in the study. The treatments used in the Cooper study included psychotherapy, muscular relaxation, provision as far as possible from the partner for optimum sex stimulation, and sex education. Acute onset cases had a better response and similar to our experience their males had a lower sexual drive. Persons in the higher social class were over-represented, and nearly all the men were sent to the clinic by their frustrated wives.[6]

Patients with sexual potency disorders have varying degrees of personality difficulties, some more susceptible to treatment and unknown constitutional factors so far unaffected by any known therapeutic techniques. Younger patients with transitory impotence or secondary impotence are more easily treated by re-training, re-education and muscle relaxing and conditioning techniques. In addition, more supportive forms of psychotherapy may also be effective in modifying such cases of secondary impotence without the use of ancillary techniques. The co-operation of the wife in the treatment plan as described by Semans[23] and later by Johnson and Masters,[13] can be most effective in the re-training and re-educative treatment procedures.

Patients with primary erectile or ejaculatory impotence nearly always have other personality disturbances which may require more intensive psychotherapy or psychoanalytic treatment. At times, such psychological treatment may need to be followed up by re-training and re-educative techniques to overcome old and difficult habit patterns. (Even patients with speech defects caused by serious emotional disturbance may still require re-educative and re-training to overcome the speech defects, despite the insight gained in psychotherapy.)

Patients with acute onset of symptoms are more easily treated than those patients whose symptoms are chronic and whose personality difficulties are also deeply ingrained. In those selected patients who have good relationships with their spouses, the prognosis is much better. Often, however, patients seen by psychiatrists and psychoanalysts are so involved in their neurotic problem, so impaired in their relations with the opposite sex, that they cannot participate in re-training and re-educative techniques. Prognosis in such cases is never as good as in younger selected cases with more co-operative spouses.

REFERENCES

1. ABRAMS, M. 1969. Personal Communication.
2. BENEDEK, T., HAM, G. C., ROBBINS, F. P. and RUBENSTEIN, B. B. 1953. Some emotional factors in infertility. *Psychosom. Med.*, **15**, 485.
3. BENEDEK, T. and RUBENSTEIN, B. B. 1942. *The sexual cycle in women.* Baltimore: The Williams & Wilkins Co.
4. BERGLER, E. 1949. *The basic neurosis.* New York: Grune & Stratton.
5. BERGLER, E. 1951. *Neurotic counterfeit-sex.* New York: Grune & Stratton.
6. COOPER, A. J. 1968. A factual study of male potency disorders. *Brit. J. Psychiat.*, **114**, 719.
7. DE WATTEVILLE, H. 1957. Psychologic factors in the treatment of sterility. *Fertil. & Steril.*, **8**, 12.
8. FERENCZI, S. 1958. The analytic interpretation and treatment of psychosexual impotence (1908). In *Sex in Psychoanalysis.* New York: Dover Publications.
9. FISCHER, I. C. 1953. Psychogenic aspects of sterility. *Fertil. Steril.*, **4**, 466.
10. FREUD, S. 1953. Contribution to the psychology of love (1912). In *Collected Papers*, **IV**, 203. London: Hogarth Press.
11. HEIMAN, M. 1955. Psychoanalytic evaluation of the problem of "one-child sterility". *Fertil. Steril.*, **6**, 405.
12. JOHNSON, J. 1965. Prognosis of disorders of sexual potency in the male. *J. psychosom. Res.*, **9**, 195.
13. JOHNSON, V. E. and MASTERS, W. H. 1964. Sexual incompatability: diagnosis and treatment. In *Human reproduction and sexual behaviour* (Lloyd, C. W., ed.). Philadelphia: Lea & Febiger.
14. KAPLAN, A. H. 1968. Male potency disorders. Paper to St. Louis Psychoanalytic Society.
15. KAPLAN, A. H. and ABRAMS, M. 1958. Ejaculatory impotence. *J. Urol.*, **79**, 964.
16. KINSEY, A. C., POMEROY, W. B. and MARTIN, C. E. 1948. *Sexual behavior in the human male.* Philadelphia and London: Saunders.
17. LEWIS, J. M. 1969. Impotence as a reflection of marital conflict. *Medical Aspects of Human Sexuality*, **3**, 73.
18. MASTERS, W. H. and JOHNSON, V. E. 1966. *Human sexual response.* Boston: Little-Brown.
19. NOY, P., WOLLSTEIN, S. and KAPLAN-DE-NOUR, A. 1966. Clinical observations on the psychogenesis of impotence. *Brit. J. med. Psychol.*, **39**, 43.
20. OVESEY, L. and MEYERS, H. 1968. Retarded ejaculation. *Amer. J. Psychother.*, **22**, 185.
21. ROTHMAN, D., KAPLAN, A. H. and NETTLES, E. 1962. Psychosomatic infertility. *Amer. J. Obst. Gynec.*, **83**, 373.
22. RUBENSTEIN, B. B. 1951. An emotional factor in infertility: a psychosomatic approach. *Fertil. Steril.*, **2**, 80.
23. SEMANS, J. H. 1956. Premature ejaculation: a new approach. *J. Urol.*, **148**, 836.
24. SENOUSSI, A. E., COLEMAN, D. R. and TAUBER, A. S. 1959. Factors in male impotence. *J. Psychol.*, **48**, 3.
25. STEKEL, W. 1927. Impotence in the male. In *Psychic disorder of the sexual function in the male. I, II.* New York: Liveright.
26. STEWART, L. 1963. Impotence in the male. Series on urology for the practitioner. *The Journal-Lancet*, **83**, 2.
27. TANNER, J. M. 1964. *Human biology; an introduction to human evolution, variation and growth.* Oxford: Clarendon Press.
28. TUTHILL, J. F. 1955. Impotence. *Lancet*, **i**, 124.
29. WOLPE, J. and LAZARUS, A. A. 1961. *Behavior therapy techniques.* New York: Pergamon.

III

PSEUDOCYESIS

TO BE AND NOT TO BE PREGNANT: A PSYCHOSOMATIC QUESTION

PETER BARGLOW

M.D.

*Dept. Psychiatry and Dept. Obstetrics and Gynecology,
Michael Reese Hospital
Lecturer, University of Chicago, U.S.A.*

and

EDWARD BROWN

M.D., B.SC. (MED.)

*Staff Psychiatrist, New Mount Sinai Hospital, Toronto,
and Clinical Teacher, University of Toronto, Canada*

1

Introduction

Pregnancy fantasies of women who are not pregnant may be accompanied by somatic compliance resulting in the psychopathological condition called pseudocyesis. Hippocrates, in 300 B.C., described twelve women "who imagine they are pregnant seeing that the menses are suppressed and the matrices swollen."[21] John Mason Good in 1823 introduced the term "pseudocyesis" (Greek *pseudes*—false, *kyesis*—pregnancy) in his *System of nosology.*[18]

The following recollection appeared in an 1889 obstetrical journal:

> A half-century ago a distinguished German surgeon was called in consultation by a very competent obstetrician to a case in which the patient had apparently been in labor for three weeks. A caesarean section was decided upon, and the abdomen opened, when, to the discomfiture of all, nothing but intestines distended with gas were found. That the professor was chagrined and in a vindictive frame of mind was demonstrated by the after-treatment, for he kept the abdomen packed with ice and applied 200 leeches to the abdominal walls, and in addition, subjected her to three bleedings. The patient recovered, and doubtless ever after desisted from trifling with the resources of surgery.[41]

Pseudocyesis has been described as an illusion, a conversion, a delusion, and a hysterical identification, but no unifying links between these concepts have been offered. A variety of key etiological factors have been suggested, the most common being a fear of, or a wish for, pregnancy. Secondary factors are said to be wishes to please a husband, to have an heir, to force marriage, to prove youthfulness, and to effect self-punishment. Different psychodynamic explanations have emphasized "penis-envy", a "masculinity complex", and an unconscious denial of femininity with a view of menstruation as a symbol of inferiority and deficiency. A number of studies describe physiological mechanisms producing the symptoms of pseudocyesis.

2

Epidemiology

Moulton[30] observed that "79 cases were reported in the literature between 1890 and 1899, and only 26 cases between 1930 and 1936." However, she pointed out that this apparent decrease may have resulted "from the obstetrician merely confirming the diagnosis and dismissing the patient as neurotic, 'psychotic' or malingering." Fischer[15] speculated that the incidence of pseudocyesis might be significantly higher than had been thought. He maintained that there were many patients with a clinical diagnosis of missed abortion who really had pseudocyesis. These patients, at the time of dilatation and curettage, had no gestational tissue.

Bivin and Klinger[8] reviewed 444 cases of pseudocyesis, some dating back to the eighteenth century. These cases ranged in age from 7 to 79 years, with an average age of 33 years. There was no significant correlation between false pregnancy and marital status, age, size of family, or socio-economic or racial factors. Fried and Rakoff[17] collected 27 cases in $2\frac{1}{2}$ years, an incidence of one studied case of pseudocyesis per 250 maternity clinic admissions. Of these patients 23 were Negro. All but one of the patients were childless. One of the authors[3] observed symptoms and signs of pseudocyesis (according to his definition, as appears below) in 152 of 190 women (80%), months and years after sterilization surgery.

Selzer[38] reported the case of a 6-year-old female with delusions of pregnancy, abdominal enlargement, morning nausea and edema. Knight[26] reported the case of a 33-year-old male with delusions of pregnancy, abdominal distention and movement felt in the abdomen.

It seems, then, that the symptoms of pseudocyesis are not an extremely rare occurrence. They appear more frequently in females suffering from sterility. They can occur before or after menarche or menopause. Males are not immune.

3

Symptomatology

The symptoms which characterize pseudocyesis, in order of frequency, as derived from the observations in the two largest patient series studied,[8, 17] are as follows:

(1) Menstrual disturbance (complete amenorrhea or hypomenorrhea). The duration of the disturbance varies but is usually nine months.
(2) Abdominal enlargement without effacement of the umbilicus. The *inverted umbilicus* may be used to differentiate pseudocyesis from pregnancy. According to Jeffcoate,[25] "the enlargement of the abdomen is not caused by gaseous distention, but by unusual use of the abdominal muscles and by an assumed lordosis; it therefore disappears under anesthesia."
(3) Breast changes consisting of swelling and tenderness, secretion of milk and colostrum, pigmentation, and increase in size of papillae.
(4) Foetal movements as reported by the patient.
(5) Softening of the cervix with signs of congestion. Enlargement of the uterus; the size varying from six weeks to eight months.
(6) Nausea and vomiting. Other gastro-intestinal symptoms may consist of aberrations of appetite and constipation.
(7) Weight gain, usually greater than in pregnancy.

Fischer[15] reported one case of toxemia in pseudocyesis. The symptoms included an elevated blood pressure, 2 to 3 plus albumin in the urine, and edema of the lower extremities. These symptoms subsided soon after the diagnosis of pseudocyesis was made.

Pseudocyesis has fooled many able obstetricians. In Bivin and Klinger's report,[8] one or more physicians erroneously had made the diagnosis of pregnancy in 161 of 444 cases of pseudocyesis. In the series of Fried *et al.*,[17] 9 of the 27 patients were told that they were pregnant by 16 of 40 examining physicians and each of the other patients "appeared" to be pregnant to at least one physician. Pseudocyesis patients have been subjected to surgery for supposed ectopic pregnancies and for suspected placenta previa. Organic pathological conditions such as tumors, ascites, uremia, or disease of the genital tract, may on occasion present as a spurious pregnancy.

The presence of an inverted umbilicus, roentgenographic evidence of absence of foetal parts, and the reversal of abdominal enlargement under anaesthesia can be used to make the definitive diagnosis of pseudocyesis. It has been demonstrated that some patients with pseudocyesis have elevated levels of urinary gonadotropin,[17, 39] and the Friedman pregnancy test may give false positive results.[17]

4

Physiology

Human Studies

Bivin and Klinger[8] speculated that "pseudo-pregnancy, a normal state in the menstrual cycle, becomes pseudocyesis, an abnormal state, because the hormones which regulate this phenomenon are thrown out of balance by physical or emotional changes or a combination of these two factors." They noted that "the symptomatology of pseudocyesis simulates in great detail that of true pregnancy, at least as far as outwardly observable indications are concerned." They stressed the importance of psychological factors in the etiology, pointing out that "psychotherapy in the form of simple categorical statements, education and re-education, hypnosis and suggestion, as well as more formal psychotherapeutic techniques, were used with success. . ."

Moulton,[30] in her review of the literature on pseudocyesis, which included both human and animal studies, suggested that the mechanism in certain cases of pseudocyesis might involve the production of a persistent corpus luteum brought about by psychological factors acting on the anterior pituitary. She cited three cases from the French literature. Each was a case of pseudocyesis in which a persistent corpus luteum was demonstrated by surgery. Excision of the corpus luteum resulted in a return of the menses in all three cases. She also reported the case of a seventeen-year-old girl whose symptoms consisted of amenorrhea and abdominal distention, but no breast or uterine changes. Urinary hormone assays and vaginal and oral smears showed a suppression of ovarian activity. This picture was not consistent with a persistent corpus luteum. There was one high gonadotropic assay. Moulton suggested that a suppression of ovarian activity by the pituitary was the mechanism in this case.

Greaves[19] presented one case of pseudocyesis in which follicle stimulating hormone (F.S.H.) assays on two occasions were within normal limits. This also was not consistent with the persistence of a corpus luteum, since the secretion of estrogen and progesterone from the corpus luteum should result in decreased F.S.H. from the anterior pituitary. Steinberg *et al.*,[39] reported three cases of pseudocyesis. In each, the 24-hour urinary gonadotropin and estrogen excretion were assayed and found to be far above normal values. In each case, when the patient was told that she was definitely not pregnant, prompt recession in physical signs took place, attended by a return to normal hormone titers.

Fried *et al.*,[17] in their study of endocrine function in pseudocyesis, presented significant evidence which corroborates the persistence of the corpus luteum. They postulated that "the psychic factor . . . is capable of affecting the pituitary, probably by way of the hypothalamus, causing the release of lactogenic hormones, the suppression of follicle-stimulating hormone and consequent persistence of lutein function with the production of estrogen and progesterone." They studied 27 women with pseudocyesis and concluded that these patients had persisted luteinization of the ovaries as indicated by: (1) varying degrees of endometrial secretory (progesteronic) activity shown on biopsy, (2) the presence of normal or elevated levels of estrogen in the urine, and (3) good estrogen effects shown by vaginal smears. Moreover, the urinary F.S.H. titers were diminished in 24 patients and normal in only 2 patients.

The many examples of reversal of symptoms[3, 8, 15, 17, 19, 26, 30, 34] and return to normal hormonal titers[17, 30, 39] following psychotherapy, provide substantial evidence regarding the presence of psychological factors in the etiology of pseudocyesis.

Animal Studies

There is an extensive literature concerned with the induction and study of pseudocyesis in animals.

Horning,[22] in 1932, described 6 cases of pseudocyesis in dogs who developed symptoms of delayed menses, hydrometra, pseudolactation, abdominal distention, and a peculiar walking gait. They manifested symptoms of maternal caring for an imaginary litter, substituting a rubber dog, slipper, or rag. This condition usually followed a period of heat.

Moulton[30] reviewed the literature to 1942. Pseudopregnancy had been induced in the rat by a variety of methods, which included:

mating the females with vasectomized males,
mechanical stimulation of the cervical canal with a glass rod,
electrical stimulation of the cervical canal,
electrical stimulation of the head,
treatment with vitamin E,
chemical depression of the nasal mucosa.

Several investigators showed that a corpus luteum persisted in the rat and rabbit during the period of false pregnancy. Moulton felt that the most acceptable hypothesis to explain how stimulation of the cervix would lead to a persistent corpus luteum was the existence of a neuronal route to the pituitary, which then acted on the ovaries endocrinologically. There is no evidence to support such a neuronal mechanism in the human.

Bogdanove[9] showed that appropriate estrogen treatment could initiate and maintain pseudopregnancy in the rat. Direct evidence that the sustained pseudocyesis reflected preservation of a single set of corpora was provided by "tagging" 2-3-week-old corpora with microinjections of India ink and allowing the rats to survive for an additional period. In the prolonged studies, when the corpora eventually underwent involution, termination of the pseudocyesis soon followed. Moreover, when the tagged ovaries were removed surgically, termination of the pseudocyesis followed. He suggested that the effect of the estrogen on extending the existence of the corpora lutea depended on its ability to suppress follicle-stimulating hormone secretion and increase luteotropic hormone secretion. The luteotropic hormone then maintained the corpus luteum. Schwartz and Rothchild[37] found an increased concentration of luteinizing hormone in the pituitaries of pseudopregnant rats.

Talwalker et al.[40] demonstrated that the rat hypothalamus contains a factor which inhibits the synthesis or release of luteotropic hormone (prolactin) from the anterior pituitary. This prolactin-inhibiting-factor (P.I.F.), it was shown, is not one of the neurohumors previously known to be present in the hypothalamus. Nikitovitch-Winer[31] presented further evidence that the hypothalamus contains a prolactin-inhibiting-factor. He demonstrated that persistent corpora lutea and pseudocyesis are induced in the rat when the pituitary gland is effectively isolated from the hypothalamus by the placement of a barrier to vascular regeneration.

Cappola et al.[12] confirmed the finding that agents such as reserpine, which act as potent depletors of brain norepinephrine, induce pseudopregnancy in rats. Their study led them to postulate that, in the absence of an endogenous store of brain norepinephrine, the synthesis or release of a prolactin-inhibiting factor in the hypothalamus is impaired. This then results in the release of luteotropic hormone from the anterior pituitary which maintains a persistent corpus luteum and induces pseudopregnancy.

Psychophysiology

Extrapolation of these findings, from animal studies to the human, is open to criticism. Reichlin[36] has pointed out that, in the human, conclusive evidence that prolactin is luteotropic has not yet been advanced. However, it has been observed[25] that, in the human, "certain drugs acting on the hypothalamus can also cause amenorrhea, sometimes accompanied by lactation. These include the phenothiazines, reserpine, and ganglion blocking agents."

Further study of the psychological and endocrinological factors in pseudocyesis should be of significant value in the elucidation of the correlates between psyche and soma. This area of investigation is the topic of a recent publication.[11]

To be and not to be pregnant—indeed a fascinating psychosomatic question.

5

Psychology

What are the criteria which define the existence of human pseudocyesis? Some investigators require the co-existence of one or more of the objective typical somatic signs with a firm, conscious belief in the presence of pregnancy. Others define pseudocyesis by any physical symptom that seems to be related to the existence of an unconscious pregnancy wish.[10]

In 1964, one of the authors[3] proposed that the classical concept of pseudocyesis be expanded to include a multitude of emotional manifestations and somatic symptoms, observed in "healthy", neurotic, and psychotic patients, following an interference with the reproductive capacity. Subsequent clinical experience suggested the usefulness of even a broader definition.

We now use the term "pseudocyesis" to describe those psychic or somatic manifestations which, upon psychiatric investigation, appear to originate from two intimately interconnected components:

(1) the awareness of a recent bodily change or disturbance, linked to
(2) a conscious fantasy about some aspect of a pregnancy wish, fantasy or fear.

For purposes of explication, these two components can be separated and each viewed as a primary etiological factor.

A. *Soma to Psyche.* Single or multiple bodily sensory stimuli may be misinterpreted to indicate presence of pregnancy. If such a subjective impression is transitory and subject to reality testing, an adaptive mourning of loss of fertility may be occurring.

Case No. 1. A 36-year-old Catholic mother of four children had a tubal ligation five years prior to a psychiatric evaluation. She had had no pain during surgery, which was done under local anesthesia with scopolamine pre-medication; but she had severe, almost constant pelvic pain for four days afterwards. Her doctor had told her that sterility was 100% assured, but for six months she continued to be sceptical, feared that another pregnancy would occur, and had many dreams of giving birth to a child. Two months after the operation, she had a delayed menstrual period, following an incident in which she lifted a heavy object; and she felt a strange pelvic sensation. This led her to believe that the "tubes had come untied". She immediately called her gynecologist, who reassured her that she was not pregnant. "For a year it seemed very strange to me that I wouldn't have any more children, and I couldn't really believe it, but gradually I got used to the idea."

Secondary amenorrhea, either of somatic or psychic origin, is the most common symptom associated with pseudocyesis. It has been suggested that many abortions are performed in which a pseudo-pregnancy goes unrecognized.[15] The threat of pelvic symptoms subjectively associated with cancer may be denied by a belief in pregnancy. Hunter[23] described a seven-year-old girl, considered pregnant after coitus, who was found on laparotomy to have a sarcoma of the ovary. The following adult patient illustrates the dynamics of denial.

Case No. 2. A 43-year-old patient with two children was sterilized five years prior to psychiatric evaluation. Following tubal ligation, she had severe menstrual cramps similar to those she had had since menarche up to the time of her first pregnancy, when cramping ceased all together, only to return again following sterilization. Two months before the psychiatric interview, she had a dilatation and curettage because of intermenstrual bleeding. Immediately following the dilatation and curettage, she thought that the gynecologist must have removed the fetus in order to perform an abortion. It could be clearly shown that this fantasy covered the more frightening fear that she had cancer, in spite of the reassurance of the doctor. When the patient was evaluated again six months after the first interview, both the reality of her fantasies and her anxiety about cancer had disappeared.

Uterine enlargement or pelvic pressure secondary to benign tumors are occasionally the causes of a mistaken diagnosis of pregnancy, by patient and even by physician. Visual or tactile recognition of an enlargement in abdominal girth secondary to ageing, or breast changes secondary to the pre-menstrual phase, or vague abdominal symptoms may become sources of pregnancy fantasies. We have noted that patients who have had illegal abortions often have intense conflicts, guilt, and fear related to pregnancy. The fluid retention and other physiological side effects of oral contraceptives often simulate the pregnant state closely enough that withdrawal of hormones produces an emotional reliving of the abortion. Such patients usually must use other forms of contraception.[4]

The child-bearing function can be visualized as part of the body image from a theoretical standpoint. This is consistent with a statement by Margolin:[29] "To the extent that one's conception of the body and its parts are derived by sensations and subjective experience, one can speak of a 'fantasy of function' or perhaps an 'illusion of function'. In general these fantasies of function undergo continuous modification under the abrasive influence of reality testing. They may become unconscious and emerge in dreams, free associations, daydreams, and neurotic and psychotic symptoms."

Consistent with this viewpoint the child-bearing function and its object (the child) are highly treasured, as well as the real or fantasied sexual parts. The individual woman's perception of sensory experiences resulting from menstruation, defloration, pregnancy, and gynecological pathology undoubtedly leaves an imprint on the mental representation of the reproductive function.[3]

This conceptualization helps to explain our observation that the duration of new psychiatric symptoms following abortion usually was 3–6 months. "The time period corresponds closely with the unfulfilled length of the aborted pregnancy, and may represent an unconscious carrying-through of the pregnancy."[32] Reports of 3–6 month depression following abortion,[33] and Dunbar's finding of the "post-abortion hangover,"[14] represent confirmatory evidence of this formulation.

B. *Psyche to Soma.* The woman's wish for a child originates from a biologically rooted primary female reproductive drive. "Pregnancy, like puberty, is a biologically motivated step in the maturation of the individual, which requires physiologic adjustments and psychological adaptations to lead to a new level of integration. . . ."[7]

Defensive pathological, pregenital motivations to become pregnant can also produce the previously described physiological changes that in turn lead to pseudocyesis. The mechanisms of conversion, or hypochondriasis, through obscure psychophysiological or psychosomatic mechanisms, can have a similar result. As will be described further, we hypothesize the syndrome of depression to be also a major etiological factor. Benedek[6] recognized that pregnancy may be an immense source of narcissistic supplies, and that the fetus itself may be a substitute for the gratification of outside object relationships. "The pregnant woman, in her placid vegetative calmness enjoys her pregnant body which is like a reservoir replenished with libidinous feelings." This condition presents a future "irresistible temptation." The woman for whom pregnancy is a major, defensive, regressive source of narcissistic gratification will relinquish this function of her body very reluctantly. The following patient illustrates such psychodynamics.

Case No. 3. A 40-year-old Swiss woman had been unhappily married for many years and often was on the brink of divorce. However, when separation seemed imminent, she would become pregnant. She repeatedly experienced the bliss of this state and the intense pleasure of motherhood for several years. However, she was severely Rh sensitized during her fifth pregnancy. The fetus barely survived through excellent pre-natal obstetrical efforts (intra-uterine exchange transfusion), but it was unlikely the next child would survive.

The patient had been unable to use oral contraceptives or the intra-uterine device. The husband opposed a post-partum sterilization for various unconscious reasons, maintaining that if he died prematurely, his wife could marry an Rh negative man and resume her child-bearing. The patient and her obstetrician agreed that they would try to enlist the husband's co-operation again a few months after delivery, and this was done successfully. Tubal ligation was scheduled to follow the end of the next menstrual period. When the next menstrual period did not come on time, the patient was convinced she was pregnant, although she had not been exposed to sperm. She experienced breast and abdominal symptoms characteristic of her previous conceptions. Eventually she had another period and telephoned the obstetrician to schedule the sterilization. Suddenly she became incapacitated by attacks of anxiety associated with a re-experiencing of the overwhelming fear and trauma associated with the danger to her last baby. There were intense, idealizing romantic wishes toward the obstetrician, making it impossible for her to see him in his office.

She related the following dream: "I was at the beautician's to have my hair cut. A younger girl friend talked to me, absorbing my attention. I suddenly realized that my favorite beautician had cut my hair far too short." From her associations it appeared that the girl friend represented her weak indecisive husband and the beautician (beauty operator) was the obstetrician whose surgery turned her into a sexless boy.

This dream and other material was utilized to explain to the patient several implications of the loss of the child-bearing capacity.

(1) Loss of fertility had the unconscious meaning that she would become a boy.
(2) Proceeding with the tubal ligation meant that she would lose her important relationship with her obstetrician.
(3) Sterility would end her conflict about leaving her husband, since without her capacity to bear children, another man would not want her anyway.

This situation necessitated a putting off of the tubal ligation, a change of obstetricians and the initiation of intensive psychotherapy.

An acute threat of annihilation may require the defence of denial supported by a belief in pregnancy. This has been observed[34] in patients with sickle cell anemia and in cases of thyrotoxicosis. However, it is important to remember that the equation between magical future protection against death and pregnancy does not necessarily reflect a pathological denial.

To illustrate this point, one could refer to Freud's comment[16] on the relationship between narcissism and the wish for the child:

The child shall have a better time than his parents; he shall not be subject to the necessities which they have recognized as paramount in life. Illness, death, renunciation of enjoyment, restrictions of his own will, shall not touch him; the law of society shall be abrogated in his favour; he shall once more really be the centre and core of creation— "His Majesty the baby" as we once fancied ourselves.

Pseudocyesis may also be a primitive "last-ditch" defence against a psychotic ego disintegration.

Case No. 4. A sobbing 46-year-old single woman was admitted to the psychiatric unit with the isolated paranoid delusion that she was pregnant, and being watched and accused by other women because she was unmarried. Four years prior to admission, she had dated a certain man for one year. According to the patient, the relationship had ended because he had wanted a huge number of children and she did not want to go along with this plan. He had married another woman but had been divorced and renewed his acquaintance with the patient. Three months prior to hospitalization she had intercourse with him and one week later "knew" she was pregnant. This was only the second time in her life that she had had intercourse, and it is even possible that upon this occasion her partner was impotent. He promised marriage when she refused his suggestion of an abortion, but then he abruptly terminated the relationship, declaring she was trying to blackmail him.

For several weeks the patient was tremendously anxious with unbearable heart pounding, chest constriction, and the belief that she would die. These symptoms were apparently replaced by concern about her pregnancy which led finally to her delusion. Somatic compliance was suggested only by a hypomenorrhea and her emotional state was characterized by a constant attitude of pained perplexity. Such unconvincing symptoms of pregnancy might be explained by the absence of any previous physical and emotional experience of pregnancy. It was noted that at times when the patient wavered in her pregnancy conviction she became more anxious and paranoid.

One day six months following admission (and nine months after the date of intercourse), the patient complained of abdominal cramps following three days of constipation. She had muscular contractions of the lower abdomen and urinary frequency, which she used as evidence that she was in labor. One day later she expressed the conviction that electro-shock therapy or medication had killed the fetus. She recovered in the following months and was discharged, with no memory of her imagined pregnancy.

In this case a massive regression was stimulated by the threat of an object loss in the unconscious. The conviction of pregnancy again, as with healthy and neurotic persons, was considered restitutive in so far as it constituted a bridge between the fragmenting self and the object world (her lover) representing reality.

C. *Depressive Dynamics of Pseudocyesis.* In any discussion of spurious pregnancy, the importance of the principle of multiple function (or over-determination) in symptom formation cannot be over-emphasized. Case reports of false pregnancy in the last few years[1, 27, 38] clearly demonstrate multiple contributants to the syndrome from all levels of psychosexual development and all phases of ego maturation. However, our review of the psychiatric literature suggests that depressive mechanisms are the single most important etiological factor.

"The 'phantom fetus' occasionally would be noted . . . as a reaction to a threatened object loss or a physical illness." "An imaginary pregnancy function seemed to provide a defensive restitution, a kind of compensation for a real or imagined loss."[3]

Greaves[19] emphasized the importance of securing the certainty of a source of affection. Bressler,[10] in his evaluation of abdominal symptoms of unknown origin (later attributed to pregnancy fantasies), was struck by the need to compensate for the loss of oral receptive gratification. Littner[28] noted the pregnancy need was exaggerated by the necessity of maintaining a relationship with the mother.

Deutsch[13] felt that imaginary pregnancy can avoid the danger of being abandoned and helpless. A patient described by Lerner[27] lost her mother at the age of three. She later wished to be pregnant to overcome depression. Turning away from objects to the self, in her identification with the fetus, she established a symbolic fusion and symbiosis with her own mother. Selzer[38] described a six-year-old girl with an imagined pregnancy and multiple psychogenic gastrointestinal symptoms. She was depressed and lonely, and had intense oral yearnings, frustrated by an impulsive, narcissistic, unmarried mother. Abram[1] described a patient who developed first a false, then a true pregnancy in the termination phase of psychoanalysis. The patient, who had been severely deprived during childhood, developed extraordinary separation anxiety and feelings of emptiness and depression during the termination phase.

To present a more balanced picture of the literature, it should be pointed out that castration— or mutilation-anxiety is also an often mentioned etiological variable.[1, 27, 38]

Amenorrhea is often mentioned as a symptom of depression,[2, 20, 35] and as a symptom of anorexia nervosa, in which the dynamics of depression are considered important. In a recent unpublished study[5] of post-partum psychosis and depression, we have made the observation that there seems to be a delayed onset of menstruation following delivery in these patients.

The reproductive function is closely connected developmentally to separation phenomena and depression. Anxiety about the loss of an imagined penis can cause childhood depression, which becomes the model for later depressions, coinciding with menses, defloration, and childbirth.[24] Benedek[7] related the psychopathology of pregnancy primarily to the oral phase of development. She felt that the characteristic manifestations of child-bearing pathology are depression and psychosomatic oral problems.

The adult fear of losing the capacity to bear a child can be intimately linked to earlier fears of the oral period such as fear of loss of love, fear of loss of body integrity, or fear of loss of sexual identity. A connection between the reproductive function and separation fear may be reinforced by menstruation. Menarche often symbolizes the termination of a girl's childhood ties to her mother, and revives the idea of the early wound representing castration. Common depressive and eliminative fantasies during the last few days of the menstrual cycle suggest that the blood flow may symbolize a loss in the sense of fecal expulsion. L. Arey, the well-known embryologist, used to describe menstruation to medical students as the "weeping of the womb in its sorrow at remaining unfertilized."

Of course we recognize that any kind of loss can produce a variety of defensive and regressive phenomena, even a psychosis. When pseudocyesis seems closely related to depressive phenomena, we assume the existence of a certain personality structure prior to a precipitating stress. Narcissistic object choice, unneutralized aggression, oral fixation, and the prominent use of incorporation and introjection, and turning against the self-mechanisms, are elements in a depressive personality predisposition.

6

Therapy

Our clinical view and broad definition of pseudocyesis both suggest the impossibility of using any simple or single therapeutic technique. A fever may equally well be a symptom of measles or the first sign of leukemia. Likewise, the manifestations of imagined pregnancy may reflect adaptive mourning activity, a defence against psychotic deterioration, or the subjective interpretation of physiological changes.

Proper diagnosis and correct understanding of contributing factors are essential for appropriate psychotherapy. The therapeutic avenues vary as widely as the underlying etiology of the symptoms. Approaches range from no therapy, or simple suggestion, to intensive psychotherapy or hospitalization.

If our hypothesis concerning the frequent relationship between false pregnancy and depression is correct, physiological connecting links may explain the symptoms in some instances. These patients should have a positive response to the administration of anti-depressant drugs. We will report further on our investigation of these organic aspects in another publication.[11]

REFERENCES

1. ABRAM, H. S. 1969. Pseudocyesis folowed by true pregnancy in the termination phase of an analysis. *Brit. J. med. Psychol.*, **42**, 255.
2. ARIETI, S. 1959. Manic-depressive psychosis. *Am. Handbook of Psychiatry* (ed. Arieti, S.), Vol. I. New York: Basic Books.
3. BARGLOW, P. 1964. Pseudocyesis and psychiatric sequelae of sterilization. *Arch. gen. Psychiat.*, **11**, 571.
4. BARGLOW, P. 1966. Some psychiatric aspects of obstetrics and gynecology. *Obst. Gyn. Digest*, **8**, 31.
5. BARGLOW, P. and WILSON, J. 1970. A control study of postpartum psychosis. (To be published.)
6. BENEDEK, T. 1952. *Psychosexual functions in women: studies in psychosomatic medicine.* New York: Ronald Press.
7. BENEDEK, T. 1970. *Parenthood, its psychology and psychopathology* (E. J. Anthony and T. Benedek, eds.). New York: Little Brown.
8. BIVIN, G. D. and KLINGER, M. P. 1937. *Pseudocyesis.* Bloomington, Indiana: Principia Press.
9. BOGDANOVE, E. M. 1966. Preservation of functional corpora lutea in the rat by estrogen treatment. *Endocrinology*, **79**, 1011.
10. BRESSLER, B., NYHUS, P. and MAGNUSSEN, G. 1958. Pregnancy fantasies. *Psychosom. Med.*, **20**, 187.
11. BROWN, E. and BARGLOW, P. 1971. Pseudocyesis. A paradigm for psychophysiological interactions. *Arch. gen. Psychiat.*, **24**, 221.
12. CAPPOLA, J. A., LEONARDI, R. G., LIPPMANN, W., PERRINE, J. W. and RINGLER, I.

1965. Induction of pseudopregnancy in rats by depletors of endogenous catecholamines. Endocrinology, **77**, 485.

13. DEUTSCH, H. 1945. *Psychology of women*, Vols. I and II. New York: Grune & Stratton.

14. DUNBAR, R. F. 1954. The psychosomatic approach to abortion and the abortion habit. In *Therapeutic abortion* (H. Rosen, ed.). New York: Julian Press.

15. FISCHER, I. C. 1962. Hypothalamic amenorrhea: pseudocyesis. In *Psychosomatic obstetrics, gynecology and endocrinology* (W. S. Kroger, ed.). Springfield, Illinois: Charles C. Thomas (p. 291).

16. FREUD, S. 1914. *On narcissism: an introduction*, Stand. edn. 14. London: Hogarth Press.

17. FRIED, P. H., RAKOFF, A. E., SCHOPBACH, R. R. and KAPLAN, A. J. 1951. Pseudocyesis: a psychosomatic study in gynecology. *J. Amer. med. Ass.*, **145**, 329.

18. GOOD, J. M. 1823. *Physiological system of nosology with corrected and simplified nomenclature*. Boston: Wells and Lilly.

19. GREAVES, D. C., GREEN, P. E. and WEST, L. J. 1960. Psychodynamic and psychophysiological aspects of pseudocyesis. *Psychosom. Med.*, **22**, 24.

20. GUTHEIL, E. A. 1959. Reactive Depressions. *Am. Handbook of Psychiatry* (S. Arieti, ed.), Vol. I. New York: Basic Books.

21. HIPPOCRATES. 1839. *Oeuvres Complètes*. Paris: Baliere.

22. HORNING, J. C. 1932. Nervous pregnancy in the dog. *Vet. Med.*, **27**, 240.

23. HUNTER, Q. W. 1905. Pseudocyesis. *Med. Age*, **23**, 326.

24. JACOBSON, E. 1968. On the development of the girl's wish for a child. *Psychoanal. Quart.*, **37**, 523.

25. JEFFCOATE, T. N. A. 1962. *Principles of gynaecology*. London: Butterworth.

26. KNIGHT, J. A. 1960. False pregnancy in a male. *Psychosom. Med.*, **7**, 260.

27. LERNER, B., RASKIN, R. and DAVIS, E. B. 1967. On the need to be pregnant. *Int. J. Psycho-Anal.*, **48**, 288.

28. LITTNER, N. 1956. The natural parent. In: *A study of adoption practice* (M. A. Schapiro, ed.). New York: Child Welfare League of America.

29. MARGOLIN, S. G. 1953. Pathophysiological processes in psychosomatic concepts in psychoanalysis. New York: Int. Univ. Press.

30. MOULTON, R. 1942. Psychosomatic implication of pseudocyesis. *Psychosom. Med*, **4**, 376.

31. NIKITOVITCH-WINER, M. B. 1965. Effect of hypophyseal stalk transection on luteotropic hormone secretion in the rat. *Endocrinology*, **77**, 658.

32. PATT, S. L., RAPPAPORT, R. G. and BARGLOW, P. 1969. Follow-up of therapeutic abortion. *Arch. gen. Psychiat.*, **20**, 408.

33. PECK, A. and MARCUS, H. 1966. Psychiatric sequelae of therapeutic interruption of pregnancy, *J. nerv. ment. Dis.*, **143**, 417.

34. POLLOCK, G. 1965. Some notes on psychological factors in contraceptive decision, choice and utilization. Paper presented at 132nd Meeting, Am. Ass. Advancement Science, Berkeley, California, U.S.A.

35. REDLICH, F. C. and FREEDMAN, D. X. 1966. *The theory and practice of psychiatry*. New York: Basic Books.

36. REICHLIN, S. 1968. Neurogenic amenorrhea. Textbook of Endocrinology. London: W. B. Saunders (p. 1003).

37. SCHWARTZ, N. B. and ROTHCHILD, I. 1964. Changes in pituitary L.H. concentration during pseudopregnancy in the rat. *Proc. Soc. exp. Biol. Med.*, **116**, 107.

38. SELZER, J. G. 1968. Pseudocyesis in a six-year-old girl. *J. Am. Acad. Child Psychiat.*, **7**, 693.

39. STEINBERG, A., PASTOR, N., WINHELD, E. B., SEGAL, H. I., SCHECHTER, F. R. and COTTON, N. H. 1946. Psychoendocrine relationships in pseudocyesis. *Psychosom. Med.*, **8**, 176.

40. TALWALKER, P. K., RATNER, A. and MEITES, J. 1963. *In vitro* inhibition of pituitary prolactin synthesis and release by hypothalamic extract. *Amer. J. Physiol.*, **205**, 213.

41. VANDER VEER, A. 1889. Concealed pregnancy: its relation to abdominal surgery. *Amer. J. Obstet.*, **22**, 1121.

IV

THE COUVADE SYNDROME

W. H. TRETHOWAN

M.B., F.R.C.P., F.R.A.C.P., D.P.M.

Professor of Psychiatry,
University of Birmingham
England

1

Introduction

The Couvade syndrome is a curious psychogenic disorder, in which expectant fathers are afflicted by symptoms which often bear a resemblance to those which their wives experience during pregnancy or labour. The condition has been given its name by virtue of its apparent similarity to some aspects of the ritual Couvade.[17, 58, 59] This is a magical practice common to many primitive peoples which has been known for centuries.[16, 51] It consists of an apparent pretence of childbirth or lying-in by a pregnant woman's husband at or about the time she is confined. The name "Couvade" was given to this ritual in 1865 by the anthropologist Sir Edward Tylor who derived the term from the French verb *couver*, to brood or hatch.[60]

Unlike the ritual Couvade, the Couvade syndrome is not a pretence. The expectant father who suffers from it does not deliberately "act out" his wife's pregnancy, but reacts to it by the unintentional acquisition of symptoms. These may either be physical manifestations of the anxiety which he experiences or, as a result of a conversion reaction, may occur without any awareness on his part of the connection between his symptoms and his wife's condition.[58]

The Couvade syndrome may therefore be regarded as analogous to, or a neurotic equivalent of, the ritual Couvade. Even so, by no means all those who suffer from the Couvade syndrome should be viewed as neurotic, although many clearly are. While certain special factors may predispose a man to become unduly anxious during his wife's pregnancy or confinement, if he is not an unduly anxious man at other times, he cannot fairly be branded as neurotic in the wider sense.

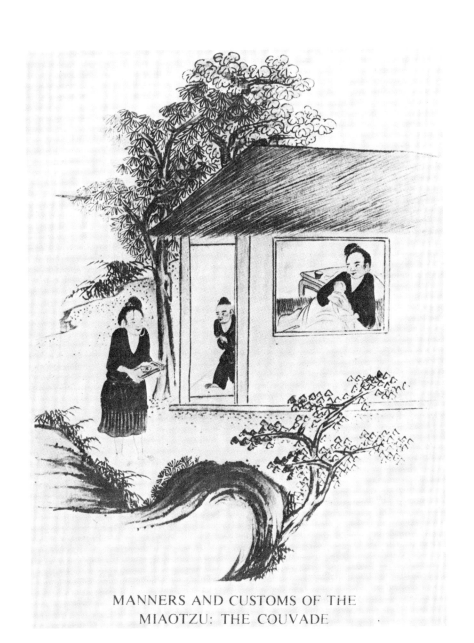

MANNERS AND CUSTOMS OF THE
MIAOTZU: THE COUVADE

2

Historical Background

Historical records of the Couvade syndrome do not extend so far back as those of the ritual Couvade, which has even found a place in Greek mythology. According to Plutarch, Theseus returning to Athens from Crete was obliged to leave Ariadne in Cyprus because, on account of pregnancy and severe sea-sickness, she could not continue the voyage. When Theseus later returned to fetch her, he found she had died in childbirth. Because of this he left a sum of money to found an annual feast in her honour. At this feast, it is said, a man lay down and cried and acted the part of a woman in labour.[4] However, this is only one version of what happened to Ariadne, this particular myth possibly arising from her role in the cult of Aphrodite.[52]

The custom of Couvade is world-wide. It was observed by Diodorus Siculus in Corsica in 60 B.C.,[37] and has since been recorded in one form or another in China, India, Assam, Borneo, Siam, Africa and the Americas. Australia is the only continent where the ritual has apparently never been observed. Marco Polo saw instances of it in his travels in Chinese Turkestan in the 13th Century.[14] This fact, according to Moore,[43] is referred to in Samuel Butler's Hudibras:

> Chinese thus are said
> To lie-in in their ladies' stead.

Early references to what is now called the Couvade syndrome, as opposed to the ritual Couvade, were made, according to Hunter and Macalpine[28] by Francis Bacon in 1627, who did not commit himself to a definite opinion as to whether the phenomenon was fact or fantasy; by James Primrose, a Hull physician, in 1650 or thereabouts, who apparently doubted its existence, and in 1677 by Robert Plot, professor of chemistry at Oxford, who, although he referred to Primrose's disbelief, professed himself "otherwise perswaded".

But even if some scientists and medical men regarded the Couvade syndrome as no more than a piece of folklore, the Restoration playwrights obviously were in no doubt of its existence and were quick to make capital out of the matter. Among others, toothache as a symptom of the Couvade syndrome appears to have excited them. The belief that the husbands of pregnant women are more than ordinarily liable to toothache has been long recorded from several parts of the British Isles.[16, 49] This then was the phenomenon referred to when the dramatists made their characters discuss the odd notion of "breeding a child in the teeth". Examples may be found in Dekker and Webster's *Westward Ho*, first published in 1607,[8] and in Thomas Middleton's *The Widdow* in 1652, and *Women Beware Women* in 1659.[35] But there are several references by other playwrights to other kinds of Couvade symptoms also. Wilkins in *The Miseries of Enforced Marriage*, written in 1607, puts the following words into the mouth of one of his characters:

> I have got thee with child in my conscience and,
> like a kind husband, methinks I breed it for thee.
> For I am already sick at my stomach and long extremely.[35]

Beaumont and Fletcher in two of their plays, *The Custom of the Country* and *A Wife for a Month*, both published in 1647, refer to *sympathy pains* in husbands. There is also a splendidly unequivocal reference to a husband *breeding for his wife*, by William Wycherley in 1672 in *The Country Wife*.[64] But perhaps an even better reference is to be found, not in a play, but in a poem by Robert Heath written in 1650:

> We observe each loving husband, when the wife
> Is labouring by a strange reciproque strife
> Doth sympathising sicken; and 't may be
> In Law they're one and in Divinity.[35]

Other more remarkable, but perhaps less insightful, explanations both of the syndrome and of the ritual Couvade have been listed by Dawson.[14] Physical explanations have occasionally been advanced, but most observers have usually recognized that the basis of the phenomenon is psychological.

Some, either in referring to the incidence or to the explanation of the disorder, have tended to confuse the syndrome itself with the ritual Couvade, as if they were one and the same; whereas they are really separate although clearly related happenings. But there are, nevertheless, what might be called transitional beliefs which appear to stand halfway between the ritual Couvade and the syndrome. The French writer Chesnel de la Charbouclais in his *Dictionnaire des Superstitions* (quoted by Lean),[35] having referred to the need for an expectant mother to make preparations in the shape of baby-clothes, etc., in anticipation of her lying-in, states:

> And to ensure an easy delivery she must put on
> her husband's clothes when the pains come on.
> *Se revêtir de la chemise de leurs maris, mettre*
> *leurs braies ou pantalons et leurs bonnets de*
> *coton Limogis.*

Similar practices have been recorded from Germany and the West of Ireland, and no doubt could be found to exist or to have existed in many other places. Such notions belong to a large class of beliefs which are essentially of a magical kind.[22] They rest on the basic notion of the omnipotence of thought,[27] i.e. that if something is sufficiently strongly wished for, it will actually happen. To reinforce the wish-fulfilment process there may also be a need to perform some appropriate ritual.

The idea that midwives had the power to transfer labour pains from their patients to their husbands, or even possibly to cast them upon some domestic animal, comes of course into the same category and is appropriate to the general class of superstitious beliefs with which midwives were at one time surrounded.[47] Indeed the local midwife and the village witch were, it appears, often one and the same person.[44]

3

More Recent Reports

Between Jacobean and more modern times there seems to have been little interest in the Couvade. Medical writers seemingly ignored it and the public, if they were aware of its existence, may have considered the matter so commonplace as to be unworthy of attention.

What might appropriately be called the modern history of the Couvade began just over a century ago with Sir Edward Tylor's reformulation of ideas concerning the ritual, together with giving it its name.[60] Following this, the custom began to attract the attention of a series of anthropologists including Frazer,[22] Westermarck,[63] Crawley, [11] and more recently Malinowski,[41] all of whom advanced somewhat different explanations of its nature. In 1929 Dawson[14] wrote a monograph in which he dealt comprehensively with the history of the subject, and in 1931 Reik, in his book *Ritual*, was the first to approach the Couvade from the point of view of psychoanalysis.[48] His interpretation of the psychodynamic factors underlying the ritual Couvade are also relevant to the Couvade syndrome and will be considered later. None of these authors, however, dealt specifically or in any detail with the Couvade syndrome, but confined themselves largely to a consideration of the ritual.

Sporadic reports, usually of isolated cases of the Couvade syndrome, began to appear in English medical literature after 1940,[18, 33, 43] but it was not until much more recently that more extensive studies were published. Freeman[23] reported 6 cases of mental illness occurring in men during and apparently in relation to their wives' pregnancies. Some of his subjects also suffered from physical symptoms. One had such severe abdominal pain that his appendix was removed on this account, apparently without relief. The first fairly extensive series of published cases with primarily physical symptoms was that of Curtis[12] who, in 1955, reported a series of 55 expectant fathers, of whom 22 developed a variety of complaints including morning sickness, increase or decrease in appetite, epigastric discomfort, constipation or diarrhoea, headache and dizzy spells. As this was an uncontrolled study, it was not possible to establish in how many cases the symptoms could be ascribed with any degree of certainty to the Couvade syndrome, and in how many to other causes quite unrelated to the fact that the subjects' wives were pregnant. A further uncontrolled study was carried out on Indian Army personnel by Bardhan in 1964.[6] This gave very similar results.

In 1965 the results of a very much more extensive and controlled study were published by Trethowan and Conlon.[59] Taking Curtis's findings as a starting point, a questionnaire was compiled and administered to a series of 327 expectant fathers at or about the time their wives were confined. Enquiry was made about the state of their own health during the previous nine months. All that the subjects were asked to do was to mark "Yes" or "No" against each of the symptoms in a check-list which, in addition to those enumerated by Curtis, also included toothache. A few simple questions were also asked about time of onset, duration and disappearance of symptoms. Each questionnaire was completed under supervision and scrutinized for completeness. A similar questionnaire was administered to 220 married men of comparable age, social and occupational class whose wives had not been pregnant at any time during the previous year. These control subjects were drawn from factories situated within the same area served by the hospital where the expectant fathers' wives were delivered of their babies.

The results of this investigation have been enumerated in detail elsewhere.[58, 59] All that need be said here, therefore, is that certain statistically highly significant differences emerged between the group of expectant fathers and the control group. Not only were a significantly greater number of expectant fathers affected by symptoms than were the control subjects, but they also suffered between them from a significantly greater number of symptoms. All symptoms with the exception of backache, which occurred in an identical proportion of men in both groups, were commoner in expectant fathers, although only in the case of loss of appetite, toothache and nausea and sickness did the difference in the incidence of individual symptoms reach statistical significance. A further significant relationship between the incidence of physical and psychiatric symptoms and a similar association between physical symptoms and anxiety felt by the subjects over their wives' pregnancies, was also observed. This relationship, however, often went quite unperceived by the sufferer.

The questionnaire method of investigation, even when supervised as in this instance (which at least produced a one-hundred-per-cent return), has its limitations as a research tool. It was possible, however, to draw several useful conclusions. Firstly, the existence of the disorder was established without doubt. Secondly, light was thrown on some of the commoner ways in which it presented itself. Thirdly, some notion was obtained of its frequency and severity. Finally, the results of the investigation together with a study of the relevant literature appeared to justify calling the disorder the Couvade syndrome.

What of course the investigation did not do was to throw light upon the psychopathology of the disorder. It was possible to discover something about this only by investigating a number of individual cases in depth, a process not too easily accomplished owing to a general unwillingness on the part of subjects to submit themselves to an extensive psychiatric investigation especially when, following the birth of their children, all symptoms have vanished. However, following a detailed account of the clinical features of the syndrome, further consideration will be given to underlying psychological factors.

4

Incidence

The exact incidence of the Couvade syndrome is difficult to determine, but there is no doubt at all that it is much commoner than many might suppose. Such estimates as have been made vary from 1 in 9 (11%)[55] expectant fathers being affected, which is almost certainly too low, to 1 in 2[15] which is almost certainly too high. Much depends on what is accounted for within the definition of the syndrome. Clearly, if very minor and transient symptoms are included, the prevalence of the disorder will be found to be greater than if symptoms considered to be characteristic are restricted only to those of a grosser and more obvious kind. The frequency of the phenomenon is also likely to be over-emphasized by those who are interested in it and underestimated by those who are inclined to dismiss it as unimportant. However, all things considered, about 1 in 4 or 5 is probably the correct figure.[58]

The author himself did not become aware of the condition until, while on active service in 1944 with the Royal Army Medical Corps, he was confronted by a husky and seemingly healthy-looking warrant officer who complained of severe abdominal cramps. Examination showed no physical reason for his complaint. It turned out however that this was about the time when his wife, from whom he had not recently heard, would have been likely to have been confined. Twenty-four hours later a telegram arrived giving news that she had been successfully delivered, whereupon all his symptoms subsided. The matter seemed then to be no more than of passing interest, although the condition was said to be not uncommon among service men. Subsequent investigation, however, has shown that the condition is certainly no less common in civilian life.

Although almost all those who develop the Couvade syndrome are expectant fathers, it appears, very occasionally, that other relatives, too, may be affected. For example some fathers may develop Couvade symptoms during their daughters' pregnancies or at about the time they are delivered. Although this seems to be a very uncommon event, it is possible that direct investigation of the matter might bring more examples to light. There are also two cases on record of children developing symptoms in such a way as to suggest that the occurrence of these was in some way related to childbirth: in the first instance during the mother's labour, and in the second, immediately following the birth of a younger sibling.[10, 13] Finally, the author has received a hearsay report of a pupil midwife who had to change her job because attendance upon women in labour apparently caused her to suffer from attacks of colic.

5

The Clinical Picture

As there are a large number and variety of Couvade symptoms, only the main ones will be discussed in detail. Those most frequently complained of are alimentary, and in many cases mimic the symptoms from which pregnant women suffer. It may be observed, however, that almost any symptom of any kind which a man develops during his wife's pregnancy but which disappears immediately after childbirth may well be a symptom of the Couvade syndrome.

Nausea and Vomiting

These are among the commonest of all symptoms and while varying in severity may affect as many as 1 in 5 expectant fathers. As in the case of their pregnant wives, nausea or vomiting tends to start at about the beginning of the third month. The symptoms may be slight and transient or, in severer cases, may persist throughout pregnancy. Actual morning sickness is not uncommon. While there are of course obviously other reasons for this event, such as gastritis due to alcoholic over-indulgence the night before, nausea or vomiting has, however, been found to be at least twice as frequent in the husbands of pregnant women as in husbands whose wives are not pregnant. It is interesting to observe that husbands do not necessarily suffer from nausea or vomiting because their wives also do.

The wife of a 38-year-old man who suffered from severe morning sickness and a large number of other Couvade symptoms during each of her six pregnancies, was never herself troubled by sickness at all. Indeed in all of her pregnancies, which were quite uncomplicated, she suffered little or no discomfort. Similarly, in a series of 90 pregnant primiparae, 17 of their husbands suffered from nausea or vomiting, while 7 of their wives were completely free of this symptom. Of the remaining 10 only 5 women suffered at all severely.[15]

Alterations of Appetite

Some degree of loss of appetite is equally common; increased appetite rather less so. Perversions of appetite, resembling the cravings or longings of pregnant women, are by no means rare. In the series of 90 cases referred to above, 6 men suffered from what seemed to be cravings although only 4 of their wives also did. The foods craved for included chocolate, ice-cream, various sweet things, doughnuts and chips—foods for which no undue preference had been shown prior to the occurrence of pregnancy. One husband developed a craving for fried eggs on fried bread. The eggs had to be carefully and symmetrically arranged and if they ruptured had to be replaced.

Toothache

This too is a very frequent symptom and appears to affect nearly a quarter of all husbands at some time or other during their wives' pregnancies. In contrast, its occurrence in a control group was found to be only about 1 in 10. This is a statistically highly significant difference. The symptom may be persistent or transient and sufferers have been known to demand extraction of perfectly sound teeth because of it.[57] In some patients the ache may migrate from one tooth to another; in others it appears to be a form of facial or palatal neuralgia rather than toothache.

A woman recounted retrospectively how when she was expecting her first baby her husband suffered very severe facial neuralgia for eight months of her pregnancy. Eleven years later, when she was pregnant for the second time, the symptom recurred though not before then or since. His teeth were said to be sound. In each instance his pain was relieved only when his wife gave birth.

A 24-year-old man who complained of toothache only developed this half-way through his wife's first pregnancy, when she was admitted to hospital for investigation of glycosuria. When she was discharged two weeks later his toothache disappeared but recurred when she was re-admitted in labour. He described the ache as migrating from one tooth to another and then finally to his hard palate, where it took on a neuralgia-like quality.

Indigestion, Heartburn, Abdominal Pain, etc.

Leaving aside sympathy pains during labour, which will be dealt with separately, some form of indigestion often occurs. Its nature varies. Backache and pain in the chest are also frequently complained of and may occur separately or together with abdominal symptoms. Collectively the prevalence of symptoms of these kinds is about 1 in 4 in expectant fathers, but it must be observed that, as they often affect men whose wives are not pregnant, the significance of the frequency of their occurrence in expectant fathers is difficult to assess. Nonetheless, in many individual instances the relationship to pregnancy is clear enough.

A psychiatrist who had just read an account of the Couvade syndrome became aware that his son-in-law's indigestion might possibly be due to the fact that his wife (the psychiatrist's own daughter) was pregnant. When he proffered this interpretation of its nature, the symptom immediately vanished.

A distinguished obstetrician suffered from vague ill-defined abdominal pain during the latter part of his wife's second pregnancy. This was investigated without any significant findings. Finally he was advised that it might be wise if he had his appendix removed. He was on the point of submitting himself to this operation, when his wife prematurely but successfully gave birth and his symptoms disappeared at once. Only then did he realise what their likely cause was.

Abdominal Swelling

This symptom, although rare, is of great interest and therefore deserves special mention. A swelling of the abdomen occurs which may mimic that of advancing pregnancy. Abdominal hysterical proptosis or bloating, as it has been called, has also been described in men in a variety of circumstances.[3, 50] Records of this happening go back at least a hundred years. Hurst,[29] who observed the symptom in soldiers during the 1914–18 war, referred to it as "Ventre en Accordeon" but did not record whether in any of his cases it was related to pregnancy. When it occurs as a Couvade symptom, it is tempting to draw an analogy between it and pseudocyesis in women, though of course in men it is not accompanied by the belief that the swelling is due to pregnancy. Like pseudocyesis, it is not caused, as is often thought, by aerophagy or the retention of excess intestinal gas, but, as Sir James Simpson demonstrated long ago, is due to forward displacement of the viscera as a result of a downward thrust of the diaphragm together with lumbar lordosis.[53]

A 26-year-old soldier on active service developed a markedly swollen abdomen which persisted for twenty-two months, until he returned home on leave and saw his wife and child for the first time since the birth. It was reported that this tumefaction disappeared when he was anaesthetized and reappeared as he regained consciousness. (Simpson demonstrated a precisely similar phenomenon in women with pseudocyesis.) Twelve years later he had a second attack—in this instance not in relation to pregnancy as on the first occasion (there were no further children), but in relation to the break-up of his marriage.

A woman pregnant with her first child started to put on a great deal of weight. So did her husband apparently. He was working away from home during most of her pregnancy and she observed that each time they met his abdomen seemed to be getting larger. Following childbirth she stated that her husband who had by this time "become very large indeed" seemed to lose so much weight that she thought he must be ill. But because on medical examination nothing was found to be wrong, both then realized that her pregnancy had probably had something to do with the phenomenon.

Sympathy Pains

Sympathy or spurious labour pains are extremely common and usually, although not absolutely invariably, occur in men at or about the time their wives start labour.[56] The symptom is commonly described either as stomachache, lower abdominal pain, or as cramps or colic, sometimes accompanied by diarrhoea. It may be severe and can cause considerable distress. Characteristically it ceases as soon as childbirth is over. The symptom may occur as an isolated event affecting a husband during his wife's labour but more often is associated with other Couvade symptoms such as have been described and which may have occurred earlier on. Sometimes these earlier symptoms do not always persist but return again when labour begins.

A woman described how during the birth of her child her husband came to visit her. He came again the following day, after the child had been born, saying, "I wouldn't like to go through that again." He described how, on leaving the hospital the previous day, pains in his stomach had started and continued until the evening, when he vomited and felt better. This coincided more or less with the time the baby was born. She also added that during both her pregnancies her husband insisted on having a tooth extracted despite the dentist's opinion that his teeth were perfectly sound.

A 29-year-old man not only complained of "labour pains" but, when he learned of his wife having undergone an episiotomy, developed perineal soreness as well. It was discovered that prior to this he had suffered from a whole series of mimetic symptoms including morning nausea, a feeling of abdominal distension and also quickening sensations. The wealth of symptoms experienced by this patient may have been in part due to the fact that he was a paranoid schizophrenic, although a well-preserved one. Apparently he identified himself remarkably strongly with his wife. Indeed it seemed as if this, together with a failure of his own ego identity, had led him to develop pregnancy symptoms as a pathoplastic feature of his psychosis.[59] It should be noted, however, that while patients with the Couvade syndrome are often demonstrably neurotic, the condition appears to be uncommon in psychotic subjects.

Miscellaneous Physical Symptoms

A large number of these have been described, though their relationship to pregnancy may be more difficult to perceive than that of the more obviously mimetic symptoms already enumerated. However, as has already been pointed out, if a symptom or some disorder affects a husband only during his wife's pregnancy and at no other time, there may be grounds in some cases for including it among the many manifestations of the Couvade syndrome. If one accepts the psychosomatic hypothesis that, given a certain kind of predisposition, a physical lesion may be due to or exacerbated by psychological stress, it may not be too far-fetched to relate it to pregnancy, especially when the lesion occurs in a man to whom, on account of certain pre-existing neurotic or emotional conflicts, his wife's pregnancy is a stressful event. There may therefore be some causal connection between his wife's pregnancy and the fact that in a man who has a duodenal ulcer this perforates during that pregnancy. However, as perforations not infrequently occur at other times, the connection may be apparent rather than real and, even if real, impossible to establish with any degree of certainty.

Apart from abdominal symptoms of various kinds, such as have been described, other recorded complaints by expectant fathers include nosebleeds, earache, swelling of the lips, cramps in the legs, skin rashes and boils. Inman[30] has described several cases of styes and tarsal cysts in husbands whose wives were pregnant. He also observed that these lesions were often associated in some mysterious way with fantasies about birth. Indeed,

Abenheimer[1] has even suggested an association between eye and egg. Inman also referred to the old folklore belief, which still obtains in some places, of the effectiveness of applying a gold wedding ring to the eye as a cure for styes.

One man recounted how, while he was on army service and when his wife was three months pregnant, he had to be excused duty on account of severe styes, a complaint he had never suffered before or since. Another, on naval service, during his wife's second pregnancy suffered severely from dental abcesses and whitlows and had to be put off duty until the child was born, whereupon he completely recovered. He also suffered severely from sickness during this time, but not apparently from seasickness.

The investigator is on uncertain ground in many of these cases not only because much of the evidence is anecdotal and even more of it is retrospective, but also because there is probably an over-ready tendency on the part of some wives to ascribe the occurrence of many minor maladies in their husbands to the fact that they are pregnant. Indeed the possibility has to be considered that some women, and perhaps some of their husbands also, feel that the latter ought to share in some of the discomforts of pregnancy. This may give rise to rationalization. Some support may be lent to this notion by the fact that, whereas in the author's original study of the Couvade syndrome[59] highly significant differences were found in the incidence of appetite changes, toothache, and nausea or sickness in a group of expectant fathers as compared with a control group, no such differences could be demonstrated in regard to a number of other symptoms about which information was also sought.

Psychiatric Symptoms

Although not properly part of the Couvade syndrome, in which the symptoms by definition are physical not psychiatric, these deserve mention if only on account of their frequency. While to some the anxious father may be a figure of fun, in many cases he certainly suffers considerable mental anguish. Of 327 expectant fathers in the author's original study[58] 130 (40%) admitted to being anxious. Over half of these (21%) also complained of other psychiatric symptoms—depression, tension, insomnia, irritability, nervousness, weakness, headaches and stuttering. As might be expected a statistically highly significant association between somatic symptoms and anxiety was demonstrable and, when considered collectively, a further significant association between the occurrence of these and that of other psychiatric symptoms also. What perhaps is of even greater interest is that there were quite a substantial number of men with physical symptoms (56 of 186), who on questioning did not admit to anxiety over their wives' pregnancies. There are of course two possible explanations for this: the first, that the physical symptoms which occurred bore really no relationship at all to pregnancy; the second, that they were the outcome of repression and conversion of anxiety and were not, as in the case of those who experienced anxiety overtly, direct somatic expressions of this emotional state. Further investigation has suggested that this is likely to have been the case in some instances.

There seems to be only slender evidence of the precipitation of psychosis in men by pregnancy in their wives (the case of the man with paranoid schizophrenia quoted earlier had obviously developed this disorder long before his wife became pregnant), but it does appear that childbirth itself may precipitate a so-called post-partum psychiatric illness in men. Several authors have described this occurrence .[9, 54, 65] As in the case of women who develop puerperal psychoses, it is presumably necessary to postulate some kind of predisposition, possibly one hereditarily determined. Nonetheless, to men who suffer in this way pregnancy must necessarily be a very significant event.

A 24-year-old man with no previous or family history of mental illness was present at the birth of his daughter. Shortly afterwards his sister gave birth to an illegitimate child. He then became hypomanic, but after five weeks passed into a state of depression during which he became preoccupied with ideas of violence and death. After ten days in hospital, during which time he was treated with antidepressive drugs, he swung back once again into a state of hypomania. On one occasion during this, he lay in bed adopting the lithotomy position and appeared to be re-enacting the birth of his child. When questioned retrospectively, however, he insisted he was "giving birth to ideas". Following this incident and further drug treatment his psychosis subsided, so that within three weeks he was well enough to be discharged to day care.

6

Other Clinical Aspects

Couvade symptoms can occur at any time during pregnancy, although usually not before the end of the second to the middle of the third month— by which time pregnancy is usually strongly suspected or has been confirmed. Very occasionally symptoms are complained of earlier than this and before either husband or wife appear to know that pregnancy is definitely established.

A 31-year-old patient still menstruating, consulted her doctor to find out if she was pregnant. This was because her husband had developed toothache. She mentioned that he suffered from this symptom only when she was pregnant. Her suspicion was confirmed. On investigation, it turned out that her husband had also suffered from toothache during each of her four previous pregnancies and not at other times, although on two of these four occasions he insisted that his toothache was due to bad teeth, which he had duly had extracted. It was clear that both the patient and her husband regarded pregnancy as a hazard. Indeed one of her children had been born anencephalic. After that there was some anxiety that a subsequent child might also be born abnormal. There was no evidence, however, to suggest that on this, the fifth occasion, her husband was consciously aware she was pregnant, although he had previously observed that when she was she tended to be irritable and anxious and to suffer from heartburn.

While the circumstances of this case are difficult to interpret, it may be postulated that both parties, although not overtly conscious of the wife being pregnant might, by reason of certain slight but familiar changes in her, have been subliminally aware of this occurrence.[12] Also, as pregnancy was regarded as a hazard and in this instance was definitely unwanted (she sought termination once it was confirmed), repression may well have played some part. In those cases in which symptoms occur early, they may persist throughout pregnancy or disappear after some months, having a tendency to recur again at about the time labour begins. Whether symptoms occur early on and persist, or occur for the first time, or recur at the time of confinement, they almost invariably disappear immediately following or within a very short time of the completion of childbirth. If they are prolonged for any appreciable time after this event, some other cause for the symptoms should obviously be suspected.

While symptoms such as nausea and vomiting tend to occur earlier on (as in the case of pregnant women), abdominal cramps and colic seem to be commoner at about the time of labour. But there are no hard and fast rules.

A 30-year-old university lecturer enjoyed good physical health during his wife's first pregnancy and confinement. Although he was anxious he did not suffer any physical symptoms. But during her second pregnancy he suffered considerably. When she was about five months pregnant, he developed colic and diarrhoea which he described as "labour after food". At about six months, he started to vomit precipitately, particularly after breakfast, although once over this did not recur during the rest of the day. These symptoms continued until his wife had been confined for a few days and had had three false starts to her labour. The patient, being unable to obtain what he considered to be adequate information about her progress from the midwife in charge of the labour ward, became increasingly frustrated and irritable to the point of losing his temper. Following this cathartic event, his somatic symptoms subsided. By the time his child was born, on this occasion by Caesarian section, he was symptom-free.[17]

Whether there is any special liability to the occurrence of Couvade symptoms during the first as opposed to later pregnancies, is open to question. The existing evidence is conflicting. One inquiry, made among a consecutive series of primiparae immediately following childbirth, revealed that 47 of their 90 husbands (52%) suffered from symptoms which their wives, having recently been pregnant, ascribed to this cause.[15] But in another study of 155 expectant fathers, who experienced symptoms during their wives' most recent pregnancies but who had previously had other children, only 46 (30%) stated that they had previously been affected in the same way.[59] This discrepancy may be in part accounted for by the fact that the first investigation quoted was uncontrolled and the wives' interpretation of the cause of their husbands' symptoms might not always have been correct, although the women concerned may have preferred to believe otherwise. In the second investigation, which was controlled, it was clear enough that in a considerable number of cases the symptoms from which the expectant fathers suffered were not due to the Couvade syndrome at all. While the nature of the investigation did not permit an exact estimate of the actual number of those with the Couvade syndrome, a further analysis of the data suggested that in about 40 subjects, who had already had other children, this was virtually certain to have been so. In at least as many more, the probability of their symptoms having also been due to the same cause seemed reasonably high.[58] However, taking the lesser number only, this may be seen to coincide fairly closely with the number of those who related having had similar symptoms on a previous occasion. This suggests some liability to recurrence in those predisposed. There are of course records of patients whose wives have had three, four, or more children who are afflicted by symptoms on every occasion.

Where symptoms occur their severity varies. In most instances they are relatively mild and, even in the case of those who do not recognize their origin, few appear to seek medical help; although toothache, it seems, not uncommonly leads the sufferer to seek dental attention.

7

Psychopathology

Neurotic Reaction

From a phenomenological viewpoint, the Couvade syndrome can be regarded as a neurotic reaction with somatic manifestations to the forefront. The physical symptoms which affect expectant fathers are therefore due to an anxiety state precipitated by concern over their wives' pregnancies. In a fair number of cases the sufferer perceives the relationship of his anxiety to his physical symptoms. Insight, however, does not necessarily bring him relief, although it may do so if initially absent and acquired at a later juncture. There are also those who, while they express concern over their wives' pregnancies and at the same time experience a variety of physical discomforts, are apparently unaware of any connection between these events. In these cases some degree of dissociation is present. But there is a third category, in which the degree of dissociation is even more complete. This comprises those who develop sometimes quite severe and obviously related physical symptoms but who, presumably due to repression and conversion, seem apparently not to be at all anxious.

From a diagnostic viewpoint, therefore, the Couvade syndrome covers a variety of reactions ranging from simple anxiety states via anxiety-hysteria to full-blown dissociative-conversion states.[17]

Apart from lack of awareness, which may be due to dissociation or something akin to it, Curtis, observing that his subjects were seldom aware that their symptoms were due to approaching parenthood, put forward the idea that this could be partly explained by the fact that in our culture there is general silence concerning expectant fatherhood. This, he pointed out, is in marked contrast to many primitive societies where the behaviour of the expectant father is strictly ritualized.[12] If this is correct, it not only points to one essential difference between the ritual Couvade and the Couvade syndrome but may also explain why those with the Couvade syndrome, who may guess what the cause of their symptoms is, nevertheless tend to conceal the fact.

If it is agreed that anxiety is the basis of the Couvade syndrome, what are the sufferers anxious about? Interestingly enough, their concern appears not primarily to be with the occurrence or threat of genuine obstetrical hazards, but with what instead might be called pseudo-obstetrical or fantasied risks. These, characteristically, are contained in such statements as: "It's her first", or "Her mother had such a terrible time" etc., or ideas so disturbing as to be impossible to put into words. Although there are exceptions, such evidence as is available does not therefore suggest, either in initial or recurrent instances, that a woman's obstetric difficulties, such as a history of miscarriage, toxaemia of pregnancy, difficulties in labour etc. are factors which play any real part in the genesis of the Couvade syndrome. Because of this, it would appear that the anxiety of expectant fathers is on the whole inherent, insubstantial, and neurotically determined, rather than due to any immediate or necessary cause.

This leads directly to a consideration of the psychodynamic background of the Couvade, both as a disorder of fathers-to-be and in its ritual aspects. Although there are points of divergence there are some common psychodynamic mechanisms.

Ritual

Tylor's explanation of the custom of Couvade was that it arose during the transition from the matriarchal to the patriarchal system of tribal organization and was therefore an act by the father carried out to emphasize the bond of blood between himself and his child. Another example of such an act of adoption was the Roman ceremony in which the husband raised the baby from the floor and thus formally proclaimed his acceptance of and responsibility for his offspring.[16, 60]

Freud, in his only reference to the Couvade,[26] carried the matter of the legitimacy of the child a stage further. He put forward the notion that the purpose of the ritual was to contradict any doubt that he, the child's actual father, might have about the paternity of the child. But there is no evidence that this explanation pertains in any way to the Couvade syndrome except possibly in a purely negative sense. No example of its occurrence has as yet been discovered in the father of an illegitimate child, who might as a general rule, presumably, be expected to want to deny rather than to affirm his paternity. Not much weight, however, should be placed on this, as there is no record of the matter even having been positively investigated.

Superstition

Quite a different explanation of the Couvade was advanced by Sir James Frazer[22] and later by Crawley.[11] Both saw it not primarily as an attempt to establish paternity but as an act of sympathetic magic carried out in order to protect the woman and her unborn child from evil influences at or about the time of birth and in the immediate post-natal period. Contrary to an apparently still popular belief, childbirth among primitive peoples is not necessarily an easy or effortless procedure but may be as difficult for an aboriginal mother as for her more civilized sister. Birth, to a primitive woman, may also be fraught with greater risk owing to her poorer nutritional state and a lack of availability of proper antenatal and obstetric care.

All primitive and unsophisticated persons tend to ascribe untoward disasters of any kind to evil spirits or other malign influences. In accord with this, rituals, religious practices, taboos and similar prohibitions are procedures put into practice to ward off evil spirits, keep away the devil, appease the gods and so on. In our own culture many everyday and relatively mundane ceremonies such as form part of weddings, funerals, prize-givings etc., all contain elements which have precisely similar purposes, although with the passage of time the magical aspects of these ceremonies have become somewhat attenuated. They may, however, be seen to be magical procedures in that they have well-wishing as their basis which, as stated earlier, is the outcome of a primitive lingering belief in the omnipotence of thought.

According to Crawley, childbirth is regarded as an occasion of religious peril by primitive peoples. At the time of labour both mother and child are believed to be particularly at risk from evil influences. In an effort to protect them, therefore, father pretends to be mother. By acting as if he himself were pregnant or in labour and about to give birth, his hope is to try to deceive the evil spirits which might otherwise harm his wife and her infant, by directing their attentions away from her and on to himself.[11]

What application does this have to the Couvade syndrome? Crawley's explanation contains two essential elements—empathy between husband and wife, and superstitious fear. While the empathetic hypothesis is an attractive one and probably a reasonable explanation of the aetiology of some cases of the Couvade syndrome, superstition, although still evident even among those in our own culture who would like to consider themselves worldly-wise, cannot be invoked as quite so potent an explanation. There are probably relatively few in Western Europe who would nowadays directly subscribe to the view that an obstetric accident is likely to be due to some form of evil influence, although in the face of disaster or some totally unexpected misfortune it is remarkable how otherwise sophisticated persons tend to revert to primitive superstitious explanations.[20] But if to modern man the devil does not exist as a corporate entity, his likeness may still be discovered lurking in that primitive instinctual part of himself which contains those deep-seated, aggressive, sadistic and other antisocial strivings which are normally kept under control.

Ambivalence and Hostility

Theodore Reik's explanation of the Couvade is based essentially upon this notion and upon ambivalence which, he states, characterizes every intimate emotional relationship between human beings. Thus the relationship between man and wife contains both tender and hostile emotions. Reik, like Crawley, was of course discussing primitives. He further emphasized that the participation of sexual wishes was accessory to the high psychic tension of the period, the hostility of the husband for his pregnant wife being enhanced by the superstitious fear which prohibited him from having sexual intercourse with her especially when she was so far advanced in pregnancy.

To what extent is this hypothesis applicable to the Couvade syndrome in modern man? In the world of the neurotic the projection of repressed hostile feelings on to others is familiar enough, particularly in those who are obsessional, sensitive, insecure, and who, under duress, are prone to resort to paranoid defence mechanisms. Reaction-formation is another case in point. A façade of meekness often masks aggression and resentment. A man who therefore appears unduly solicitous over his wife's pregnancy may be trying to conceal from himself more or less buried but completely contrary feelings towards her and her unborn child. On close examination there is evidence that in some cases such ambivalent attitudes can play a part in the production of the Couvade syndrome. However, the difficulty about psychodynamic formulations based on the concept of ambivalence is that they are as difficult to disprove as they are easy to assume.

But why should a man be hostile towards his pregnant wife? There are several possibilities, the first being that he already contains feelings of antagonism towards her which existed before she ever became pregnant. When she does become pregnant, he may therefore entertain the fantasy that she is in jeopardy and that he himself is responsible, the fantasy being that in making her pregnant he has acted out his hostile intentions towards her, with the possible result that if some misfortune actually does overtake her the responsibility will be his. A second, and more likely, possibility is that owing to pregnancy his wife may become more inward-looking and as a result may withdraw some of the affection she previously expressed towards her husband. As an extension of this, there are some husbands who are so immature, narcissistic and demanding of attention that they tend to regard their offspring, even before birth, as siblings, i.e. as rivals for their wives' attention which they themselves in childhood demanded of their mothers, and after marriage continue to demand of their wives. In such cases an obvious equation between wife and mother is operative.

Parturition Envy

Quite a different explanation of the Couvade rests on the supposition that man is envious of woman's ability to bear children.[7, 18, 31] This notion has been given the ungainly title of *parturition envy*. Some doubt may, however, be cast on the idea that it is the actual process of parturition which is envied, despite the fact that it is this which may be acted out. If there is any substance to this hypothesis, it would appear to be likely that it is the creative act of bearing a child rather than childbirth itself which is envied; for, in real life, the role of the father in this comparatively long drawn out process is relegated to a more or less momentary act of procreation, essential though this is. Ernest Jones[33] has written:

"... envy of the female's capacity to give birth to children is less recognized than its counterpart. It seems to find adequate indirect expression in the creative productivity widely open to man, but traces of it are often to be found in its unaltered form. It may well contribute to the various motives at work in the curious custom of couvade, in which the husband up to the last moment acts the part of the wife in labour."

Jones went on to suggest that the treatment of husbands during labour was much neglected and that some of their distress might be alleviated if it were better recognized that much of it originated in remorse at the sadistic elements that were operative in bringing about their wives' happy but painful state. This notion is clearly reminiscent of Reik's hypothesis of ambivalence with its basis of hidden hostility. Wessel[62] also advanced the suggestion that the occurrence of the Couvade syndrome indicates a need for more attention to be given to the emotional impact of childbirth upon expectant fathers.

The possibility that the Couvade syndrome may originate from a husband's jealousy of his wife's ability to bear children follows the observation of some clearly selected patients undergoing psychoanalysis. It has been postulated[7] that this jealousy is the outcome of the persistence of maternal trends in young boys, which usually disappear following the resolution of the Oedipus complex but may, in certain circumstances, persist. The most striking case on record is that quoted by Evans[18] who described how a male patient during the course of analysis simulated childbirth while on the couch. He gave a history of a previous Couvade reaction which had occurred during the first stage of his wife's labour. Evans interpreted this happening as the culmination of events which had their origin in the patient at the age of three first witnessing sexual intercourse between his father and mother, when the former returned from the war. The patient's fantasy of being pregnant and later acting this out was interpreted as a dramatic identification with his mother whose supreme claim to womanhood was seen by him to lie in her possession of a baby.

Psychosis

But if parturition envy, or jealousy by men of the ability of women to bear children, is an important contributing factor to the genesis of the Couvade, it might be expected that this would be something which would be encountered very much more frequently in everyday psychiatric practice than appears to be the case. Even psychotic patients only very rarely suffer from a delusion of being pregnant. This has been observed both in single and in married men, although in the latter apparently without bearing any definite relationship to their wives' pregnancies.[5, 21, 45]

Although the delusion may occur independently of diagnosis, rather more of the few reported instances seem to have occurred in patients with schizophrenia. This is not surprising, owing to the common occurrence of a confusion of sexual identity in this disorder.[55]

Jenkins and his associates[32] reported a case of a 19-year-old single white American male who was admitted to hospital believing that he was not only pregnant but in the first stage of labour. He was a schizophrenic of limited intelligence who believed he was controlled by his mother, whom he regarded as a witch. A speculative interpretation was advanced that his delusional belief of carrying a male baby represented not only a rebirth fantasy but a playing out of the role both of the good child-bearing mother and the reborn self.

In another schizophrenic reaction affecting a young African male in which, once again, the main symptom was a delusional belief of pregnancy, Alliez and his colleagues[2] considered whether this could in any way be related to femininization, gynaecomastia being apparently a common abnormality among certain African native tribes of one of which their patient was a member. Consideration was also given to the supposition that the symptom might be a reflection of guilt feelings arising from latent homosexual desires. They observed that some of the reported cases were apparently sexually inverted.[21, 45] Despite this, their final conclusion was that cultural determinants were probably of greater significance.

Psychoanalytic Aspects

Freud, of course, had something to say on the subject of latent homosexuality and procreative fantasies, both in his paper entitled *A neurosis of demoniacal possession in the seventeenth century*[25] and in his earlier discussion of the famous Schreber case,[24] on which the psychoanalytic concept of covert homosexuality as a basis of paranoia appears to rest.

While there is no evidence to be gleaned from the records that the "possessed" Bavarian painter Christoph Haitzmann ever regarded himself as pregnant, from some of his coloured drawings which portray the Devil as having both male and female sexual characteristics (a large penis and pendulous breasts) Freud concluded that Haitzmann was struggling against a feminine attitude to his own father culminating in the fantasy of bearing him a child. On the whole, the evidence for this conclusion seems slender.

In the much better documented case of Judge Schreber, who suffered from an involutional paranoid psychosis coloured by a delusional belief that his sex was changing and that he would or could bear children, Freud also postulated that the exciting course was a passive homosexual wish-fantasy.[24]

More recently the Schreber case has been re-analysed by Macalpine and Hunter[39] who, after a critical scrutiny of the prodromal phase of the worthy judge's illness, advanced a somewhat different view. They did not see Schreber's psychosis as explicable in terms of an outburst of homosexual libido repudiated by his ego, nor the delusion of turning into a woman as a wish-fulfilment of homosexual desires. Instead they interpreted the illness as a reactivation of unconscious, archaic procreation fantasies accompanied by ambisexuality expressed in Schreber's uncertainty in regard to his own sex identity. In support of the latter notion clinical experience indicates that disturbed sexuality is an extremely common early symptom of schizophrenia.[55]

While a delusion of pregnancy in psychotic male patients may pathoplastically be determined by some of the same factors which give rise to Couvade symptoms in non-psychotic subjects, there would appear to be no other very close relationship between the incidence of these two phenomena. For one thing, although a psychotic episode may apparently be precipitated in a man by his wife giving birth, the occurrence of a delusion of pregnancy in men does not appear to bear any direct relationship to this event. Likewise those who develop Couvade symptoms, however vivid these may be, are never deluded that they are pregnant or about to give birth.

Discussion

To recapitulate: if the ritual Couvade can be explained as an act of sympathetic magic designed to protect mother and child from malign influences and at the same time to establish the paternity of the child, no such relatively simple explanation can be advanced to account for the Couvade syndrome. The three most likely hypotheses are, therefore, firstly, that it is the outcome of ambivalence in which the symptoms which occur can be regarded as a reaction-formation against concealed or repressed hostile or sadistic wishes felt by a man towards his pregnant wife; secondly, that it is due to identification[46] and empathy; and finally, that it is due to jealousy of her ability to bear a child. None of these three possible explanations necessarily excludes the others. All could be operative in varying degrees of intensity in any single case, although it might be expected that an explanation which invokes ambivalence based on repressed hostility, and one which depends on intense empathy would tend to exclude one another.

The study of individual cases certainly illustrates the complexity of the matter. For example a patient seen by Pryse-Phillips whose case has been reported at length elsewhere,[17] who was both over-attached to and dominated by his mother, seemed to have transferred some of the ambivalence he felt towards her on to his wife. This became especially evident when his wife became pregnant. On each of the six occasions when this happened he suffered severely from Couvade symptoms. His anxiety during his wife's pregnancies, all of which were quite uncomplicated, was striking, this being associated with self-blame and guilt for putting her, as he felt, in jeopardy. But in addition to this, strong feelings of empathy were evident with a need to protect his wife from danger and discomfort from which, paradoxically enough, she never suffered at all. He also exhibited some evidence of frustrated creativity.

This was a particularly complex case. Two others reported below are fairly representative of the type of Couvade reaction which occurs in those with neurotic problems which, unlike the case of the patient just quoted, extend outside pregnancy but tend nevertheless to be exacerbated in relation to this occurrence.

K.J., a 31-year-old carpenter, complained of fatigue, phobic anxiety and a desire to hit out. He was the youngest of three sibs. His childhood was said to have been happy; but his father deserted his family during the patient's adolescence. His relationship with his mother was close and dependent. He married when aged twenty-seven, his wife being six years younger. The marriage was said to be happy though sexual adjustment was very poor. His wife was apparently completely frigid and developed cystitis following each attempt at intercourse. He himself gained little sexual satisfaction on this account. He also described himself as intensely jealous. Despite their sexual difficulties, his wife first became pregnant soon after marriage. She suffered severely from pregnancy vomiting and later on from toxaemia. He had no physical symptoms during this pregnancy though admitted that he worried greatly about her condition. Two years after the birth of their first child she became pregnant again. On this occasion her pregnancy was uneventful but he suffered from Couvade symptoms. He stated: "She didn't have anything actually. I seemed to have it all for her. She had it all with the first baby." At two months he lost his appetite and developed morning sickness (his wife had none on this occasion). This became so severe that he was actually admitted to hospital for a short time. He also suffered from backache and seemed to feel the baby moving in his own abdomen; this phenomenon coinciding with his wife's experience of quickening. During her labour, however, he was free from symptoms. As she had her baby in hospital, she was out of sight and presumably out of mind to a large extent. As he himself had already observed, his symptoms were much more liable to occur when they were together and she was under his direct observation.

This appears to be a fairly simple straightforward example of the Couvade syndrome, occurring in an anxious, insecure and somewhat narcissistic man. It would appear, that being alarmed by his wife's difficulties during her first pregnancy, during her second he himself developed symptoms as if to protect her from a recurrence of her previous difficulties. There was no convincing evidence of any other psychological mechanisms at work, although his jealousy and her frigidity may have been contributory factors. However, the overall degree of disturbance exhibited by this patient was much less severe than in the next example.

M.C., a 24-year-old tool-setter, was seen on account of recurrent attacks of depression, irritability, lack of confidence and irregular attendance at work. He was the second of nine sibs and had been reared in an atmosphere of severe domestic strife. In childhood he suffered from frequent nightmares, fear of the dark, and nocturnal enuresis. He did poorly at school and was several times delinquent. This gave rise to chronic anxiety and persistent self-consciousness. He was clearly a man of inadequate personality and of dull normal intelligence. He married at age twenty-two, having known his wife for three years. They had had fairly frequent premarital sexual intercourse without difficulty. She was two months pregnant at marriage. He later became partially impotent, fearing that his wife might become pregnant again. At the same time he became fiercely possessive and jealous and refused to let his wife have a coil fitted because this would entail a medical examination. In contrast to his behaviour before marriage, which was said to be considerate, finding he could no longer satisfy his wife sexually he started to beat her on frequent occasions. During his wife's pregnancy, and almost from the start, he appeared afraid that something might happen to her. He followed her everywhere. At two-and-a-half months he developed morning sickness and indigestion. Shortly afterwards he complained of "cravings" which induced in him an overwhelming compulsion to eat chocolate first thing in the morning, a substance he normally disliked and never ate. Also, during the night he would sometimes wake, get up, cook and eat potato chips. His wife suffered from none of these symptoms. Later during her pregnancy, he suffered from quite severe attacks of abdominal pain, and on one occasion when he was said to be "rolling around" on this account his wife told him she had just felt the baby move for the first time. His pains immediately ceased, though he did not see the significance of this. At about this time also he began to feel that his stomach was swollen and hard. His wife noticed this also though this phenomenon apparently did not persist for long. When his wife was about seven months pregnant he became so anxious that she and the child might die that he made a suicidal gesture, taking 30 tablets of chlordiazepoxide, as if by this act of self-sacrifice he could protect them. When she went into labour he again suffered pains, this time intermittently and in the lower part of his abdomen, as if he were in labour too. After the birth of his daughter his Couvade symptoms vanished but he became so attached to her that his wife, in her turn, began to feel jealous in that her husband clearly preferred the child to her.

It is difficult to escape the conclusion that this man was in an infantile way jealous of his wife's ability to bear a child and in going through a mock pregnancy was indulging in a primitive act of wish-fulfilment. At the same time his ambivalence towards his wife was clear enough. He both attacked her physically but feared for her safety; thus it is likely that his symptoms could be construed not as empathy but as an act of sympathetic magic designed to protect her from the disasters which he, on account of his own hostility towards her, fantasied might overtake her. It is again worth noting that this patient, like the last, was of an intensely jealous nature. It is also interesting to observe that his fear of her again becoming pregnant led to him becoming at least partially impotent.

The mimetic symptoms of pregnancy—nausea and vomiting, vagaries of appetite, colic, cramps, and other varieties of abdominal symptoms—have a symbolic aspect which makes it easy to relate them to the pangs of pregnancy. But there is one commonly occurring symptom—toothache—which seems to have a much more mysterious origin and on this account is worthy of special consideration. In 1856 Levison in a book entitled *Obscure nervous diseases popularly explained*, wrote:

> "During foetal gestation there is often . . . great irritation of the nervous system . . . including active inflammation of the mouth generally, and the teeth in particular, frequently causing some of them to become carious."[36]

This clearly ties in with the old saw "For every child a tooth", in which so many pregnant women and their husbands still believe, but which apparently has little foundation in fact. Even on a low calcium diet teeth do not—like bones—decalcify, nor is there apparently any special liability to dental caries during pregnancy. There is, however, it is said, a tendency towards a troublesome gingivitis.

What is of greater importance is: firstly, the persistence of the belief that pregnancy harms the teeth, and secondly, the fact that there is a strong sexual symbolism surrounding teeth, organs which have from the earliest time been regarded as objects of special veneration. [34, 38] Every,[19] discussing the importance of teeth as weapons to kill for protection and for food, stated that "the only other factors of comparable survival significance involving morphology, behaviour and intense feeling are those related to procreation." Add to this the once firmly held belief that to extract a tooth from a pregnant woman might cause her unborn child to die[33, 61] and the observation by the Manholds of a high correlation between decayed, missing, or filled teeth and neuroticism. [40, 42] the occurrence of toothache as a Couvade symptom becomes much more easily understandable.

8

Conclusion

How important is the Couvade syndrome? It is very unlikely that any expectant father ever died of it, and there are relatively few who suffer from it severely. If then it has any importance, this is not the outcome of it being even relatively rarely a severe source of discomfort or because it occasionally leads to diagnostic confusion. Rather it is important in that it occurs at all and, in its occurrence, helps to throw some light upon the dynamics of family relationships. As Malinowski stated:

"It is of high biological value for the human family to consist of both father and mother, if traditional customs and rules are there to establish a social situation of close moral proximity between father and child; if all such customs aim at drawing man's attention to his off-spring, then the *couvade* which makes men simulate the birth pangs and the illness of maternity is of great value and provides the necessary stimulus and expression for paternal tendencies."[41]

In writing those words Malinowski was referring to the ritual Couvade not to the Couvade syndrome. But could not his words apply equally to those fathers who by reason of their own personality problems must, like their wives, suffer a little in order better to accept their paternal role?

REFERENCES

1. ABENHEIMER, K. M. 1946. A note on the Couvade in modern England (and Scotland). *Brit. J. med. Psychol.*, **20**, 376.
2. ALLIEZ, J., COLLOMB, H. and VIDAL, G. 1956. Idées délirantes de grossesse, chez un Africain de race Ovolof. *Annls. med-psychol.*, **114**, 845.
3. ALVAREZ, W. C. 1949. Hysterical abdominal bloating. *Arch. Int. Med.*, **84**, 217.
4. *Annotation.* 1953. *Brit. med. J.*, **2**, 1105.
5. BAONVILLE, H., LEY, J. and TITECA, J. 1953. Les Idées de grossesse chez l'homme à propos de deux cas. *Annls med-psychol.*, **1**, 138.
6. BARDHAN, P. N. 1964. The fathering syndrome. *Armed Forces Med. J.*, **20**, 200.
7. BOEHM, F. 1930. The femininity complex in man. *Int. J. Psycho-Anal.*, **11**, 456.
8. BOWERS, F. (ed.) 1955. *The dramatic works of Thomas Dekker*, p. 329. Cambridge University Press.
9. BUCOVE, A. 1964. Post-partum psychosis in the male. *Bull. N.Y. Acad. Med.*, **40**, 61.
10. CLYNE, M. B. 1964. Thirty-seconds psychotherapy. *Med. World*, **100**, 9.
11. CRAWLEY, E. 1927. *The mystic rose*, Vol 2, p. 177. London: Methuen.
12. CURTIS, J. L. 1955. A psychiatric study of 55 expectant fathers. *U.S. Armed Forces Med. J.*, **6**, 937.
13. DALLY, P. J. and MULLINS, A. G. 1954. A mysterious pain. *Brit. Med. J.*, **2**, 757.
14. DAWSON, W. R. 1929. *The custom of Couvade.* Manchester University Press.
15. DICKENS, G. and TRETHOWAN, W. H. 1971. Cravings and aversions during pregnancy. *J. psychosom. Res.*, **15**, 259–268.

16. DRIVER, H. E. 1969. Couvade. *Encyclopaedia Britannica*, **6**, 674.
17. ENOCH, M. D., TRETHOWAN, W. H. and BARKER, J. C. 1967. *Some uncommon psychiatric syndromes* (p. 56). Bristol: John Wright & Sons.
18. EVANS, W. N. 1951. Simulated pregnancy in a male. *Psychoanal. Quart.*, **20**, 165.
19. EVERY, R. G. 1965. The teeth as weapons. *Lancet*, i, 685.
20. FLUGEL, J. C. 1921. *The psycho-analytic study of the family* (p. 164). London: Hogarth Press.
21. FOCQUET, P. 1935. De la grossesse chez des sujects masculins. *Annls. med-psychol.*, **93**, 328.
22. FRAZER, J. G. 1910. *Totemism and exogamy*, Vol. 4 (p. 245), London: Macmillan.
23. FREEMAN, T. 1951. Pregnancy as a precipitant of mental illness in men. *Brit. J. Med. Psychol.*, **24**, 49.
24. FREUD, S. 1911. Psychoanalytic notes upon a case of paranoia (dementia paranoides). *Collected Papers*, **4**, 436.
25. FREUD, S. 1923. A neurosis of demoniacal possession in the seventeenth century. *Collected Papers*, **4**, 436.
26. FREUD, S. 1946. *Collected Papers of Sigmund Freud*, Vol. 2 (p. 72) ed. by E. Jones. London: Institute of Psychoanalysis.
27. FREUD, S. 1950. *Totem and taboo*. London: Routledge and Kegan Paul.
28. HUNTER, R. and MACALPINE, I. 1963. *Three hundred years of psychiatry* (p. 207). London: Oxford University Press.
29. HURST, A. F. 1944. *Medical diseases of war* (p. 195). London: Arnold.
30. INMAN, W. S. 1941. The Couvade in modern England. *Brit. J. Med. Psychol.*, **19**, 37.
31. JACOBSON, E. 1950. *Psychoanal. Study Child.*, **5**, 139.
32. JENKINS, S., REVITA, D. M. and TOUSIGNANT, A. 1962. Delusions of childbirth and labor in a bachelor. *Amer. J. Psychiat.*, **118**, 1048.
33. JONES, E. 1942. Psychology and childbirth. *Lancet*, i, 695.
34. KANNER, L. 1928. *Folklore of the teeth*. New York: Macmillan.
35. LEAN, V. S. 1904. *Collectanea*. Bristol: Simpkin, Marshall & Co.
36. LEVISON, J. L. 1856. *Obscure nervous diseases popularly explained*. London: Effingham Wilson.
37. LICHT, H. 1935. *Sexual life in ancient Greece* (p. 522). London: Routledge.
38. LINDSAY, L. 1933. *A short history of dentistry*. London: Bole & Danielson.
39. MACALPINE, I. and HUNTER, R. 1955. *Schreber; Memoirs of my nervous illness* (p. 416). London: Dawson.
40. MCCARTNEY, J. L. 1951. Psychosomatics in dentistry. *J. Canad. Dent. Assc.*, **17**, 3.
41. MALINOWSKI, B. 1937. *Sex and repression in savage society* (p. 285). London: Kegan Paul.
42. MANHOLD, J. H. and MANHOLD, V. W. 1949. Preliminary report on study of relationship of psychosomatics to oral conditions. *Science*, **110**, 535.
43. MOORE, L. H. G. 1952. The Couvade. *Brit. Med. J.*, **2**, 677
44. MURRAY, M. 1921. *The God of the witches* (p. 145). London: Sampson Low.
45. NEVEU, P. and BOYER, R. 1950. Délire paranoide de grossesse chez un encephalitique. *Annls med-psychol.*, **108**, 275.
46. NOYES, A. P. and KOLB, L. C. 1963. *Modern clinical psychiatry* (p. 44). Philadelphia: Saunders.
47. PENNANT, T. 1772. *A Tour of Scotland and voyage to the Hebrides*. Quoted by J. G. Frazer, 1910.
48. REIK, T. 1931. *Ritual* (p. 27). London: Hogarth Press.
49. ROLLESTON, J. D. 1945. The folklore of toothache. *Br. Dent. J.*, **78**, 225.
50. ROUSSAK, N. J. 1951. Hysterical abdominal proptosis. *Gastroenterology*, **17**, 133.

51. RUBEL, A. J. and SPIELBERG, J. 1966. Aspects of the Couvade in Texas and Northeast Mexico. *Summa Anthropologica en Homenaje a Roberto J. Weitlaner* (p. 299). Mexico City. Instituto Nacional de Antropologia e Historia (Secretaria de Educaion Publica).

52. SALE, W. M. 1969. Ariadne. *Encyclopaedia Britannica*, **2**, 381.

53. SIMPSON, J. 1872. *Clinical lectures on diseases of women* (p. 363). Edinburgh: Black.

54. TOWNE, R. D. and AFTERMAN, J. 1955, Psychosis in males related to parenthood. *Bull. Menninger Clin.*, **19**, 19.

55. TRETHOWAN, W. H. 1958. Early manifestations of schizophrenia. *Med. J. Austral.*, **2**, 722.

56. TRETHOWAN, W. H. 1965. Sympathy pains. *Discovery, Lond.*, **26**, 30.

57. TRETHOWAN, W. H. 1965. Expectant father's toothache. *Mother and Child Care*, **1**, 53.

58. TRETHOWAN, W. H. 1968. The Couvade syndrome—Some further observations. *J. Psychosom. Res.*, **12**, 107.

59. TRETHOWAN, W. H. and CONLON, M. F. 1965. The Couvade syndrome, *Brit. J. Psychiat.*, **111**, 57.

60. TYLOR, E. B. 1865. *Researches into the early history of mankind and the development of civilization* 2nd. ed. (p. 301). London: Murray.

61. WEINBERGER, B. W. 1948. *An introduction to the history of dentistry*, Vol. 1. St. Louis: Mosby.

62. WESSEL, M. A. 1963. The prenatal pediatric visit. *Pediatrics*, **32**, 926.

63. WESTERMARCK, E. 1921. *The History of human marriage* 3rd ed. Vol. 1 (p. 287). London: Macmillan.

64. WYCHERLEY, W. 1672. "The country wife" Act IV, Sc. IV (p. 58). *Famous plays of the Restoration and eighteenth century*. New York: The Modern Library.

65. ZILBOORG, G. 1931. Depressive reactions related to parenthood. *Amer. J. Psychiat.*, **10**, 927.

V

THE PSYCHOLOGY OF HUMAN SEXUAL BEHAVIOUR

ALFRED AUERBACK

M.D.

Clinical Professor of Psychiatry, University of California
San Francisco, California, U.S.A.

At the beginning of the twentieth century, sexual attitudes reflected the thinking of the Victorian era. It was believed that sexuality did not appear before puberty, that sexual intercourse was for the pleasure of the male and few women enjoyed the sexual act. The emphasis was on the innocence of women, a profound preoccupation with modesty and morality, and great concern about immorality in the adolescent and the unmarried.

1

Psycho-Sexual Development

Infancy

A few years later Sigmund Freud's writings shook the complacency of this puritanical thinking. Freud pointed out that sexuality is present at all periods of life, that unsatisfactory relationships are related to the development of mental, emotional and physical illness. Sexual life does not begin at puberty but shows clear manifestations soon after birth. Sexuality is not limited to the genitals but involves obtaining pleasure from other parts of the body. These phenomena are intimately related to the child's personality development. He believed that the events of the first five years of life are critical during this development. In his formulation of this psychosexual development there are three phases, which he named *oral, anal* and *phallic.* These bodily activities show a steady increase during the early years of life and normally are integrated at maturity into genital sexuality. These three phases do not follow one another in a clear-cut fashion; they might overlap or they might be present simultaneously.[7]

During the first year of life the child's existence revolves around the obtaining of food, and his oral activities colour his personality. The extent of satisfaction or dissatisfaction with the feeding experience will affect his later human relationships. If the feeding experience is satisfactory, he will feel friendly and outgoing to the environment. If not satisfactory, the child will react with anger and become either demanding or clingingly dependent. In addition to food, the child learns about the world through his mouth—everything goes into it. The mother's attitude to this will begin to influence the rightness or wrongness of mouth activities. In the early months of life, passive sucking is the primary oral activity; later this gives way to active biting. The degree to which these are pleasurable will affect kissing and other mouth activities in later years.

The infant finds pleasure in body contact, in rocking and rhythmic movement. This skin and muscle erotism will have profound effects in adult life. If the body contact is unpleasurable to the infant, as an adult he may find intimate physical contact disturbing and unpleasant with no conscious awareness of the reason.

During the second year of life attention is focused on the child's acquisition of bowel control. The parental permissiveness or demand for conformity will influence the child's later development. Being trained too early or under too much pressure will cause the child anxiety. Attitudes of cleanliness or dirtiness, of giving or retaining, are in large measure established at this time. If a predominant feeling of dirtiness colours the toilet training period, it will inevitably influence the sexual sphere owing to the anatomical proximity of the genital and excretory areas.

Soon thereafter attention is focused on acquiring bladder control—the phallic phase. The male child becomes increasingly aware of his penis. Masturbation is a universal phenomenon at this age, and the parental reaction to it profoundly affects his later sexual life. Reproaching, scolding or threatening the child produces feelings of guilt, shame and anxiety. The verbal threat to cut off the penis or even the implication of such a threat as a punishment becomes a major factor in what is called "castration anxiety". Even if no such threats arise, this form of anxiety will still be present in some degree, because children becoming aware of the anatomic difference between boys and girls assume that the penis can be lost.

Childhood

Castration fears are increased between the ages of three and five, a period when the boy has feelings of attachment for the mother and hostility for the father. This has been called the oedipal period. He has guilt feelings and concerns about punishment. If the home environment is relatively stable and healthy, the boy will break away from his maternal attachment and shift to a masculine identification with the father. During these same years the girl has a feeling of attachment to her father and is competitive with her mother. Freud postulated that the girl has a period of wishing to have a penis but is finally forced to accept its absence and develops what he called "penis envy". According to Freud, this is a source of disappointment to the female causing her to turn away from an interest in sexuality for some years.

How the child, male or female, handles the anxiety and disappointments of the oedipal period depends in a large degree upon its relationship with the mother and father. If the parents accept the child's gender at birth and provide a warm, loving and consistent environment, the child is able to incorporate the norms, rules and social values of the parents and to learn his or her place in the world. If a loving, trusting relationship is absent between the parents or in their dealings with the child, the development of healthy identifications will be distorted and the seeds for possible deviance, sexual, emotional and physiological, planted. If the father is rough, cruel or violent in action, the boy will be afraid and unwilling to identify with him, while the girl will develop a fear of men. The mother who is over-affectionate or over-possessive attempts to keep her child close to her and consciously or unconsciously thwarts attempts to achieve independence. Where the mother dominates the household and is contemptuous and belittling of her husband, the boy fears the mother and has no desire to identify with the weak, ineffectual father. The little girl may unconsciously compensate for her feelings of inadequacy by adopting the mother's dominating attitude and contempt for the male. Rejection, over-protection or over-indulgence by either parent impairs the child's acceptance of his or her identity. The struggle between love and hate and the patterns of self-assertion or submission established at this time, colour the child's subsequent emotional and sexual life and determine his adult object relationships.

Freud believed that by the sixth year there was a marked decrease in the intensity of the psychosexual development. He called this the "latency period", during which the child's activities centre on socialization and acquiring friends and new authority figures outside the home. With the hormonal changes of puberty, sexuality once more arises. The pre-teen years find boys playing together and manifesting hostility towards girls, a feeling girls share towards boys. This homosexual phase, as Freud termed it, ordinarily is followed by heterosexual interest during the mid-teens and the development of normal male-female courtship.

While there has been criticism of various aspects of Freud's formulation of psychosexual development,[3, 18, 25, 27] it has won acceptance in its general outlines. It constitutes the framework for explaining the emotional and mental development of the human personality and provides an explanation for sexual deviations. There is no question that the emotional interactions in the child's family during the formative years are pre-eminently important. However, in recent years, there has been increasing awareness of biological factors. It is now recognized that biologically the female is superior to the male, and better equipped for her role in life. Female sex is primal, the male is not. The embryo is morphologically female, and only after the fifth or sixth week does the male growth pattern begin. Despite Freud's concept of penis envy, the clitoris being considered a defective penis, it would appear that the penis is a clitoris that has been hormonally enlarged.

Another important biological factor is related to Lorenz's[16] studies on imprinting in animals. Lorenz showed that an animal develops a profound and lasting attachment to its species by virtue of exposure to the species at critical periods in its life. This carries over to the human. The presence of the mother at such a critical period in the child's early life establishes the love relationship of mother and child. The illness of the child or mother, the mother's death or other family tragedies during the first year or two, can traumatize the child and impair his developing healthy love relationships as an adult. It has been suggested that mal-imprinting may be a factor in the development of homosexuality and other sexual deviations.

The development of normal sexuality for every male and female is coloured by a complexity of events which consciously and unconsciously colours his or her self-image and self-acceptance. The boy is taught from earliest years to be "a little man"—meaning that crying or showing emotion are unmanly. He is encouraged to be aggressive, outgoing, but emotionally detached in human relationships. The girl is conditioned to be shy and retiring, with much emphasis on her attractiveness. There is more social acceptance of her emotionality. Her fantasies of romantic love are too often doomed to failure, since the male is conditioned to be non-romantic.

Childhood illness may prolong infantilization and make such a child accustomed to a passive, dependent role. Disruptions in the family due to illness, death, or change of residence, mobilize anxiety and increase the child's feelings of unimportance and impotence. For nearly every child the birth of siblings is an anxiety-provoking event which affects relationships within the family. While some degree of sibling rivalry is normal, it may be so intense as to interfere with healthy interpersonal adjustment.

Adolescence

While some degree of sex play is quite common amongst children, the male-female relationship begins in the teens with the onset of courtship. By the age of fifteen the average male has developed an intense sexual drive with a pressing need for immediate gratification. Ordinarily he is masturbating a great deal, with some degree of guilt for this activity and his nocturnal emissions. He has strong desires for intercourse and fears about his sexual competence, possible rejection by the girl, the possibility of pregnancy and venereal disease. Generally today there is less concern about the last two. The male is genitally centred, desirous of relieving the pressure in his pelvis. From a physiological standpoint he has a need for some form of sexual release every two or three days. Recognizing this biological drive, society condones his seeking pre-marital outlets.

The teenage girl, on the other hand, has been taught over the years to repress her sexuality. She is romantic, with desires for body contact and kissing. She is body-centred and enjoys being fondled, but ordinarily has no desire for intercourse. Physiologically the female has surges of sexual interest only a few times during the month. In the teenage courtship the boy is trying to go as far as possible, while the girl is torn between her desire to please him and her own needs, which are not in themselves directed primarily toward intercourse.

When a teenage girl has premarital intercourse it may be for a variety of reasons. She may love the boy and therefore desire intercourse with him. If she has intercourse with more than a few men, it probably represents her way of being popular, of winning acceptance, and does not necessarily mean that she enjoys the act in itself. For other girls it is a form of rebellion, of acting-out, of defiance against parental control or religious training. In a small number of cases the girl may have developed psychosexually to the point where she may enjoy intercourse itself. Ordinarily girls have learned to repress their sexuality and do not begin to enjoy sexual activity fully until the age of twenty. However, even in the absence of orgasm the feelings of intimacy with the male can be extremely satisfying, meeting—both consciously and unconsciously—her physical needs for body contact and her fantasies of being loved.

Schofield[26]* in a survey of premarital intercourse in Great Britain found that 11% of boys and 6% of girls in his sample had had intercourse by the age of seventeen, and 30% and 16% respectively by the age of nineteen. He found that by seventeen some 13% of boys and 16% of girls had had some contact, short of intercourse, with the genitalia of the opposite sex, rising to 21% and 28% by nineteen years. There were 15% of the boys and 10% of girls who by the age of nineteen had had no contact at all with the opposite sex. He found a high percentage of intercourse without the use of contraceptives. Only 0·5% of boys and 0·1% of girls had ever been infected by a venereal disease. Promiscuity was not a prominent form of behaviour, most intercourse being with "steadies".

Young Adulthood

Kinsey's study of sexual activity in the American adult found that it depended on biological maturation and educational level. The earlier the male matured, the greater the probability of his engaging in intercourse. Counterbalancing this is the finding that sexual intercourse is inversely related to scholastic levels. In the lower classes there is less masturbation and more frequent early intercourse. The better educated resort to masturbation and extensive sexual play, while intercourse occurs later. The studies by Katz[12] in 1968 of twenty-year-old university students at Stanford and the University of California, Berkeley, showed that 62% of the men and 78% of the women were still virgins. Other studies[6, 24] corroborate these findings. Lowry's[17] studies of 122 Air Force recruits with 11th or 12th grade education, most leaving high school to join the Air Force, showed that the majority had had their first intercourse at the age of sixteen with a girl about the same age. On the average, they had been going steady for six months. The initial coitus was in the girl's home or in the boy's car. No contraception

* See also Volume 4, Chapter III.

was used in 44% of the cases. Kinsey found that lower-class women began their sexual life earlier than better-educated women and had a wider range of sexual partners.

Upper middle-class women generally had premarital sex only with one partner before marriage. Only 13% had six or more premarital partners. Women associated closeness, fidelity and love in their relationships; the male was ordinarily casual, opportunistic and basically pleasure-seeking.

Reiss[23] studied approximately 2,000 young adults and found that those with a liberal philosophy tended toward early intercourse, while those who were more conservative tended to abstain. Katz found that 40% of the colleage men he studied never had a meaningful relationship with a girl. Most of the students reported conflicting thoughts and feelings about their sexual attitudes. Sexual abstinence in college men was frequently related to an inability to achieve closeness.

Adulthood

The sexual makeup of men and women is the resultant of the biological, physiological and psychological events during the formative years. The differences between the male and female also reflect in large degree the socio-cultural setting. Mead's studies[20] in New Guinea showed that different tribes had different sexual patterns and gender roles, even though they were only a few miles apart. The Kinsey studies[13, 11] have shown that in the United States there are marked differences in the sexual behaviour of working-class, middle-class and upper-class men. Women appear to have a greater consistency of sexual behaviour. This reflects to a large degree the cultural pressures to conform put on women in nearly every society throughout the world. In much of the world the female is considered a secondary creature, the property of the male. Consequently, men have generally sought to control the sexual behaviour of the female. This has been a source of continuing male-female friction. Anthropological studies have shown that those cultures which encourage women to respond sexually produce women who have a sexual response equal to that of the man. Those societies which discourage the expression of sexual drives in women produce women whose sexuality appears to be inferior to that of men. In most Western societies many women have strong anti-sex attitudes and instil these ideas in their daughters.

The Aged

The studies of Masters and Johnson[19] have shown that, while sexual responsiveness diminishes in the male by the age of sixty, men in good physical health with a healthy attitude regarding the ageing process are capable of a satisfying sexual life well beyond the age of eighty. These studies indicate that there is no time limit for sexual response in the female despite her age. The ageing female is perfectly capable of orgasmic response if she is regularly exposed to effective sexual stimulation. All studies on sexual activity in ageing individuals indicate that there is a continuation of sexual needs, interest and ability into late years, despite a gradual diminution in the male's sex drive with the passage of time. This decrease in the male does not occur precipitately, but develops at the same gradual rate throughout his lifetime. There is no point at which old age suddenly enters the picture.

2

Female Sexuality

Sexual Interest in Women

The female interest in sexual activity develops more slowly because of the difference in her sexual anatomy and function and also because of the strong restraints traditionally put upon girls. The boy has an external genital which is easily touched, so that he begins to masturbate at an early age. The girl learns about masturbation at a later date and fewer girls masturbate than boys. Girls are taught to be careful about sex and to protect themselves from exploitation by the male. Their attention is focused on romance, falling in love, being a wife, having a baby and raising a family.

At the present time our culture shows an increasing concern about the possibility of frigidity in women and their ability to achieve a satisfactory orgasm. All women are physically capable of orgasmic response, but whether they can do so depends upon many complex, interacting factors. While all women have the physical potential for sexual response, not all achieve it. The orgasm is a learned response and does not occur automatically, as has so often been assumed.

Studies by the Kinsey group indicate that only 30% of women have sexual drives roughly comparable with those of men; there are women who are interested in sex, have many fantasies, and can respond rapidly and with intensity in intercourse. Another 30% have less sexual interest than men but, when aroused adequately, can achieve orgasm most of the time. Another 30% have still less sexual interest and fantasies, but when adequately stimulated can have an occasional orgasm, although their need for this seems to be less. The remaining 10% of women practically never have an orgasm, largely because of psychological blocks.

Since only one-third of women have sexual interests comparable with those of the male, it is obvious that in the majority of marriages differences in sexual needs of the husband and wife will cause greater or lesser strains upon their relationship.

The Kinsey figures are not absolute. A woman may be frigid with her husband yet quite sexually responsive with a lover. On the other hand, a wife who ordinarily enjoys intercourse with her husband may become angry with him and go through a period in which she is completely unable to respond, no matter how he tries to stimulate her.

Women generally have to learn how to respond to sexual stimulation, disregarding their former inhibitions. This learning is tied up in large degree with their feelings of love, trust and respect for the male. They must forgo the inhibitions about their genitalia, permitting the man to put his hands on them and welcoming intrusion by the penis.

Because girls are reared with ambivalence concerning genital sexuality many wives have a lower orgasmic response level than their husbands. While men reach orgasm virtually 100% of the time, only between the ages of thirty-one and forty do women approach this level (at 90%). Wives from sixteen to twenty report orgasm only at a 71% level. This means that about 30% of brides are not sexually responsive. With the passage of time marriages that last report a gradual improvement in orgasmic response. Gebhard[9] suggests that marital happiness may be positively correlated with sexual adjustment. He found that the majority of "very happy" wives had orgasms at least 90% of the time. Only 4·4% of "very happy" wives did not experience orgasm in marriage. Those who reported unhappy marriages also found their sexual life unsatisfying.

Whether a woman can become sexually aroused to the point of being sexually responsive depends to a large degree on the lovemaking skills of the husband and the sexual attitudes of the socio-cultural setting. The average woman requires from five to thirty minutes of lovemaking if she is to be adequately aroused to the point where she can be sexually responsive. Most men are unaware of this fact. Being aroused quickly themselves, they assume that the wife has an equal degree of arousal and they become anxious to consummate the sexual act.

Women ordinarily desire languorous lovemaking and are dismayed or angered by their husbands' impetuosity. The most common complaints are that husbands are either too fast, clumsy, or too limited in their sexual technique. Gebhard quoting the Kinsey studies found that marital coitus preceded by twenty minutes or longer of foreplay produces orgasm for 92·3% of the wives. Where penile intromission lasts fifteen minutes or more, only 5% of wives fail to experience orgasm.

Other cultures educate the young in the skills necessary for enjoyable sexual activity through erotic dances, pictures, puberty rites or other rituals. In the Western societies we have subdued overt eroticism. It is believed that the biological drive in itself is sufficient to permit satisfactory sexual functioning. Thus most men assume that putting the penis in the vagina after a few minutes of stimulation is all that is required to bring the female partner to a satisfactory level of arousal. Kinsey found that 75% of men have orgasm in less than two minutes, many within ten or twenty seconds after coital entrance, some even before entrance. This quick performance by the average male is unsatisfactory for the wife, and in most cases leaves her sexually unsatisfied.

Female Sexual Response

For years there has been much talk about vaginal and clitoral orgasms, stressing the importance of the former and decrying the latter. The studies by Masters and Johnson[19] have shown that all female orgasms produce the same physiological responses, whether they are brought about by hand, mouth or penis. Most women can have intense orgasms through clitoral stimulation, but the sexually experienced woman prefers an orgasm with the penis in the vagina, which gives her a subjective feeling of greater satisfaction.

The male orgasm is a simple reflex phenomenon, whereas the female orgasm involves a number of learned responses which may be developed or inhibited by the cultural pattern. Any woman can be brought to orgasm if effective stimulation is applied. Whether or not a woman will develop an orgasm depends on her own psychosexual development, her anatomical and physiological makeup, the sexual attitudes of the social-cultural setting, and —perhaps most important—the male's attitudes of tenderness, patience and emotional involvement.

The Four Phases of Female Sexual Response

Masters and Johnson found that a woman's total sexual response can be divided into four phases: excitement, plateau, orgasm and resolution. During the excitement phase there is vaginal secretion due to an actual sweating or weeping of the vaginal lining. At the same time the vagina elongates and becomes two or three times wider. The cervix pulls up at the top of the vagina, the clitoris becomes enlarged, and the labia majora pull back, making the vaginal opening more accessible. During this excitement phase the breasts enlarge and the nipples become erect.

With continued effective stimulation, the plateau phase develops. The sweating in the vagina continues, a diffuse blush like a measles rash appears over the breasts, the labia minora change from bright pink to cardinal red, and the outer one-third of the vagina becomes grossly distended with blood. This engorgement of the vagina and labia minora is the anatomic foundation for the vagina's physiological expression of the orgasmic experience. Masters and Johnson refer to this plateau-phase vaso-congestion as the "orgasmic platform". This venous engorgement of the vagina is anatomically comparable to the venous congestion which brings about the penile erection.

The intensity of orgasm is directly proportional to the degree of sexual excitation the woman has developed during the excitement and plateau phases. With orgasm there is a generalized tonic spasm followed by clonic spasms of the entire body. The face becomes contorted as though in pain. There are four to ten rhythmic vaginal contractions about a tenth of a second apart in the area of the orgasmic platform.

The number of contractions depends on the orgasmic platform's excitability and determines the strength of the orgasm. Three to five contractions produce a mild orgasm; five to eight provide a satisfying orgasm. More than eight produce an intense orgasm. The intensity of orgasmic response may vary with repeated coitus, depending on the time spent in preliminary lovemaking, the emotional attitudes of husband and wife, physical or mental fatigue, and other factors.

Many women are capable of multiple orgasms if stimulation is continued during or shortly after the first orgasm. If the orgasm does not occur, the unrelieved sexual tension in the pelvis may last as long as twelve hours before returning to normal. After the orgasm there is a filmy perspiration over the body. In the resolution phase, the measles-like rash disappears and the breasts return to normal size. Within one or two minutes the labia return to normal size and colour. The vagina returns to its normal size in five to ten minutes.

Frequently in our culture the woman goes through normal excitement and plateau phases only to become stuck, unable to reach orgasm. This reflects some psychological inhibition due to conscious or unconscious hostility towards the male, guilt feelings about the pleasure she is having, or over-concern about achieving orgasm.

The woman's orgasm is somewhat longer in duration than the male's and has a wider range of intensity. Many women have mild orgasms which are only partially satisfying. An intense orgasm following adequate stimulation brings them the most complete gratification.

Foreplay, Fantasy and Experimentation

Until a woman has achieved orgasmic experience she finds her greatest pleasure in the sexual foreplay rather than in the sexual act. When she feels the male is interested in her she can indulge in her own conscious and unconscious, romantic, fantasies. Men generally are more responsive to stimuli and fantasies than women but become bored faster by repetition of stereotyped sexual activity. They have a need for novelty and experimentation.

As a result of our Puritan thinking most men and women have little or no knowledge about the anatomy and function of the genitals. This is reflected in their limited foreplay. Few pay much attention to the erogenous areas elsewhere in the bodies of both, including lips, ears, neck, armpits, breasts, buttocks, anus, thighs, back and shoulders. The eroticity of these areas varies from individual to individual. Husbands and wives should explore and experiment in lovemaking, but regrettably most do not. Too often the usual foreplay consists of a few embraces and perfunctory kissing, and the male begins to stimulate the woman's genitals. Men tend to move quickly while women prefer a firm pressure and slow stimulation.

Most women feel inhibited about their role in the sexual foreplay. Touching the husband's genitals or even touching their own appears to be improper. In the love relationship the partners should feel free to touch or kiss any part of the mate's body. Praise, commendation, or thanks for a particular stimulation serves as an aphrodisiac to stir the partner to even greater efforts. There should be some playful talk since love made in silence is a mechanical act. Happy sex should have a playful element to give it sparkle and vitality.[15]

Body hygiene is very important, since undue body odor of mouth, armpits, or genitals can be repulsive to the partner. A wife with curlers in her hair or wearing a layer of facial cream is not very stimulating. Men generally like to make love with the lights on while women prefer dark. Sexual drives are eliminated or impeded by fatigue, illness, or emotional tension. Worry of any sort will interfere with a satisfactory relationship.

3

Sexual Adjustment in Marriage

With so many variables in the attitudes of the male and female towards sex, adjustment within marriage is for many an ongoing struggle. For the young bride her initial experiences are uncomfortable, disappointing and in many cases confusing. During the early months of marriage many brides rarely experience orgasm or even much satisfaction. Her husband is prone to uncertainty and nervousness which in turn interferes with his sexual function. Some degree of impotence or premature ejaculation is common for the male, while some degree of frigidity or non-response is almost inevitable for the female. However, if the young couple do not become upset by early failures, and if they mutually love and respect each other, patient effort on the part of both will bring increasing success. With more awareness of the mate's needs the average husband can overcome his tendency to be precipitate and with patience can help his wife develop orgasmic response.

However, adjustment is a continuing problem in most marriages. During the early years, some men are in a constant state of sexual excitement, at a higher peak than their wives. They recurrently want intercourse at times when sex is farthest from the wife's mind. If he tends to rush the foreplay she may develop the feeling that her body is a vehicle for his pleasure and her desires carry little weight.

Unless the wife achieves adequate stimulation in foreplay to reach the orgasmic platform, she is going to find the sexual act recurrently disappointing and will become increasingly resentful. With the passing of years, sexual foreplay tends to become routine and stereotyped—in many cases actually boring. Only by continuous courtship and experimentation can the sexual life retain its sparkle and fun. Most marriages are coloured by concern about the wife's ability to respond sexually. This is a common complaint when the husband and wife consult the physician.

However, recent years have seen an increase in marital friction arising from the wife's complaint that her husband no longer desires her sexually or does not seek intercourse often enough to meet her needs. The woman who has become accustomed to a satisfying orgasm is disturbed when her husband can no longer provide adequate sexual gratification. This phenomenon of sexual apathy in the male, described by Greenson,[11] arises for many reasons. Sometimes the wife's sexual needs may appear as expressed or subtle demands and the husband may feel threatened by her pressure for his performance. If there is competition between the marital partners, increasing sexual strain may develop. Unless these areas of friction are eliminated domestic quarrels, emotional or physical illness, impotence or infidelity may arise. A recent development in some marriages, where the partners have become bored with each other, is wife- or partner-exchanging. Here the marital partners sanction mutual involvement with other partners in their search for new sexual thrills.

With the passage of time there is a slow decline in the male's sexual drive. This decline in physiologic capacity is also influenced by psychological fatigue due to stereotyped repetition of the sexual act in the absence of new techniques, new contacts and new situations. After twenty or thirty years of married life, sex no longer brings excitement or passion as in earlier years. If the couple have a good interpersonal relationship, their sexual life now brings tenderness, closeness and a more complete sharing of experiences. However, if their sexual life has been characterized by open or concealed hostility, this gives rise to arguments and friction. The wife who has found the sexual experience unsatisfying may express openly or covertly a desire to discontinue. The husband who has felt his wife's resistance may develop impotence as an unconscious device to resolve this dilemma. Other reasons for loss of interest in sex are preoccupation with career or economic pursuits, mental or physical fatigue, overindulgence in food or drink, physical and mental infirmities in the individual or spouse, or continuing fear of failure in performance of the sexual act.

The degree of sexual pleasure in marriage is closely linked to social class. The Kinsey studies showed that women who have low educational levels experience less erotic arousal and have fewer orgasms than women in high educational levels. This is probably associated with the fact that lower class males are less interested in sexual foreplay or variations in technique. Lower class men have less interest in their wives as partners in the marriage and consequently the wives are less sexually responsive.[22] Their husbands rarely evince concern about the presence or absence of orgasm for them.

Middle-class and upper-class marriages show a greater sense of sharing and togetherness. There is more concern about the partner and consequently a higher degree of sexual pleasure for both than is found in lower-class marriages.

The study of college-educated women married not more than ten years revealed that 58% found their sexual life to be what they had anticipated before marriage.[1] 20% believed that they had over-estimated its importance, and 13% had under-estimated. 79% considered the sexual relationship very satisfying to them and their husbands. In the sample 69% said the frequency of intercourse was about right, and 25% complained it was too infrequent.

The degree to which people enjoy their sexual life in marriage is variable. A study of apparently happily married Americans by Cuber[4] showed that most American marriages are not very happy. For most there are elements of competition, hostility and exploitation in the relationship which inevitably colours their sexual life. However, he found a small percentage who had a mutually complementary relationship and enjoyed every aspect of their marriage. Where partners are able to entrust themselves to each other without fear of hurt, shame or embarrassment, a satisfying sexual life follows as a natural development.

4

Sexual Deviations

Man's sexual drive is a potentially disruptive force, and every society has attempted to socialize and control the sexual impulses of its members. The norms and standards governing sexual behaviour have varied widely among different groups. Most societies have agreed that certain sexual behaviour is socially disruptive to some extent. Those activities not conforming to the rules of a particular social setting are labelled as sexual deviations. Some are more serious than others. The deviations to be considered here include pathological expressions of normal sexual drives (exhibitionism, voyeurism, sadomasochism, rape and incest), homosexuality, transvestism and transsexualism and pedophilia (sexual activity between adult and child).

Pathological Expressions of Normal Sexual Drives

In many societies only certain forms of marital intercourse are considered normal. Yet it has long been recognized that unorthodox sexual play, using unusual objects or different parts of the body to obtain or enhance sexual enjoyment, is frequent in the normal heterosexuality of happily married couples. Watching or exhibiting the naked body is a healthy stimulus to sexual activity. Hurting or being hurt, including biting, scratching or hitting, as attenuated forms of sadism, add to the mounting excitement in preliminary lovemaking. Most people can contain these impulses within social bounds. However, some persons feel compelled to perform these acts outside of marriage and in ways that society regards as threatening.

(1) Exhibitionism. In exhibitionism the exposure of the male genitals is the sexual act in itself; the exhibitionist derives his gratification from the victim's reaction and does not attempt any further sexual contact. The exhibitionist usually performs the act in unexpected places, and with rare exceptions directs it toward a female with whom he has no personal relationship. Situation and impulse, rather than any special stimulus, determine when he will perform the act, which may range from partial exposure to

open masturbation. The conscious and unconscious purpose is to arouse a strong emotional reaction in the female victim.

The exhibitionist is a male with strong inhibitions about sex and doubts about his masculinity. Exhibitionism generally reflects a restrictive, puritanical childhood. Although many exhibitionists may marry, they usually have serious difficulties in the marital relationship. At times of stress the exhibitionistic act tends to occur. Exhibitionism is one of the commonest sexual offences brought to the attention of the authorities.[21]

(2) *Voyeurism.* Normal children have considerable sexual curiosity and wish to learn about sex. Small boys and girls often examine each other and sometimes attempt to emulate coitus. The environment that is unduly repressive about sexual matters and permits no questions is prone to produce sexual problems in the child. He may hear his parents having intercourse or may walk into their bedroom during the sexual act. Consciously or unconsciously excited he may develop a compulsive desire to repeat the experience. He may wish to watch the sexual act or to see a member of the opposite sex in some stage of undress. While the average man may enjoy the occasional opportunity of observing a woman undressing, the voyeur has a compulsive need to repeat this experience. For him a lighted window is a stimulus for looking. Whenever he thinks that he might see a woman undressing or a couple engaging in sexual activity, he cannot resist the temptation.

(3) *Sadomasochism.* Sadomasochism is a form of erotic behaviour in which inflicting or experiencing pain is a substitute for, or the predominant source of, pleasure in the sexual act. Often a seemingly normal man must beat his partner or be beaten himself as an essential preliminary to, or sometimes as a substitute for, the sexual act. Psychiatric study of such an individual indicates that as a child he was often beaten, usually on the buttocks, and experienced mixed feelings of pain and sexual excitement.

This impulse to beat or be beaten is common in upper-class individuals. Often they were brought up by governesses or housemaids, who spanked them when they were naughty. As children, spanking had an erotic quality that they enjoyed, and as adults they attempt to repeat the experience.

Ellis[5] has said: "Sadism has variations ranging from the innocent 'love bite' to the antisocial acts of 'Jack the Ripper'." The "lust killer" is usually a quiet, well-behaved man who has episodes of killing women he does not know. He often mutilates their bodies, but rarely performs the sexual act. Frequently he is an impotent male, for whom the stabbing symbolically represents intercourse. Sometimes the victim is a prostitute, suggesting that the lust-killer equates sex with evil and in killing a "bad" woman he is trying to deny his own sexual drives. When the victims are older women, they serve as unconscious substitutes for a hated mother figure.

(4) *Rape.* In the U.S.A., sexual aggression against women eighteen years old or more is considered rape. Sexual aggression against girls less than 18 years old is statutory rape, the law assuming that the girl is not aware of

what is happening and thus is not responsible no matter how seductive or willing she might be.

Society is apt to be sceptical of the woman who accuses a man of raping her. Too often she is sexually provocative, either consciously or unconsciously, and arouses the man to the point where he pushes the sexual play to intercourse despite the woman's protests. Many women with repressed sexual desires unconsciously wish to be raped. This unconscious wish, often reflected in dreams, may cause them to be unduly anxious about being home alone and to compulsively check windows and lock doors. Psychologically these women are ambivalent about their sexual impulses and they unconsciously hope that someone will break in when they are alone.

The Kinsey[10] studies indicated that about 30% of rapists are unduly aggressive physically, and many appear to enjoy the physical assault more than the sexual act. Often sexual contact does not occur; the man may be impotent. Another 15% of rapists do not care what outlet they use for their sexual desire. The victim may be old or young; she is simply a means for sexual release. Usually the rape occurs when the aggressor is drunk.

Another 10 to 15% of rapists are otherwise conforming citizens, who explosively react to their sexual urges by assault. A common example is the "nice" high school boy who walks into a neighbour's home and tries to have intercourse with her. When she fights him off, he may assault her and even kill her. Usually these persons are sexually repressed and mother-dominated.

About 10% of rapists divide women into good and bad categories. They will not molest a "good" woman; however, any woman they consider "bad" is fair game.

About one-third of convicted rapists do not fall into a clear-cut category. They may be mentally ill or retarded, or they may represent a combination of the types described here.

In the last few years there has been a new form of rape. In those social settings where racial strife is present the rape of a woman belonging to a different ethnic group or social class is an increasingly common occurrence. The rapist is an individual who feels socially or economically deprived, and the assault is a form of revenge against society itself. At times a gang of such individuals may attack the female victim and conclude the gang rape by beating, mutilating or killing her.

(5) *Incest*. All societies, no matter how primitive, have an incest taboo. The only known exception was ancient Egypt, where the royal family was considered divine and was not to mix its blood with that of commoners. It has been suggested that societies banned incest because they believed it to be biologically harmful due to a possible transmission of hereditary defects. However, this theory has not proved valid. We now believe that the taboo against incest persists because the rivalries between father and sons for the female members of the family or between females for the father would disorganize the family structure.

Psychological studies have shown that little boys compete with their father for the mother's love and attention; similarly girls seek to win their father's approval. The extent to which the child resolves this oedipal struggle determines how much incestuous attachment persists in later years. The male troubled by unresolved incestuous drives may become promiscuous or impotent; a woman with a father fixation may become promiscuous or frigid in her struggle against incestuous impulses.

Incest is more common than is generally believed. Accurate statistics are impossible to obtain because in most cases knowledge of the incest is kept within the family. About 80% of reported cases involve father-daughter relationships.[28] About 18% involve brother and sister, and only 2% mother-son relationships.

Fathers who become involved in an incestuous relationship are generally of normal intelligence and have a good work record. They become increasingly frustrated in marriage and find the sexual relationship not going well. The presence of an adolescent daughter evokes feelings the father had for his wife during their courtship. Often the father forces or threatens the daughter into intercourse, but in some cases the daughter has been mutually seductive with the father so that the sexual act consciously or unconsciously gratifies her. The mother is often aware of the situation but refuses to admit it to herself. She does not love or sexually desire her husband, and allows the incestuous relationship to continue.

In the few reported cases of incest between mother and son, the mother was consistently seductive and at times was openly sexually stimulating.

How the family and society react to a known case of incest determines the extent of its destructive force. Incest can trigger a psychotic or hysterical reaction, but a surprising number of the children involved appear to grow up with a relatively normal sexual adjustment. However, a careful history often reveals that the incestuous relationship has left scars in their sexual makeup.

Homosexuality

Kinsey[13] estimated that 4% of white males are exclusively homosexual throughout their lives; 18% are exclusively homosexual for three or more years; and 37% have had at least one homosexual experience, Kinsey estimated that 2 to 6% of unmarried women and about 1% of married women are homosexual.[14] Studies in the United States and elsewhere have not refuted these general patterns of homosexuality. These findings suggest that homosexuality is one of the most common known psychological disorders.

No biological basis for homosexuality has been found. Studies have not shown any hormonal variations from normal, even in extremely effeminate men. No measurable physical characteristics differentiate homosexual and heterosexual men. Most homosexual men function in society as normal persons; only a small percentage are markedly effeminate. The effeminate male has a strong need to renounce his biologic sex and a conscious or unconscious desire to identify with women.

Psychologic studies indicate that homosexuality arises from a distorted psychological development. During a child's formative years the absence of a parent, overattachment to a parent, lack of identification or overidentification with a parent, and conscious or unconscious parental seduction may all contribute to later homosexuality. When the father is weak, absent from the home, or psychologically displaced by the mother, the boy may become overly attached to the mother. If the father is brutal and abusive, the boy will not identify with him. If either parent is blatantly promiscuous, the child may develop a fear of or distaste for sex.

If the mother is antisexual she instils in her children the feeling that sex is wrong. When adulthood is reached, such a child is afraid to seek a relationship with a member of the opposite sex.

The female homosexual (lesbian) also reflects a disturbed childhood. Fear of men may develop in the girl who is terrified by her father's violence or alcoholic outbursts. The mother who dominates the household and shows her dislike for men can instil similar attitudes in her developing daughter.

Until very recently the law has been most punitive to the male homosexual but has not concerned itself with the existence of the female homosexual. Now society has begun to recognize that homosexuality in itself is not criminal. In England, Canada and the state of Illinois, homosexual relationships between consenting adults are not illegal if conducted in private. There is an increasing question whether homosexuality is really a psychological illness or merely a way of life for much of our population. In most cases psychiatric treatment is unsuccessful. Despite increasing acceptance of the fact that homosexuality between adults is not a sex crime, society has consistently frowned on the seduction of the young or adolescent.

Transvestism and Transsexualism

The *transvestite* finds his strongest sexual gratification in wearing women's clothing. Usually he is heterosexual rather than homosexual, as has been commonly believed because of his feminine dress. In many cases the transvestite is married and has children. However, as a child he closely identified with his mother, and as an adult he finds gratification in appearing as an attractive woman. Yet at the same time, he performs as a man in the sexual act and has no desire to sacrifice his external genitals. While society becomes concerned about the male dressing as a female, it is accepting of the female who wears male attire. Consequently the female transvestite, a woman attempting to pass as a man, rarely becomes a clinical problem.

The *transsexual* male desires a sexual transformation operation to remove the penis and testes and construct a vulva, and takes hormones to produce enlarged breasts and a feminine body. The presence of external genitals and the possibility of having an erection disturb the transsexual; he wants to appear as a normal woman in both habitus and external appearance, and he will sacrifice all male sexual outlets, in order to live as a woman in all respects.

Pedophilia

Pedophilia is a desire for immature sexual pleasure with a pre-pubertal child. It can be heterosexual or homosexual.[21]

Heterosexual coitus with children is rare since generally it is not anatomically feasible. If the child is over fourteen years old, the act ceases to be pedophilia and becomes statutory rape or carnal knowledge. Most pedophelic sexual acts consist of sexual play such as looking, showing, fondling or being fondled. The nature of the sex play is related to the victim's rather than the offender's age.

Pedophilia reflects an arrested psychosexual development; the offender either has never passed the prepubertal stage or has regressed to this level because of stresses in adult life or the changes of old age. The adolescent pedophile is characterized by poor social relationships and immaturity. Because his relationships with girls are virtually absent he turns to younger children as a sexual outlet. Fondling is the most common expression of his sexuality.

The middle-aged pedophile is usually a married man whose family relationships have deteriorated due to serious marital conflicts. He tends to drink excessively, and many of his pedophilic acts occur when he has been drinking. Ordinarily these men have a strong liking for children, which, under the influence of alcohol, leads to immature sexual play.

The elderly pedophile is lonely and isolated. Contrary to popular belief, he is not markedly senile but rather is emotionally deprived. Seeking a close human relationship, he becomes involved with little children, usually at the level of fondling.

Contrary to popular belief, the offender is seldom a total stranger to the victim; often he is a neighbour, family friend or stepfather. In only one-fifth of cases is he a stranger. The offence most commonly occurs in the home of the offender or victim; movie theatres and automobiles are relatively uncommon sites.

Often the child wittingly or unwittingly acts as the seducer or triggers the relationship. Emotionally deprived children tend to be charming and responsive, often to the point of being flirtatious, with all persons. These children enjoy the offender's attention, affection and approval, which compensate for their neglect at home. A study of sexual offences in California in 1950[2] indicated that in a majority of pedophilic offences the child consciously or unconsciously was emotionally involved.

However, Gagnon's study[8] of girls who had been victims of sexual offences found only a small percentage involved collaboration by the victim. Only 5% involved physical force. About 85% of the cases involved exhibitionism or genital fondling, and the child was almost always an innocent participant. Gagnon found that about 25% of all females experience some sexual incident at least once during childhood.

The overt sexual act does not in itself lead to subsequent sexual maladjustment in the victim. Only 5% of the women reporting a prepubertal sexual incident had serious sexual maladjustment as adults. The permanent effects depend largely on the reaction of the parents and other adults. If they react with fear, anger, disgust or hysteria, the effects are more likely to be lasting. The harmful effects are compounded if a child has to talk to police officers or testify in court.

Sexual murder of children is rare. The killing is not the sexual aim but occurs after the sexual act, most often as a frantic effort to cover up the episode. Often such a killer is psychotic. In general, murder rarely follows a pedophilic offence, and the child molester is no more homicidal than the average person. The pedophile is not interested either in hurting the child or in making sexual connection. His interests are at a more primitive level such as fondling.

Sex Crimes

The public is always disturbed about the individual labelled as a "sex criminal" or "sexual psychopath". Who is the sexual offender?

As the Kinsey studies point out, a truck driver may pat a waitress on the buttocks in a roadside cafe and no one pays attention. A woman treated this way on a city street would call a policeman to arrest the offender for a sexual attack. Kinsey also cites the following illustrations: If a man walks past an open window and watches a woman undressing, he can be arrested as a peeper. If a woman looks through a window and sees a man undressing, he can be arrested as an exhibitionist.

Most sexual behaviour between adult men and women would be illegal under statutes in many parts of the United States. Oral-genital activity between consenting partners, even married couples, can result in a jail sentence despite the present recognition that such activity is normal. In his report to the California legislature, Bowman[2] concluded that the laws forbid nearly all of the known voluntary sexual acts. In California only marital intercourse, solitary masturbation and fornication are not specifically outlawed, provided these acts are done in private. Kinsey has stated that most men in the United States could be imprisoned for sexual acts they have performed sometime during their lives.

The voyeur may go through life repeatedly watching women undress, yet carefully avoiding arrest. He is never classed as a sexual deviant. On the other hand, a normal man passing a lighted window may impulsively look in and be arrested as a "peeping Tom". Homosexuals engaged in sexual activity can be imprisoned as sexual psychopaths.

Whether or not an individual will be labelled a sexual deviate or sexual criminal depends on the sexual mores of his society and whether or not he is punished for the act. The punishment may be legal action or public condemnation. Not the act, but society's reaction, determines whether a sexual deviation or specific behaviour is considered a sex crime.

The standards of sexual conduct have constantly changed throughout history. Most of the sexual activities that are now considered deviations are usually thought to be only socially disruptive. Generally these deviations cause little physical or psychological harm to the persons involved. Only a small percentage involve physical force. The social setting determines whether a particular behaviour will be considered sexually deviant or criminal.

REFERENCES

1. BELL, R. R. 1967. Some emerging sexual expectations among women. *Med. Aspects of Human Sexuality*, **1**, 65–72.
2. BOWMAN, K. M. 1954. Final report on California sexual deviation research. Assembly of the State of California: Sacramento, California.
3. CHODOFF, P. 1966. Critique of Freud's theory of infantile sexuality. *Amer. J. Psychiat.*, **123**, 507–518.
4. CUBER, J. F. and HARROFF, P. B. 1965. *The significant Americans: a study of sexual behavior among the affluent.* New York: Appleton Century.
5. ELLIS, H. 1945. *Psychology of sex.* New York: Emerson Books.
6. FREEDMAN, M. B. 1965. The sexual behavior of American college women. *Merill-Palmer Quart.*, **11**, 33–47.
7. FREUD, S. 1954. *Origins of psycho-analysis.* New York. Basic Books.
8. GAGNON, J. H. 1965. Female child victims of sex offenses. *Social Problems*, **12**, 176–192.
9. GEBHARD, P. H. 1966. Factors in marital orgasm. *Social Issues*, **22**, 88–95.
10. GEBHARD, P. H., GAGNON, J., POMEROY, W. and CHRISTENSON, C. 1965. *Sex Offenders.* New York: Harper & Row.
11. GREENSON, R. R. 1968. On sexual apathy in the male. *Calif. Med.*, **108**, 275–279.
12. KATZ, J. *et al.* 1968. *No time for youth.* San Francisco: Jossey-Bass.
13. KINSEY, A. C., POMEROY, W. B. and MARTIN, C. E. 1948. *Sexual behavior in the human male.* Philadelphia: Saunders.
14. KINSEY, A. C., POMEROY, W. B., MARTIN, C. E. and GEBHARD, P. H. 1953. *Sexual behavior in the human female.* Philadelphia: Saunders.
15. LISWOOD, R. 1969. Variety: The spice of marital sex. *Med. Aspects of Human Sexuality*, **3**, 105–112.
16. LORENZ, K. 1952. *King Solomon's Ring.* New York: Crowell.
17. LOWRY, T. P. 1964. Initial coital experiences—where and with whom. *Milit. Med.*, **129**, 966–967.
18. MARMOR, J. 1954. Some considerations concerning orgasm in the female. *Psychosom. Med.*, **16**, 240–245.
19. MASTERS, W. H. and JOHNSON, V. E. 1966. *Human sexual response.* Boston: Little, Brown and Co.
20. MEAD, M. 1939. *From the South Seas.* New York: Morrow & Co.
21. MOHR, J. W., TURNER, R. E. and JERRY, M. B. 1964. *Pedophilia and exhibitionism.* Toronto: University of Toronto Press.
22. RAINWATER, L. 1960. *And the poor get children.* Chicago: Quadrangle Books.
23. REISS, I. 1968. How and why America's sex standards are changing. *Transaction*, **5**, 26–32.
24. RUBIN, I. 1963. Sex and the college student. *J. nat. Ass. Women Deans and Counsellors*, **26**, 34–39.

25. SALZMAN, L. 1967. Recently exploded sexual myths. *Med. Aspects of Human Sexuality*, **1**, 6–11.
26. SCHOFIELD, M. 1965. *The sexual behaviour of young people*. London: Longmans Green.
27. SHERFEY, M. J. 1966. The evolution and nature of female sexuality in relation to psychoanalytic theory. *J. Amer. psychoanal. Ass.*, **14**, 28–128.
28. WEINBERG, S. K. 1955. *Incest behavior*. New York: Citadel Press.

VI

PREGNANCY IN ADOLESCENTS

HELEN M. WALLACE

M.D., M.P.H.

Professor and Chairman
Division of Maternal and Child Health
University of California School of Public Health
at Berkeley, U.S.A.

1

Introduction

General

One part of the present American scene has to do with recent problems in the activities of our youth. On the positive side, it is clear that the great majority of them are fine young people. On the other side, there are signs that a minority of them have symptoms of serious or potentially serious underlying problems which we have not yet learned to prevent or help— such as the continuing rise in juvenile delinquency, the hippie culture and the basic withdrawal of some of them from society, the rise in out-of-wedlock pregnancy, the use and abuse of drugs, the increase in venereal disease, and the problem of school dropouts. Theories about the basic causes of these types of atypical behavior include such factors as general dissatisfaction with our society as a whole, the Vietnam war, inability to give more help to the disadvantaged minority groups, inability of parents to rear their children and youth more adequately, and the previous general permissiveness of child rearing advocated by experts in the children's field.

In countries in developing parts of the world, early marriage has been the traditional custom, with its concomitant pattern of pregnancy among teenagers. In more "developed" countries, there has been a gradual trend in this same direction.

General Demographic Background in the U.S.A.

The marriage rate in the United States rose rapidly in the immediate post-World War II years (early and middle 1940s), and then declined in the 1950s. It has again risen in the 1960s, to a present peak almost as high as that immediately after World War II. Thus, it is clear that marriage has remained and is continued to be regarded as the significant pattern of modern society in the United States. Along with this is the tendency to marry younger, have children earlier, and have their last child sooner.[9]

The divorce rate in the United States has followed a trend similar to the marriage rate—a rise in the middle 1940s, a decline in the late 1940s and the 1950s, and a gradual rise in the 1960s. In 1968 there were approximately 2,100,000 marriages and approximately 600,000 divorces in the United States; in other words, approximately one in every four marriages ended in divorce.[13] Teenage marriage is frequently accompanied by marital complications. The highest divorce rate occurs among couples married in their teens. The divorce rate of this group is three to four times higher than that for couples who marry at a later age.

While the marriage rate has risen in the 1960s, the birth rate has declined since the latter 1950s.

Because of the baby boom in the 1950s, the population in the late teens is now increasing in the United States. This increase in population of the late teens has resulted in certain phenomena—a larger number of teenagers in secondary school and in college and a larger number of teenage marriages. Furthermore, more babies are being born to teenage mothers.[13]

The Illegitimacy Rate

This is the number of illegitimate births per 1,000 unmarried women aged 15–44 years. This rate is used to measure the likelihood that an unmarried woman will give birth. The illegitimacy rate has risen steadily in the United States from 1940 (7·1) to 1965 (23·5). In 1965 it was approximately nine times higher in the non-white (97·6) than in the white (11·6) population.

In the age group 15–19 years, the illegitimacy rate rose from 7·4 in 1940 to 16·7 in 1965. For white girls, 15–19 years of age, there was an increase from 3·3 to 7·9, and for non-white girls there was an increase from 42·5 to 75·8 from 1940 to 1965. Non-white teenagers have shown a slight decline in the illegitimacy rate in the middle 1960s.[4]

The Illegitimacy Ratio

This is the number of illegitimate births per 1,000 total births; it pictures the role played by illegitimate births as a proportion of total births.

Data from the United States in 1965 reveal that 79% of all live births born to girls under 15 years of age were illegitimate; 21% of those born to girls in the 15–19 year age group were illegitimate. These proportions have been increasing since 1955. The respective proportions in the white and non-white groups are as shown at the top of the next page.

The illegitimacy ratio has been highest at the youngest ages. Very few teenagers are married in comparison with older women. Therefore, a smaller proportion of teenage girls are in a position to have a legitimate child. The result is that even though only a very small percentage of girls aged 15–19 years have an illegitimate child (1·7% in 1965 in the U.S.A.), a

*Proportion of live births
born to mothers under twenty years of age
which were illegitimate*

	1955		1965	
	Under 15 Years	15–19 Years	Under 15 Years	15–19 Years
	%	%	%	%
Total	66·3	14·2	78·5	20·8
White	42·1	6·4	57·3	11·4
Non-white	80·1	40·7	86·4	49·2

Source: Reference 4.

much larger percentage of all births to teenage mothers are classified as illegitimate.

In the United States, at least 40 percent of teenage pregnancies are known to be delivered out of wedlock. This figure does not include some other categories of teenage pregnancies—those whose pregnancies are delivered out of wedlock and are concealed from reported statistics, and those pregnancies which are aborted.

Number of Illegitimate Births

The number of illegitimate births in the United States in 1965 was 291,200. Of this number, 123,200 were born to girls aged 15–19 years, and 6,100 to girls under 15 years of age. The color and age breakdown are as follows:

Number of illegitimate births—U.S.A.—1965

	All ages	Under 15 years of age	15–19 years of age
Total	291,200	6,100	123,200
White	123,700	1,400	50,700
Non-white	167,500	4,600	72,400

Source: Reference 4.

The number of illegitimate births has been growing rapidly in the United States.

Premarital Conceptions ending in Legitimate Births

Not all conceptions occurring before marriage result in illegitimate births. In the United States in 1955–59, estimates reveal that 16·0% of white women had a first birth within eight months of marriage, compared with 41·3% for non-white women. There has been a consistent increase in this since the early 1900s.[4] (See table on page 118.)

Landis has found that between 44 and 55% of marriages in California between two high school students involved premarital pregnancy. In a preliminary study of responses from 176 public high schools in California, 764 girls and 96 boys had married, and many of these marriages were forced by pregnancy. By mid-March 1964, 739 boys and girls had dropped out of

*Estimated per cent of women married in specified years
where first child was born within eight months of marriage,
By color—U.S.A.*

Marriage cohort	White	Non-white
1955–59	16·0	
1950–54	11·9	
1950–59		41·3
1940–49		29·4
1945–49	10·3	
1940–44	8·0	
1930–39		25·5
1935–39	8·6	
1930–34	9·0	
1920–29		21·8
1925–29	8·1	
1920–24	8·3	
1910–19	8·9	20·7
1900–09	7·4	11·8

Source: Reference 4.

school because of marriage. Thirty per cent of the schools reported an increase in premarital pregnancies during the past ten years, and only 9% reported a decrease.[2] It is clear that in some teenagers, marriage occurs as an aftermath of premarital conception. It is also evident that pregnancy in teenagers has serious implications regarding opportunity to continue their education.

2

Health Aspects of Teenage Pregnancy

General

From the health point of view, some teenage pregnant girls represent one of the high risk groups. Hassan and Falls[1] in January 1964 published a study of 159 young primiparas (12 to 15 years of age), compared with a control group of 22-year-old primiparas and with a group of all patients delivered at two hospitals in the Chicago area. The outstanding findings in the group of young primiparas were: excessive weight gain, increased frequency of prolonged labor in the 14-year-olds; increased frequency of toxemia in the 14-year-olds; increased Caesarean section rate in the 12- and 13-year-old groups compared with the others; higher incidence of prematurity in the 14-year-olds; higher neonatal and perinatal mortality rates. The authors also summarize studies on young primiparas of nine other authors. In general, these other authors confirm the increased incidence of toxemia, prolonged labor, prematurity, and neonatal mortality. Most authors have pointed out that the young primipara is less likely to receive adequate prenatal care for several reasons—efforts by the girl to prolong the concealment of the pregnancy, difficulties in receiving adequate prenatal care, inadequate services available to the teenager, etc. One important factor causing prolonged labor in teenagers is the occurrence of inadequate pelvic capacity. Hassan and Falls quote another author (Bochner) who found that the incidence of pelvic contraction among primigravidas was higher than that among older women and was higher in the 12- and 13-year-old group. This point is related to the incidence of Caesarean section; the authors found that the combined incidence of prolonged labor and Caesarean section was higher in the young; the 12- and 13-year-old girls had the highest section rate. The well-known relationship between adequacy of pre-natal care and toxemia, prematurity and perinatal mortality is pointed out.

Osofsky[6] correctly points out that the bulk of teenage pregnancies, especially those within the unmarried category, occur in members of the lower socioeconomic class. In the reported out-of-wedlock group in the United States, 60% are non-white and 40% are white. Because of these facts, the unmarried pregnant teenager is doubly at risk from a health point of view. Because she is a member of the lower socio-economic class, the incidence of pregnancy complications and perinatal wastage is increased. Not only have health and other services been fewer for the unmarried pregnant teenager of lower socioeconomic status, but it is this group who have also been deprived of the opportunity to have contraceptive services to prevent pregnancy and to have an abortion if pregnancy occurs.

Stein has reported[11] higher neonatal mortality rates, the younger the girl.

Neonatal death rates by race and age of mothers,
Baltimore residents, 1961

Age of mother	White	Non-white	Total
		Neonatal death rates	
16 years & under	23·0	42·8	35·8
17–19	20·3	33·8	27·5
20 & over	16·9	27·4	21·7
Total	17·4	27·4	21·7

Source: See reference 11.

Stein also reports: the younger the teenager, the higher the incidence of low birth weight.

Number and per cent of single live births weighing less than 2,501 grams,
by race and age, Baltimore residents, 1960

Age	White No.	White %	Non-white No.	Non-white %	Total No. of Premature infants	% of Premature infants
16 years & under	23	11·1	136	20·3	159	18·1
17–19	138	8·6	335	17·3	473	13·9
20–24	311	7·8	468	13·6	779	10·5
25–29	193	6·6	292	11·9	485	9·0
30 & over	225	7·3	321	13·1	546	9·9
Totals	890	7·6	1,552	14·2	2,442	10·8

Source: See Reference 11.

Stein reported that in Maryland pregnancy is the most frequent single physical condition causing adolescents to drop out of school.

Semmens and Lamers[10] have reported the health picture for teenagers cared for by the U.S. Navy 1961–1964, a somewhat different socioeconomic group. Weight gain in excess of 25 pounds was recorded in more than one-third of the group. There was an increased incidence of toxemia. The incidence of prematurity of 8·97% was higher than that of the control group (7·67%). There was an increased incidence of either precipitate or prolonged labor. The perinatal mortality rate was higher.

Osofsky[6] has reported preliminary data on the results of setting up a special program for pregnant teenagers. At the time of his report, 175 girls participated in the medical program; 100 girls had delivered 102 infants. The majority of the girls were seen early in the course of their pregnancy; 47% received medical care by the twentieth week of pregnancy, and only 8% had had no care prior to the last ten weeks of pregnancy. In spite of this intensive care, 24% of the girls required antepartum hospitalization because of complications of pregnancy. Incipient or early toxemia, excessive weight gain, and anemia were frequent problems. The incidence of prematurity was 14·7% In spite of these complications, Osofsky reported the absence of any perinatal deaths in his series.

Nutrition

The nutritional aspects of teenage pregnancy deserve serious consideration and emphasis. Adolescence itself is a period of rapid physical growth, and hence the teenager has increased nutritional needs for herself alone. Pregnancy is also a period of increased nutritional needs because of the growth of the fetus. Thus, pregnancy places increased nutritional stress upon the girl, who already has increased nutritional needs. Nutrition in pregnancy is of importance, because the diet of the pregnant woman, especially protein, can influence the birth weight of the newborn infant. In spite of this knowledge, studies have shown that many teenagers have an inadequate diet. The need for increased emphasis on nutrition education for all teenagers is evident.

Venereal Disease

Reported data[3] show a marked increase in the incidence of venereal disease in the United States since 1962. The overall reported increase has occurred in gonorrhea mainly.

For all teenagers aged 15–19 years in the United States, the reported incidence rate of primary and secondary syphilis has been relatively stationary. For both white and non-white males aged 15–19 years, there was a small reported increase in incidence, while for females aged 15–19 years there was a reported decrease in incidence in 1967 over 1966. In the case of gonorrhea, there was an increase in the reported incidence in all teenagers, in both sexes, and in both whites and non-whites in 1967 compared with 1966.

3

Educational Aspects of Teenage Pregnancy

Pregnancy is the primary physical cause for girls to leave school. Until very recently it has been the general policy for public schools to exclude pregnant girls from school, as soon as the pregnancy is known. The significance of such exclusion has been that it is demoralizing to the girl; her education is interrupted; she may never return to school and complete her education; and her potential for future employment is thus more limited. The threat of school exclusion has meant that girls tend to try to conceal their pregnancy as long as possible; thus the possibility of securing adequate early prenatal care is reduced. Generally, public school systems have excluded the girl when her pregnancy has become obvious, or when her condition has been judged to be "detrimental to the morale of the school". The girl is sometimes excluded until an adequate plan has been made for her baby.

From an educational point of view, many of the girls are of lower socioeconomic status, and frequently are under-achievers. They may be 2–4 years behind the usual grade in school for their age and frequently have been unable to compete successfully in school. Frequently the girls in the lower socioeconomic status belong to the inner city school group in the United States where the pupil-teacher ratios may be high and where the physical facilities may be poor. A significant proportion of the girls have a history of school attendance problems and difficulty with school authorities. Many had low I.Q. scores on testing.

Because of these multiple serious difficulties, some school systems in the United States are now developing comprehensive school programs for pregnant teenagers. A composite picture of 35 such programs is as follows. The programs are intended to provide the girls with continuation of regular school courses during pregnancy, thereby increasing the likelihood that they will go back to and continue school following childbirth. They attempt to ensure early and continuous prenatal care, thus improving the chances of a healthy outcome of childbirth for both mother and child. They attempt to help the girls solve personal problems that may have led to, or been caused by, their pregnancy, thereby improving their potential for a more satisfying future. Most of the programs involve several participating organizations, largely the public school system, the health department and one or more community voluntary agencies. A large number of services is offered, including health care for the girl before and after delivery, pediatric care of the baby, welfare services, psychological services, adoption placement, vocational training, homemaking, child care training, family planning information, and cultural activities. Among those services least likely to be offered are contraception and financial assistance. A multi-disciplinary team is usually provided, consisting of teachers, a social worker, nurse, psychologist, physician, counselor, nutritionist, psychiatrist, and non-professional aides. Some programs offer service to the putative father as well.[12] One of the other services needed is a child-care facility for the baby, if not adopted.

One of the important services needed within any school system is family-life education. While it is generally agreed that primary responsibility for this rests with the family, nevertheless it is true that this is frequently inadequate and needs to be supplemented by other instruction. The content of this includes such aspects as responsibilities of marriage; social behavior (including dating, going steady, necking, petting, premarital sex); drinking; drug addiction; venereal disease; human reproduction (including sexual anatomy and physiology); parental roles; prenatal care, and infant care.[10]

4

Psychosocial Aspects of Teenage Pregnancy

Residential Care of Pregnant Teenagers

Maternity homes provide care for only a small percentage of pregnant teenagers in the United States. They are more likely to care for white girls from middle and higher income classes. While their role is proportionately small, nevertheless it is essential that it be made effective.

Standards need to be set for maternity homes. Licensure, consultation and supervision in them are necessary by qualified interdisciplinary professionals from one or more official agencies (welfare, health). A wide variety of services need to be provided for the girls, including health services (prenatal, intrapartum usually in a good affiliated maternity hospital, postpartum, family planning; adequate nutrition; care of the baby); social service for the girl, her family, and the father of the child; counseling and psychiatric service; continuation of the girl's education; vocational training; recreation; assistance to the girl in trying to help her think through the future plan for her baby (whether to retain or adopt him); foster home placement service; adoption service. While there would be agreement that these services are needed, nevertheless it has been most difficult for maternity homes to provide all or most of these services, largely due to lack of adequate community support for the maternity homes. This lack of adequate support may be one manifestation of the community's attitude toward the problems of out of wedlock pregnancy.

Adolescents and Contraception

In the United States, although family planning services are becoming generally more available, nevertheless for unmarried minors who are poor such services are very limited. In a number of communities, they are eligible for service, only if they have had at least one out-of-wedlock pregnancy.

Much of the reluctance to make contraceptives available on a community basis to teenagers is based on long-standing community prejudice, which feels that providing such a service will encourage sexual promiscuity, venereal disease and illegitimacy. There is little, if any, evidence to support this point of view; on the contrary, it is evident that, if such a service is withheld, it may lead to abortion, unwanted babies, and illegitimacy.

Frequently parental consent is required, prior to prescribing a contraceptive to a teenager in a community program. Failure to obtain such consent may make the physician liable for damages arising from a civil suit.

In the past few years, some states in the United States are beginning to permit family planning services to be provided to the public in general, including public welfare recipients over the age of fifteen years via a physician; some states have no restrictions. At the same time, some states have also made it possible to provide for the examination and treatment of minors for venereal disease without parental consent.

In steps being taken to liberalize policy regarding contraception for teenagers, it has been suggested that certain precautions should be taken. These include (1) inquiry about the feasibility to obtain parental consent; (2) taking a full history; (3) informing the minor about policies of the service, and about the nature of possible consequences of information and treatment prescribed; (4) having the minor sign a consent form; (5) providing follow-up treatment and supervision.

Because the alternatives to providing family-planning services for teenagers have serious implications (too early pregnancies, out-of-wedlock pregnancies, illegal abortion, battered infants, increased welfare burden, interrupted education, lessened potential in gainful employment, and emotional and social trauma), there is need to consider carefully the need to remove restrictions and to make family planning service to teenagers.[8]

Abortion and the Teenager

Abortion represents a potentially serious health hazard for anyone, including the teenager. Although the full extent of induced abortion in the United States is unknown, estimates indicate that it is a not infrequent method of termination of pregnancy. Some estimates indicate that for every four pregnancies terminating in a live birth, an induced abortion is performed. Induced abortion has emerged as one of the major causes of maternal mortality in the United States.

The entire picture of induced abortion is in need of review and revision. As a whole, it presents a picture of a serious health hazard, a procedure performed at considerable expense, a procedure carried out under unsavory circumstances, and a method of terminating pregnancy with legal implications and complications. For this reason, laws regarding induced abortion are gradually being revised. While formerly the indication for induced abortion was largely limited to protection of the life of the mother, there are now being gradually broadened to other indications, such as (1) protection of the health of the mother; (2) evidence of incest or rape; (3) potentiality of birth of a defective or deformed child.

Abortion is of course a negative method of family planning. It is more desirable that positive methods be used including intensifying efforts at family life education, including sex education; making family-planning services more freely available; providing premarital and pre-conceptional counseling and guidance services, including mental health; efforts to identify earlier "problem" children and "problem" families, and making available more constructive and helpful services for them.

Pregnancy out of Wedlock

Data available provide the following composite picture of the teenager who is pregnant out of wedlock. Frequently, she may come from a home which is broken, or in lower socioeconomic status. She may have a poor relationship with one or both parents. There may be signs of social maladjustment, regardless of socioeconomic status. In general, it may be said that the unmarried girl, her family, and the unmarried father are in a state of crisis and in need of considerable help. Counseling is needed for the girl, her family, and the baby's father. Unmarried teenage pregnant girls have been divided by Semmens into three categories as those having an intentional pregnancy, those having an accidental pregnancy, and those "unknowing".[10] Reactions to the pregnancy on the part of the girl may consist of desire to run away, to commit suicide or to have an abortion performed. Among the decisions which need to be made are whether to marry the father of the child, and whether to retain the child or place him for adoption.[5]

Among the major needs is that of case work and counseling for the girl (in regard to her course of action for herself, her future, marriage); for the child (adoption, placement in a foster home, or keeping the baby at home); and for the girl's family. There is frequently a need for financial support—for the girl's maternity care, for the support of the child, and for the child's education. There may be need for legal assistance in order to gain support from the child's father. There is need for protection of the child born out of wedlock so that he may have equal rights. There may be need for housing. There may be need for day care or group care for the infant. There is need for classes on family life and sex education.[5]

In general, more community services have been available in the United States for white girls of middle class than for non-white girls of lower socioeconomic class. The middle-class white girl receives the most help—i.e. she is more likely to receive care in a maternity home, counseling, better medical care, and a better diet; it is easier to have her baby placed for adoption or in a foster home. It is very difficult for the non-whites to qualify as adoptive or foster homes because of insufficient incomes, inadequate living conditions; non-white girls have received less medical care, less counseling and help, and poorer diets; it is less likely that a non-white girl will be able to enter a maternity home, because of the cost involved.[5]

A recent trend has been to be more concerned about, and to provide services for, the father of the child.[5] Among the significant findings in studies of the fathers of children born out of wedlock are their feelings about their own parents (of being dominated by their mothers and of hostility toward them, and of being deserted in one way or another by their fathers). Many of the young men have a diminished feeling about their own worth. Most expressed a desire to marry the mother of their child in order to avoid their child's hatred. Some have a fear of deserting their child. As a group, they present a picture of immaturity and irresponsibility. They seem to lack ability to engage in a mature relationship with others. They have not been able to establish a strong masculine identity, and their experience of pregnancy out of wedlock is an example of effort to prove their masculinity. As a rule, they do not present a picture of previous delinquency; they have been able to hold jobs effectively. In general, there was a failure to use contraceptives, as must be self-evident. Pannor[5] reports that, when the father is seen, the unmarried mother can be helped more effectively to cope with the problem of unwed parenthood. From the experience of Pannor, and his colleagues, it is clear that there is need for case-work services for the fathers, and that they can be helped by such services. There is also a need for contraceptive information and service.

Maternity homes play a role for a small percentage of unwed mothers. A recent report in the United States indicates that these homes care for 20,000 women a year, or 7% of the total.[5]

A study of out-of-wedlock births in New York City by Pakter[7] showed that the unmarried mothers under 18 years of age were predominantly nonwhite. Among 259 pregnant girls aged 12 to 17 years of age attending school, two-thirds came from broken homes. 12% were reported as behavior problems. Intelligence testing of the group revealed that one-third had an I.Q. of less than 75, another third had an I.Q. of 75–90, and the remaining third an I.Q. of 90 or over. About half of the girls were known for a pattern of truancy, and were reported as having an unfavorable attitude toward education. The study revealed a picture of delayed or absent prenatal care.

5

Conclusion

The Need for a Broad Spectrum of Community Services

Teenage pregnant girls and teenage boys clearly are a high risk group in any community, in great need of a broad range of services, both preventive and management. This range includes such preventive services as steps to strengthen family life, including family-life education and sex education. It includes early identification of problem children and families and bringing services to them. It includes provision of health services of at least safe, and preferably high, quality—including family planning. It includes social, counseling, and psychiatric services. It includes provision of ways to continue their education, and vocational guidance, training, and job placement. It includes recreation. It includes assisting the girl in planning for the future of her baby—retention at home, placement in a foster home, for adoption, or in a day care center. It may include the provision of a safe induced-abortion program. It includes provision of follow-up services to prevent repetition of an unwanted pregnancy. In the opinion of this writer, the time is long overdue for the provision of family centers or parent-and-child centers in communities, where such comprehensive assistance is freely and readily available for anyone needing it.

REFERENCES

1. HASSAN, H. M. and FALLS, F. H. 1964. The young primipara. *Amer. J. Obstet. Gynec.*, **88**, 256–269.
2. LANDIS, J. T. 1964. Statement for the Asilomar Conference on "The Teenage Parent", sponsored by the Governor's Advisory Committee on Children and youth.
3. Metropolitan Life Insurance Company. 1969. Patterns of venereal disease morbidity in recent years. *Statistical Bulletin*, April, pp. 5–7.
4. National Center for Health Statistics. 1968. U.S. Department of Health, Education and Welfare. *Trends in Illegitimacy—United States—1940–1965*. Washington, D.C.
5. National Council on Illegitimacy. 1968. *Effective services for unmarried parents and their children*. New York. See especially the chapters by Edith Garmezy (pp. 7–27); by Patricia G. Morisey (pp. 27–44) by Sister Margaret Mary (pp. 63–70); by Reuben Pannor *et. al.* (pp. 44–57) and by Robert Perkins and Ellis Grayson (pp. 57–63).
6. OSOFSKY, H. J. 1968. *The pregnant teenager*. Springfield, Illinois: Charles C. Thomas.
7. PAKTER, J., ROSNER, H. J., JACOBZINER, H. and GREENSTEIN, F. 1961. Out-of-Wedlock births in New York City. *Amer. J. publ. Hlth.*, **51**, 683–696, 846–865.
8. PILPEL, H. F. and WECHSLER, N. F. 1969. Birth control, teenagers and the law. *Family planning perspectives*, **1**, 29–36.
9. Population Reference Bureau, Inc. 1969. Population Profile. Washington, D.C.
10. SEMMENS, J. P. and LAMERS, W. M. 1968. *Teenage pregnancy*. Springfield, Illinois: Charles C. Thomas.
11. STEIN, O. C., RIDER, R. V. and SWEENEY, E. 1964. School leaving due to pregnancy in an urban adolescent population. *Amer. J. publ. Hlth.*, **54**, 1–6.
12. U.S. Children's Bureau. 1968. *The Webster school*, Washington, D.C.
13. U.S. Children's Bureau. 1968. *The nation's youth*. Chart 20. Washington, D.C.

VII

CHILDBIRTH IS A FAMILY EXPERIENCE

JOHN G. HOWELLS

M.D., F.R.C.Psych., D.P.M.

Director, The Institute of Family Psychiatry,
The Ipswich Hospital, Ipswich, England

1

Introduction

The family is a complete organism, a unity in its own right, as real as, an individual. The individual is an organized system; so too is the family. The family has a structure, paths of communication, characteristics, elements, as any organized system has. Like an individual, it has a psyche—the family group psyche. An event in any part of this organized system impinges on every part in the rest of the system; every experience within the organized system belongs to the system. Thus childbirth and its attendant pregnancy is an experience that belongs to the family as a whole.

Family psychiatry[8] takes the family rather than the individual as the optimum unit for clinical practice. It regards the family as the most significant and meaningful unit in the understanding of emotional events. Society is made up of a large number of clustering individuals, the family. These organized systems, families, beget more families and these units carry emotional health or ill-health as the case may be into the future. In sickness, the family is sick rather than the individual. Indeed the patient, as it were, is the family. The family's psyche, rather than the individual's psyche, is the target for assessment and treatment. Fortunately the family is a manageable unit in clinical practice.

The psychiatry of pregnancy is concerned with abnormal psychopathology produced at this nodal point in the life history of the family. Thus this chapter will briefly look at the family group and the main tenets of family psychiatry. It will then proceed to exemplify those emotional stresses that can arise within and outside the family group during its experience of pregnancy and childbirth. The chapter then moves to a consideration of the symptomatology indicative of disturbed family functioning at this period and closes with a brief discussion of the implications of this approach for the management of pregnancy.

The Family

Humanity flowing in a stream from the Past, through the Present into the Future, might appear at first glance to be made up of a multitude of unrelated individuals. Closer observation, however, shows that human beings coalesce into groups. These groups, the families, expand; individuals split off and new groups are formed. Families beget families, a fundamental truth in family psychiatry. But for the coalescing groups, the families, the flow of humanity would stop; through these groups humanity propagates itself and nurtures and trains its new members. It is these units that determine health or sickness in society. Hence the family is the most significant unit in society. In his life span the individual usually takes part in two groups, his family of origin as a child, and the family he creates later.

A family exists for a particular purpose in the social context in which it finds itself, and is shaped by this fact. The unit may be a small or large nuclear family, a nuclear family extended laterally or vertically or both, or an extended family large enough to merit the term "clan". In psychiatry, concern should be with individuals who have emotional significance as a group. This is, most commonly, the nuclear family. But a blood tie is of secondary importance to an emotional tie, e.g. a servant given intimate care of the children may have more significance for them than the natural parents. Thus, in clinical practice, the concept of the family may have to be widened to take account of this.

Every family is the product of two previous families, the families of orientation. The families of husband and wife send them as their representatives into the family they form together. Thus the group psyche of the new family is a combination of the family group psyches of the two families of orientation in the past. If there is harmony now, it is not only because the two adults are harmonious, but because their two families or orientation are in harmony. Disharmony equally springs from the clashing of the families of orientation; psycho-pathology is created here. Conflict affects the whole family unit and its effects will be found in every dimension of the family. Medicine, however, being individual-orientated, will observe it in the individual only—in the one being seen by that particular medical agency at that moment in time.

Within the family, this organized system, all the elements are equally important. In the life of the family, however, pre-eminent place has been given to the mother, with consequent neglect of the contribution of the father, children and other relatives. Such is the neglect of father, and the rest of the family that, to redress the balance, further brief discussion of their role must be made here.

Some psychoanalytical writers do not regard fathering as an element in family life so distinct as mothering. Proponents of this point of view regard any tender, kind, solicitous care of the infant by father as "mothering". This carries the implication that such behaviour by men is not masculine—yet is regarded as a virtue in the marriage relationship. They further regard these qualities as borrowed from, or an imitation of, the mother and not intrinsic to the father. Clearly, fathering is as definite an entity as mothering. Again, this viewpoint tends to emphasize the biological function of the mother in child care—that she alone bears and breast feeds the child. Furthermore, it is assumed that father is a latecomer to the child's life—important only when the child begins to talk and be independent. All these views can be challenged.

The author asserts that fathering is an element in family life as significant as mothering. Fathering and mothering may have many components; most are common, a few are dissimilar. There are more likenesses in mothering and fathering than there are differences. Both are the product of an intimate emotional experience with their own parents of both sexes; they must absorb components from both. Both also have much in common with relatedness elsewhere—foster parenting, adoptive parenting, marital relatedness, grand-parenting, etc. A child in his tender years requires this protective related-ness from any source; normally it is given equally by father and mother, sometimes better by father or mother, and sometimes better by others. Each situation is unique.

Again, to emphasize mother's biological role in bearing the infant is to overlook the psychological climate of conception and pregnancy. The acceptance of father by mother may be the predominant factor in leading to the acceptance of a child from him, and uniquely from him. Thereafter the parents become a pair linked in a common endeavour, in which, how-ever, only one of them can physically bear the yet unborn child. The father's thoughts, feelings and actions influence the mother's regard for her child and thus indirectly the child. Striking evidence of the father's involvement is seen in the couvade syndrome. The first child emerges into an already formed psychological group situation of father, mother and itself. The group of a second child is a larger one consisting of four people.

The child may be introduced to the group in any order—often he meets father first, if the mother is incapacitated. Thereafter, what he receives from each member of the group is dependent on their feelings for him, their capacity for relating, and the roles given them. This is infinitely variable, and unique for each family. The one thing that a father cannot do for his child is to breast-feed him—although there are isolated instances of the child being soothed at his father's nipples. In the contemporary bottle-feeding society, this is not the handicap that it might appear. All else the father can do directly for the child. When not directly participating in his care, the father still influences his child through his intimate relationship with the mother; after all, a father usually regards a child as a tangible evidence of his own union with the mother. The child is fortunate in the insurance of two parents, whereby one can compensate for the other. Father supports mother and child. Equally, mother supports father and child. The part played by a particular father, or a particular mother, is dependent on his or her own previous family, clan and social experiences.

It is maintained, then, that in parenting, fathering is as distinct an entity as mothering. But, while the importance of this truth is accepted, it must be understood that mother and father are but two elements to which must be added the children to make a nuclear family. Each parent relates to the other and each child to them and to one another. The family is a complex polydynamic system. Furthermore, in at least 20% of instances,[9] families are further enlarged to make an extended family. Every element in this larger group too responds to the whole system.

The Sick Family

Emotional symptoms in the family spring largely from the clash of the families of orientation of the past represented by the two adult members of the family. An emotional symptom is always the expression of the psychopathology of the whole family. Symptomatology for which obscure and symbolic explanations have been given becomes startlingly comprehensible in realistic terms when seen in the context of the family. The following example will help to make this clear. A boy of twelve suffers from anorexia; for the first few years of his life he was brought up by two grandmothers who lived with his family. The maternal grandmother was permissive and did not believe that a child should be forced to eat. The paternal grandmother held as firmly that a child should eat what was put before it. The strict grandmother forced the child to rebel against her, the other grandmother offered him a way to express his rebellion. So the child refused to eat. When the strict paternal grandmother left the family, her son, the boy's father, inherited her role and tried to force the child to eat the food he did not like. Thus his symptoms continued. A family creates the emotional stress, the emotional disorder and the particular manifestation of the disorder—the choice of symptoms.

The instance just related concerns a symptom, a manifestation of dysfunction, in an individual. But, equally surely, symptoms can show in any facet of the family. By tradition, interest has been focused on the individual. Stress may arise in the family in any of its dimensions and at any point in a dimension. As clouds gather in the sky due to a complex of variables, so do stresses within the family. Thus symptomatology can appear in any or all of the five dimensions of the family—the individual, the relationship, the group, the material circumstances and the family community interaction. Careful examination may show that they invariably appear in all the dimensions. However, a family group may not manifest dysfunction equally throughout its system. One dimension, or one aspect of it, may show disproportionate dysfunction due to the "set" of the emotional events at that time.

Pregnancy and childbirth may nurture and enhance the gay and joyful functioning of a family group. It may, on the other hand, evoke in a particular set of circumstances the opposite—hurtful, destructive dysfunction. Its consideration as a sick emotional unit at this time is the concern of family psychiatry.

Family Psychiatry

Family psychiatry is based on the principle that the family, not the individual, is the optimum unit for clinical practice. It asserts the existence of a group psyche or "collective psyche" of the family; the family collective psyche is as real an entity as the psyche of an individual. In family psychiatry, the procedures of investigation are aimed at exposing the collective family psyche; the processes of treatment have as their target the repair of dysfunctioning in the collective family psyche. Thus, throughout, family psychiatry is concerned with the family 'group psyche'. The family is the focus of endeavour throughout; the aim is to produce a harmonious, healthy and well adjusted family.

In family psychiatry, the presenting member, irrespective of age, is regarded merely as an indicator of family psycho-pathology. Thus, after the presenting member is accepted, all the remaining family members are investigated and later treated with the aim of producing an emotionally healthy family. Some of the main features of family psychiatry will emerge from a consideration of a typical clinical situation.

An adolescent of sixteen presents in April with a story of abdominal pain dating from the end of August of the previous year. The pain is such that his father decides to take him to his doctor. As they are about to leave the house, the mother calls out, "And while you are there you might get yourself sorted out." This refers to the fact that father has suffered from migraine from early August. The son is referred to a physician, and is admitted to hospital; after an extensive investigation no pathology is discovered, and the physician refers the boy to a psychiatrist. In the meantime, father, is referred to a neurologist and undergoes extensive investigation as an outpatient. The parents are invited to attend the boy's initial interview with the psychiatrist and father talks of his own migraine. Mother reveals that she has been depressed and frigid since August. Why do three family members present with pathology originating in August? Consideration of the whole family reveals that there is an absent member, a student of nineteen at a university.

Briefly, the family situation is as follows. The student member returns home in early July from the university. Father regards him as a "layabout". Tension develops between them to the point when father says, "He did everything except knock me down." Father develops migraine. Mother is torn between them and becomes depressed, loses appetite for life and becomes frigid. Father does not dare "take it out of" his elder son, and so directs his wrath at the disliked younger son instead. The younger son develops abdominal pain. It is not any one family member who is sick; the whole situation, the family, is sick. The family is regarded as a sick unit and is accepted for treatment as a unit—elder boy included.

Many lessons can be drawn from this brief illustration—choice of symptoms, the common occurrence of psychosomatic symptoms, the seasonal precipitation of a family problem, etc. Here we can consider some of the advantages of regarding the family as a sick unit. Looking on the family as a whole revealed a pathological situation involving all four members of it. The "situation" was sick. To have accepted the boy of sixteen alone for treatment would merely have resulted in an improvement in his abdominal pain and a probable worsening of father's migraine and of mother's symptoms, i.e. the boy would have been treated at the cost of the rest of the family. By accepting the family as a unit, the situation is dealt with, to the advantage of all the family members, i.e. measures are aimed at the desirable target of a healthy family.

Again, support to one member of the family (for example the adolescent) could easily antagonize other family members (for example father) with the result that part of the family is antagonistic to treatment. Acceptance of the whole family, and loyalty to it, leads to the collective co-operation of the whole family—with evident profit.

Again the remarkable cost of treating individuals separately is revealed. Failure to explore the family dynamics from the start leads to expensive investigation. Even after the revelation of a psychiatric problem the wastage could be continued had each member of the family been treated by a different psychiatrist. It is economical to treat this as a single situation, as most of the information required to help one member of the family is precisely the information required to help the others.

The obstetrician is likely to observe symptomatology in the family member under his observation—the mother. However, when emotional sickness arises in pregnancy, an evaluation of the whole family will add to its understanding. Pregnancy may result in new emotional implications stressful to the family psyche. Some of these special stresses are now described.

2

Family Stresses Precipitated by Pregnancy

It is necessary to remember that pregnancy is part of the continuing life experience of the family, which, during this time, is not specially protected from the usual stresses of living. However, in addition to the usual stresses, others can occur due to situations provoked by the experience of pregnancy itself. Some of these situations will now be discussed. The list is not exhaustive; in a particular family a unique atypical situation may arise not covered here.

Emotional stresses have one feature in common: they come from an emotional source—another person or group of persons. The persons most capable of being the source of stress are usually other members of the family, who are close and significant. Only after an accurate examination of the family should measures to elicit the source of stress move outside the family, and even then it is wise to consider the extended family before exploring sources outside the family.

Increase in Size of the Family Unit

The family unit starts off with a membership of two, which later becomes three and builds up to four, five, or more. There is no exact knowledge as to the desirable optimum number of family members. However, an increase in family membership has significance in itself. The whole psychodynamic situation changes each time a new member is added. For example, it means having to make relationships with a greater number of people, and it means sharing both emotional contacts and material commodities. Again, if the family group is large enough, the older children can take on parenting roles towards the younger. Furthermore, there can even be split-off groups within the larger family. For instance, any gap between having children tends to lead to splitting within the family, the older group of children making one group and the younger children another. Again, special partnerships or alignments may develop within the larger family group.

The Parenting Role

When the family first starts, the man has a role as a male and a role as husband. The woman has a role as a female and a role as wife. With the advent of children, the male becomes a father and takes on his fathering role; the female becomes a mother and takes on a mothering role.

In taking on any role in life, an individual lacks experience and is forced to fall back upon imitating the behaviour of others. Thus, a father will tend to take on the attitudes of the only father he previously knew—his own father. Equally, the mother will tend to take on the attitudes of the only mother she knew hitherto—her own mother. Again, the father has an idea from his own childhood of what a mother should do. This may, in reality, clash with the image of mother which the mother has garnered from her own family. Again, a wife or mother has an idea of what to expect of a father from experience with her own family. This image, again, may clash with her husband's actual performance. Thus, there is room for conflict within the family.

Sexual Guilt

In some families, sexuality in young people is taboo. There may be no discussion of it, as it is regarded as distasteful and undesirable. A pregnancy asserts that intercourse has taken place. There can no longer be any denial. Thus, guilt may be precipitated in a partner or partners at the point of pregnancy. Newton[11] exemplifies this phenomenon by quoting the work of Harvey and Sherfey.[7] Harvey and Sherfey had a psychiatrist spend five to six hours interviewing each of 20 New York women hospitalized for severe vomiting, along with their relatives. A control group was used. These authors feel that the most striking finding of their study was the relation of vomiting to sexual disorders. Every one of the patients studied expressed strong conscious aversion to coitus. Half of the total group reported pain on intercourse, and half reported vomiting provoked by coitus and at times by the anticipation of it. All reported coitus made them "upset" and "very nervous and tense". One told of vomiting when her husband came home at night, saying, "I can't stand looking at him." In contrast to this, none of the 14 control patients had experienced coital nausea and none had an aversion to intercourse during the pregnancy being investigated.

Accidental Conception

Intercourse inside or outside marriage can sometimes lead to unexpected or unwanted pregnancies. An unexpected pregnancy does not mean that the pregnancy is necessarily unwanted. But unexpected pregnancies can be stressful, although less so than unwanted pregnancies. An unexpected pregnancy outside marriage may lead to a forced marriage or unexpected marriage, which may or may not be successful, depending upon circumstances. If unsuccessful, this ultimately may lead to the rejection of the ensuing children.

A truly unwanted pregnancy carries the risk of marital stress where a marriage already exists, and the rejection of the child later. From material in Chapter 10, the grim outlook for unwanted children is seen. From the same material it can be seen that the number of unwanted pregnancies is very high.

Unexpected Pregnancy

Pregnancy can result unexpectedly in partners who have long given up any expectation of parenthood due to their apparent frigidity. There is much to suggest that these pregnancies occur with an uplift in the family fortunes. Indeed, in neurotic families, occasionally there are reports of pregnancies resulting when, due to some reason or another, the tension in the family is reduced. The mechanism for this is not clear, but it has nothing to do with frequency of intercourse. It may well be that in states of tension the conception mechanism fails in one or the other partner. With less tension there is more efficiency, and conception takes place, the barriers that produce infertility are raised. (See Chapter II).

The above is illustrated by the following transcript between doctor and an intelligent patient (Mr. S.).

Mr. S.: It is significant that every child we have had has started soon after we have had a change.

Doctor: Yes; does it produce another child?

Mr. S.: I'm sure it does! It is the attitude of life, the pleasure of life, feeling more on top of the world, instead of feeling the standard gloom, which I normally feel, of being necessarily the underdog and always being so because there is so little to look forward to—when we start a new home, it is a new life all together, and I feel much more active in every way. I don't feel lazy, I don't sit about so much in the house.

Doctor: So you then say to yourself, "Let's have another child"?

Mr. S.: No, no, it doesn't happen like that! But I just feel so much happier in life, I feel . . . all that act, anyway, seems a much more pleasurable experience, so much more longed-for, I think. It is completely . . . I don't know, just being on top of life.

Doctor: I see. Do you mean that you are more likely to have intercourse or that conception is more likely?

Mr. S.: Conception is more likely.

Imposed Pregnancy

Occasionally a pregnancy may come about with one partner's intention of tying down the other. This is more likely to happen when there is inadequacy on the part of one parent. The fear of losing the partner may end in an attempt to subdue the partner by pregnancy, either the husband forcing a pregnancy on his wife or a wife contriving to become pregnant despite the wishes of the husband. This is especially likely to happen when an older individual wonders at his or her capacity to retain the affection of the younger. Inevitably, such a forced pregnancy ultimately leads to resentment, with the possibility of rejection of the offspring.

This is illustrated by the following transcript of a discussion between doctor and a patient (Mrs. P.).

Doctor: You got married?

Mrs. P.: Yes.

Doctor: What did you do that for?

Mrs. P.: Well, I had to get married.

Doctor: Yes. I see.

Mrs. P.: I threatened to give him up, you see, and he threatened me. He told me he wouldn't be responsible, you see, if I didn't marry him, and I was so afraid I might be pregnant that I agreed to see him again.

Doctor: Yes.

Mrs. P.: But I didn't want to see him again, not really.

Doctor: I see; and when did you realize that you were pregnant then?

Mrs. P.: Well, directly when I got back with him, you see. It was all deliberate. This night he threatened me I was fool enough to get back with him and he deliberately done it. Now, he said to me, if you're all right you won't get married to me will you. I didn't answer him, but if I'd have been all right, I shouldn't have got married to him.

Doctor: How do you know he did it deliberately?

Mrs. P.: Afterwards he said, "Well there you are, you can get rid of that if you can." Of course I did try, but it was no good.

Doctor: Yes.

Mrs. P.: He said to me, "Now if you can, if you can get rid of that, you won't get married to me, will you?" I didn't say "No I wouldn't get married to you"; I just thought, no, that I won't. I was going to get clear of him.

Doctor: Anyhow you found yourself pregnant, didn't you? And then what did you do?

Mrs. P.: Well, we just got married as quick as we could—special licence.

Doctor: Yes.

Mrs. P.: I think that I just missed that first period and then I think we were married about three weeks after. You see he badly wanted to get married. I should say that he wanted to take a wife back with him.

Attention-seeking

Some persons are denied affection and interest by their own family. These individuals wherever they may find it. Some find the cuddling experience with infants a situation from which they derive affection. Thus children are sought when there is affectional need, however undesirable the family circumstances. However, later, when the infant begins to make demands on the parent, the child may be rejected and the parent seeks for a new infant.

This phenomenon is illustrated in the case of a mother of a problem family who had two children by different fathers. She took a mental defective into her house, married him, and intended to have a third child by him. No child came, and so she threw her husband out of the house. He went to live with another woman and produced a child with her. His wife promptly had him back and produced her third child. Thereafter the marriage broke down. Later she succeeded in persuading the authorities to allow her to adopt a fourth child.

Solution of Marital Tension

Given marital tension, some couples allow themselves to think that the tension arises from the absence of children. They may even receive professional advice on similar lines. Thus children are sought as a means of improving the marital situation. Unfortunately, this is an undesirable and unproductive situation, because rarely is the marital situation improved. This is a particularly undesirable practice from the point of view of the children, who find themselves in an unstable milieu and in a family situation which is likely to fragment.

Solution of Neurosis

Marital partners may suffer from neurosis. Either the partners themselves or their advisers may be persuaded into experimenting with pregnancy as a solution. Rarely does neurosis improve with the advent of children. Indeed, it is an undesirable and stressful situation for the children to find themselves in a neurotic family.

Responsibility

The hold of some individuals on life is tenuous. They find that to cope with their own requirements is as much as is possible for them. The advent of an extra member of the family may be a responsibility which they feel is beyond them. This leads to a feeling of dread, failure and stress.

This situation is exemplified by a transcript of a brief discussion between doctor and a patient (Mrs. M.).

Mrs. M.: I was pleased to have her but, well, it was just the awful depression that I had.

Doctor: What was it, do you think, that bothered you? Was it having so much responsibility to carry, or was it the fact that perhaps you felt that your husband wasn't exactly with you in the project?

Mrs. M.: I suppose it was a little of each. I know I suddenly realized what a responsibility it was. I had rather a sheltered life. My father was rather strict with me and then I suddenly left home, got married and started a baby. It all seemed to happen in five minutes. The house we'd got to rent and the baby to look after, and then I knew my husband wasn't very happy about it, and I hadn't sort of seen that side of him before. You know, you don't when you're engaged and everything is quite smooth and happy; and I think it was everything, you know, together.

Doctor: And did he feel the responsibility of his home?

Mrs. M.: Yes, I think he did because he came home one day and said what a responsibility it all was. He'd got a wife, and a family, and a house that he was suddenly responsible for and it suddenly seemed to come to him all at once. I know he takes the responsibility of it very seriously, that he must sort of work to have enough money to let the children have what they want.

Rivalry

Every extra member of the family is a potential rival. Some individuals not only have a marital relationship with a partner, but at the same time they are the partner's child. Thus, the advent of a child carries with it the possibility of rivalry. They may resent the resulting diminished attention and the exclusive interest of their mother-figure in the new child. In turn, this may lead to rejection or hostile attitudes towards the child by the rejected partner. This is exemplified by the following transcript between doctor and patient (Mrs. M. again). Her extract in the last section above has hinted at jealousy in her husband and this emerges clearly here.

Doctor: What was his first reaction when he found that you were pregnant?

Mrs. M.: He wanted me to take something to try to get rid of it, and of course I didn't. He gave me some gin at the time which probably started the sickness and kept on the whole time.

Doctor: What was the change in your husband Mrs. M.?

Mrs. M.: Well, I don't want to give a bad impression of him, but of course he was rather possessive, especially if I went home in the afternoon to see my mother and my father. Of course I wasn't working once I started being so bilious, and sometimes, if I felt a little bit better, I'd go to my home about two miles away and see them, and he didn't seem to like me going.

Doctor: Why do you feel that your husband was so reluctant to have a baby just then?

Mrs. M.: Well, I think it was because he didn't want to share me with anybody. I won't say he wasn't fond of her when she first came, but he couldn't bear it if she was in the garden while I was still in bed, and I was worried as to whether my sister-in-law who looked after me had brought her in or not. He got awkward about it, he wouldn't go and see, and, you know, he wouldn't have the cot beside the bed. He'd move it over by a far wall, you know the sort of thing, rather inclined to be jealous.

Further, we have to ask, "What does this new pregnancy mean to the children in the family?" To one, it may be a welcome partner or welcome support in family adversities, but to another, an unwelcome rival.

Phobias and Myths

Patients can have all sorts of unlikely and irrational notions about childbirth. These are garnered either due to wrong teaching within their own family, or sometimes because of silence which left ignorance and speculation. Acute anxiety at the time of childbirth may exaggerate misunderstanding. These notions may lead to a fear of pain or fear of the whole birth process, which in turn becomes stressful.

How anxiety leads to misinterpretation is exemplified by the next transcript of a discussion between doctor and patient (Mrs. P. again). In a previous extract she has referred to an unwanted child due to the pregnancy imposed on her. She now refers to her misconceptions and to the delay in labour due to her anxiety.

Doctor: What sort of time did you have when you were carrying him, would you say?

Mrs. P.: Well I suppose I was worried a lot.

Doctor: Yes, worried in what way?

Mrs. P.: Well, I mean my life wasn't very settled. You see, I didn't marry the fellow because I wanted him.

Doctor: Yes, I see. And the birth of the child, what was that like?

Mrs. P.: Well, I was very nervous. I sent for the nurse on the Tuesday. It was a false alarm that was only through me being very nervous. She said to me, "You want to make sure it is the labour before you send for me again." We had to send for her again on the Friday night, and she went away and she gave me a tablet to take to make me sleep, and I took it, but I didn't sleep. I walked about all night and, when she came in the morning, I told her and she 'phoned through to the doctor and he told her to give me an injection. So I had an injection. So you see I didn't know the worst part of it. On the Saturday afternoon before he was born, she moved everything in the room, all small photographs, everything, and put them away in drawers and drew the curtains. What did she do that for? Did she think I was going to get violent?

Doctor: Oh no, I don't think so.

Mrs. P.: Well, what did she want to move everything in the room for?

Doctor: To keep the dust out of the way, I expect, wasn't it?

Mrs. P.: Well, afterwards I thought she took them out of the way because I suppose she thought I was going to get violent and start throwing things about.

Doctor: Anyhow, what happened then?

Mrs. P.: Well, as I say, I don't know the worst of it. Roger was a long time being born. He wasn't born until eight o'clock at night. So let's see, she gave me the injection on the Saturday morning. I went right through the Saturday, you see. He was ever such a long time. I can remember the doctor sitting beside me ever so long and he got rather angry because he wanted to get back to his surgery and he told me I wasn't trying. Well, I don't know, I just couldn't do anything to help myself.

Doctor: Well, what happened then?

Mrs. P.: Well, he was born at 8.0 p.m. When he was born he was shrieking like mad.

Doctor: Yes, so it wasn't too bad was it?

Mrs. P.: No. But it said on the birth chart it was a normal birth, but I was all that trouble.

Rejection

Following childbirth, a child may be rejected as unwanted. There are degrees of rejection and acceptance. Whether a child is accepted or not depends upon its meaning to the parents at that moment in time. Normally the child is accepted as an extension of a loved partner and as a miniature of the partner. The reverse, however, can be true; it may be regarded as an extension of a hated partner and thus be rejected.

Newton[11] lists a number of social factors associated with rejection of a child. These include the following:

(a) Children of first pregnancies are more likely to be accepted than children of later pregnancies.

(b) There is a steady increase in the acceptance of pregnancy as the space between children lengthened.

(c) "Planned" babies are on the whole more accepted than "unplanned".

A child rejected at first awareness of pregnancy may gain acceptance when there is adjustment to the inevitability of the pregnancy. A further opportunity of acceptance comes at the moment of first seeing the child after birth. Unfortunately, apparent acceptance is sometimes covert rejection.

The normal reaction of a mother at the first sight of her child is discussed fully by Wolff,[22] Phyllis Greenacre[5] and Szurek.[17] Similar patterns of acceptance or rejection are seen in fathers. Rejection by fathers are discussed by

White et al.,[21] Bucove,[1] Kaplan,[10] Towne[18] and Curtis.[2] Bucove quotes the following incident:

> After thirteen years of marriage, a man's wife gave birth to a son, who, the patient felt, displaced his position with his wife. The "rage" thus evoked threatened to erupt into overwhelming hostility toward son and wife. F.E. could not even hold his son, lest his destructive impulses ascend to consciousness and action.

Identification

Either parent may see in the child extensions of the self or parents or husband or wife or relatives or acquaintances. These identifications may be benevolent or destructive. Thus attitudes to, and management of, the children may be determined by these identifications. Conflicts with parents, for instance, may be carried on into the future through the identified child.

Grandparents

Again, we need to ask, "What does this pregnancy mean to the grandparents on both sides?"

Investigation may reveal upset at the final loss of the parent as their child, or a realization that they must take second place to the new grandchild, or the final awareness of an unwelcomed marriage, or an antipathy to the offspring from an unadmired relative.

Indeed, emotional factors may prevent potential parents from ever reaching childbirth. A husband recently presented with impotence and his wife with frigidity. It emerged that the husband could not allow himself to have a child since his father, with whom they were living, was strongly opposed to it. He thus "held back' as he had when avoiding making his girl friends pregnant before his marriage. His wife feared to have children lest they should suffer from the insanity which she thought had afflicted her mother. She had also been sexually assaulted by the husband's father and had an irrational suspicion that people might think that any child of hers would be assumed to be his. Conception was a threat to both potential parents.

Robertson,[12] studying vomiting of pregnancy, noted that when the mothers of vomiters were removed from the patient the vomiting tended not to recur. He quoted a case of a mother who was a persistent vomiter in five pregnancies but who was free of it at her sixth pregnancy, which followed her mother's death. Robin[13] quoted Haas, who illustrates the strong influence of grandmothers on mothers: Haas discussed the "complexity of the reactivated conflict between mother and daughter", which "is confirmed by the frequent occurrence of peculiar apprehension over the grandmother's first visit". Haas further said, "It is significant how much pregnant women talk about their mothers' . . . pregnancies and deliveries. Not only do they know their own birth weight, but they claim to know all the particulars of their own delivery. It is striking how often this latter event is related to a danger situation in which mother or baby 'nearly died'."

Anxiety

Due to their childhood experiences, some individuals are predisposed to chronic anxiety. This anxiety may be transferred to children in the family, who are regarded as particularly precious objects. Thus children may be loved and yet over-protected. In states of anxiety a parent may be hostile and at the same time loving.

Gender Preference

Due to previous experiences in their own family, a parent may have different attitudes to the two sexes; for example, boys may be loved and girls disliked. This factor may determine parents' attitude to, and management of, their children. This phenomenon is studied at length by Wolff.[22]

Sex-identification of Parent

This may be weak in either parent, and make for difficulty in accepting their role as parents. Train[19] gives a vivid example of the effect of forced feminity on a mother.

"The only problems she suffered, before womanhood, was in keeping up with the best of the boys, a task she relished.
She stated:
'Before I began to menstruate, I was one of them. Everything I did I loved. I felt strong, immortal and secure. No disease could touch me. Then one day on the handball court, while I was beating the pants off this guy—suddenly this damned cousin yells, "Hey, you're bleeding". I got panicky, then hateful, then angry. I could have killed someone. I thought I would never "fall off the roof". Suddenly, I realized I can't do what I want. Now it was to be monthlies and pads, marriage and babies. No more ball-playing, no more kidding around. For a while, I was a sport about it and fought the feelings and forgot it. But then I began to dream. It was frightening. No longer was I daddy's favorite. His presence thrilled me like dancing and I grew to hate him and gave up dancing for a while. I joined the girls, although I hated them. They are not to be trusted and all they thought of was getting a man. When I was whistled at, I was pleasantly startled. If I shook my hair or wore slacks, the girls said I was sexy. But when, at times, I felt drawn to the boys, it shook me. Monthly mess and tensions drove me wild. Marriage was only a thing to do. Sex was a dirty meal. Later, I got satisfaction only when I imagined my husband a woman and myself a man. It's not sex, but power I feel. He sucks from me. Sometimes I get the urge to bite him, my mouth waters and instead I grind my teeth and I dig my nails. I feel I want to swallow him with my vagina. I clam up and pretend an orgasm. It is all so terrifying.
'Womanhood means pain, blood, pads and perfume, diaphragms. Pregnancy is a duty, a disfigurement and a way of getting ungrateful brats. That's what mother and her fancy ladies taught me. I could

never use diaphragms; I couldn't touch that disgusting part of me. I could take the first pregnancy—it was a boy; but the second was a nightmare. I vomited and felt like killing it. The fact it was a boy didn't help. Then I lost interest.'

This abstract presents the superficial problems and awareness of an allegedly "normal" woman who was capable of control until the stress of a second birth. Beneath this façade, however, is a long-suffering individual whose personality rejected the woman and was contaminated by infantile confusions, interpretations and reactions."

In conclusion, it must be emphasized that, even when one member of the family suffers the major impact of stress, the whole family inevitably has a changed experience; it is invariably implicated in the situation that produced the stress; the result of the stressful situation influences the whole family; its resolution is a matter for the whole family.

3

Family Symptomatology

When stress impinges on a family from within or without, it has an effect upon the whole family. Characteristically, however, in medicine and in psychiatry we pay attention to the symptomatology of the individual only. In fact, a family is influenced in every one of its dimensions. Elsewhere[8] an attempt has been made to construct a fifteen-dimensional model for the family. There are five dimensions in three sequences of present, past and future. These five dimensions are the dimension of the individual, of the relationships, of material circumstances, of general properties and of family-community interaction. The family then will be affected throughout its system, although we may be paying attention only to one facet—a particular individual.

In addition to signs in the individuals the stresses of pregnancy may, for instance, give rise to a faulty husband-wife relationship—symptomatology in the dimension of relationships. Again, some families react to stress by excessive spending which may lower their financial state—symptomatology in the dimension of material circumstances. In some families stress may result in a hostile attitude towards others and even in outbursts of delinquency—symptomatology in the dimension of family-community interaction. Lastly, the dimension of group properties may be affected; for instance, a mother may use her privileged position in pregnancy to become a destructive leader within the family.

It cannot be denied, however, that obstetricians are usually only in a position to detect symptomatology in an individual. Thus, the way in which individuals may react will be briefly outlined. It must always be borne in mind that at least three people are involved, the father, the mother, and the child. It may be of value to consider the symptomatology as it affects these three individuals in the three periods—the ante-natal, natal and post-natal. Once symptomatology has been ascertained in one individual, it behoves the clinician to understand it by reference to an exploration of the whole family. One's duty thereafter is to adjust the whole family.

Ante-natal Period

The mother may, and does, display any psychosomatic symptoms usually met with in clinical practice. Symptoms particularly associated with pregnancy are spontaneous abortion and miscarriage (Chapter XI), cravings and aversions (Chapter XII), hypertension and toxaemia (Chapter XIV) and hyperemesis gravidarum (Chapter XIII). Furthermore, the mother may develop any of the whole range of mood changes, which can end in severe depression and even in a suicidal attempt. Lastly, there may be changes in the mother's behaviour. This may result in an attempt to rid herself of the unwanted pregnancy through induced abortion (Chapter X). If such attempt is unsuccessful, it may precipitate feelings of guilt due to the possibility of having damaged the foetus. Should the foetus subsequently be damaged by accident, the mother is again liable to blame herself.

The father may also display any of the symptomatology of psychosomatic disorder. A particularly vivid example of the involvement of the father is to be seen in the couvade reaction (Chapter IV). Furthermore, he too can suffer cravings and aversions of pregnancy (Chapter XII). Furthermore, he may develop any of the symptomatology of mood changes, which again may extend to depression and even suicide. Lastly, there may be a change in the father's behaviour. Striking examples of this are two fathers seen by me, who have always involved themselves in delinquent behaviour or criminal behaviour on each occasion that their wives have become pregnant, i.e. the switch of attention from themselves to the unborn child has resulted in a feeling of rejection and the re-awakening of hostility, their response to rejection in childhood.

Emotional stress from the mother, or indeed the family, can put the child at hazard in the uterus.[16] Sontag[14] has shown that the children of anxious neurotic mothers are smaller and more active than those of placid mothers. Again, Spelt[15] has been able to condition the child *in utero* to noise externally. Indeed, this phenomenon was well known to Shakespeare, who referred to the hazards of the child *in utero* on more than one occasion, as for instance lack of love for Richard III by his mother:

> "Why, love foreswore me in my mother's womb.
> And, ...
> She did corrupt frail nature with some bribe
> To shrink mine arm up like a wither'd shrub."
> *(Henry VI, Part 3,* III, ii, 153–6).

Natal Period

In the mother there may be uterine inertia leading to delay in labour.

Ferreira[3] regards anxiety as a potent producer of delay. The example of Mrs. P. (page 138) exemplifies the role of anxiety in delay.

It is well known that the reverse can occur—there may be a precipitate birth. This is illustrated by the following example.

A mother attended our children's intake clinic with a disturbed spastic child aged three. Investigation showed that she had married her second husband in a considerable hurry at the death of the first. She was quickly disappointed with her marriage. Her unwanted husband forced pregnancy upon her. After a turbulent pregnancy, at the first signs of uterine pain, she pushed out the repellent object with the result that the child suffered cerebral haemorrhage resulting in the spastic condition. The child remained a rejected child, hence his emotional disturbance later.

Furthermore, there may be any of the signs of change of mood in the mother which can lead to acute distress. Lastly, there may be a change in behaviour, which may make her agitated, awkward and hostile, or passive and withdrawn.

The father too may develop acute physical changes at the time of childbirth and, again, the couvade reaction is a most startling example. Furthermore, there may be any signs of change of mood. Lastly, there may be a change of behaviour.

The child, too, may suffer due to emotional stress at his birth. He may suffer from the consequences of delay in delivery or from a precipitate birth. Furthermore, birth may be premature, leading to all the dangers of prematurity; these premature infants are termed "shock babies" in some localities, i.e. the result of emotional shock.

Post-natal Period

The mother may suffer any of a large number of psychosomatic symptoms. A particular example of physical involvement may be the loss of milk in the breasts (Chapter XXI). There may even be transfer of symptomatology from mother to the child. For example, a woman who had nursed her father with a carcinoma of the colon and with resulting constipation, became constipated on his death. At the birth of her child, she lost her constipation but her child became constipated instead. Furthermore, there may be any of the signs of mood changes, of which the most common and evident are those of anxiety and depression (Chapter XX). These will be demonstrated below. A central factor in post-puerperal depression is the meaning of the infant to the mother, in which again may be reflected the meaning to her husband. Lastly, there may be a change of behaviour in the mother. If this takes the form of hostility towards her infant, it may in an extreme case lead to infanticide (Chapter XXII).

Examples of post-puerperal depression are seen in the transcripts of discussions between a doctor and two patients, Mrs. P. and Mrs. M., each of whom had stresses in pregnancy, as seen in transcripts in the previous section. Mrs. P. suffered a forced marriage and an infant imposed on her by an unwanted husband. She tried to abort the foetus. She had a complicated pregnancy with delay in labour.

Doctor: Well, what did you feel like afterwards—after the birth?

Mrs. P.: Well, I think I was rather sort of low after it. I can remember crying a lot. When one of the neighbours came in one morning, I just seemed as if I couldn't help it.

Doctor: Why did you think that you were low?

Mrs. P.: Well, I suppose it was the marriage. As I say, I didn't get married because I wanted to get married.

Doctor: Why did having a baby make you feel low?

Mrs. P.: Well, I suppose it was because it was a forced marriage and I didn't want him.

Doctor: You didn't want the baby?

Mrs. P.: No, I didn't. I was anaemic and I used to attend the clinic and they used to give me tablets, but I never used to take them. I suppose I just got better myself, and didn't take no more notice of it.

Mrs. M. wanted her child and husband, but his jealousy and rejection of the baby drove her to depression and thoughts of suicide.

Mrs. M.: Well, I suppose it was rather a disappointment because it was his baby as well as mine, and I thought he would feel about her as I did.

Doctor: Did you find yourself rather miserable?

Mrs. M.: Yes.

Doctor: Depressed?

Mrs. M.: Yes, that's right.

Doctor: Did you feel that life wasn't really worth living?

Mrs. M.: I did after Mary was born. I really did. I felt, when I was terribly low, that if it hadn't been for the baby I'd have thrown myself in the river or something.

Doctor: Yes.

Mrs. M.: I don't suppose I ever should have done, but that's what I felt like.

Doctor: Yes. But you didn't feel any desire to take the baby with you. Did you feel antagonistic towards the baby or not?

Mrs. M.: Oh no.

Doctor: You felt the reverse?

Mrs. M.: Yes. I said to myself, well I must just carry on because I've got her.

Doctor: In effect she kept you going.

Mrs. M.: Yes. Sort of feeding her and looking after her. Of course I got more and more fond of her, although I was fond of her right from the start. She got more interesting as she got older.

The father, as in the other periods of pregnancy, may develop signs of psychosomatic disorder, mood changes, or a change of behaviour.[1, 2, 4, 6, 10, 18, 20, 21, 23]

The child also may have evident symptomatology. From the moment of birth, indeed perhaps before birth, the infant may manifest signs due to emotional stress. There may be physical disorders, such as feeding, weaning and habit problems. Mood changes, such as apathy and dejection. Lastly, behaviour problems such as crying, restlessness and awkward behaviour. Handicapped children have their own set of special problems (Chapter XXIV).

An example of a child disturbed from birth, if not before, emerges from the following brief transcript of a discussion between doctor and Mrs. P. again. It might have been expected that this unwanted child of an unwanted husband would be disturbed by the situation and so it was—from birth or even before.

Doctor: Did you feed the baby yourself?
Mrs. P.: Yes.
Doctor: How did he take to feeding?
Mrs. P.: Well, he was a bit of trouble at first. And he used to cry a lot during the night. He was a lot of trouble, like that when we used to take him out he used to shriek. I've never heard a baby shriek like it before. I should say he was very highly strung.
Doctor: That the baby was?
Mrs. P.: Yes.
Doctor: How early or late did he start doing that? I mean, was it during the first few weeks?
Mrs. P.: All the way along.
Doctor: From the very first?
Mrs. P.: Yes.
Doctor: From the first few days?
Mrs. P.: Yes.
Doctor: Would you say he was very highly strung, from the first few days?
Mrs. P.: Yes.

4

Family Management

Once an element in the family has shown signs of psychopathology, it is then necessary to proceed to an exploration of the family dynamics. In obstetric practice it is usual to start with the mother or with the infant, thereafter the rest of the family should be involved so as to make it possible to get a total picture of the functioning and dysfunctioning of the whole family. Problems of pregnancy cannot be regarded as exclusively concerning the mother alone. Every problem of pregnancy concerns the whole family. Its elucidation will only be possible in the light of family dynamics. Treatment should lead to a healthy family unit, which is essential to the nurturing of healthy children and, in due course, the begetting of further healthy families.

The means of exploring the family have been discussed elsewhere.[8] Sufficient to say here that the following techniques are available: exploration of individual psychopathology through individual interviews, exploration of couples through dyadic interviews, and, lastly, a direct exploration of the whole family through family group diagnosis. This last is the procedure of choice. There methods can be supplemented by special procedures, such as psycho-drama and projective techniques, such as the Family Relations Indicator (Fig. 1).

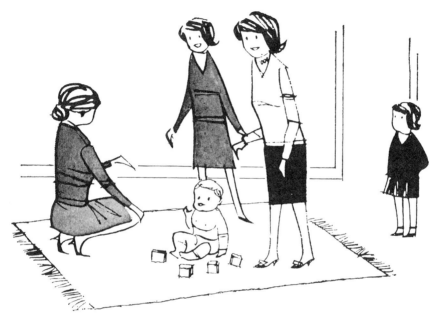

Fig. 1. A card from the projective test "Family Relations Indicator" (J. G. Howells and J. R. Lickorish 1967. *Family Relations Indicator*, Edinburgh: Oliver and Boyd).

Diagnosis leads to treatment. There are two main techniques of family therapy: (1) the direct approach of family psychotherapy; (2) vector therapy.

In family psychotherapy the psyche of the therapist is employed in a direct effort to improve the group psyche of the family. The method of choice is that of family group therapy, when the family meets as a group for therapy. This technique can be supplemented in a flexible programme of individual therapy, and dyadic therapy, the treatment of two members within the family, not necessarily husband and wife.

Vector therapy, often a more potent technique, involves work with the vectors in and without the family, a vector being a force which has direction; and thus the important emotional forces that interact within and without the family are vectors. The purpose of vector therapy is to outline the pattern of the emotional forces and then to change this pattern to the advantage of the family. For example, a full knowledge of a family will reveal that a woman's dangerous hyperemesis gravidarum is reactive to her husband's attitude; removal to hospital replaces husband's negative attitude with the supportive positive attitude of the hospital staff. Here vector therapy is an immediate necessary approach, which brings urgent relief and ameliorates the marital problem that can be dealt with by dyadic psychotherapy later. On the other hand, in a different situation, vector therapy may be long-term in its effects; for example, a careful appraisal of a family situation may reveal that the infant is unwanted and the object of damaging hostility. A family interview can, if successful, lead to acceptance of its hostility, a desire to help the infant (and so relieve its guilt) and end with acceptance of adoption. Negative emotional forces in his natural home in this uncommon instance are replaced by positive constructive forces in an adoptive home. Careful assessments of families can lead to many varying adjustments in the pattern of vectors.

The family approach can also influence obstetric practice. Preparation for childbirth should be given not only to mother, but to the whole family; imagine what one would learn about grandparents' or children's attitudes from such a procedure! Children should be prepared for the next child and so sibling rivalry be reduced. Fathers should be prepared for the coming child. Home confinements are popular with families and the home is the milieu of choice; childbirth is truly a family event when conducted at home. Economic and social considerations may make home confinements less possible. In this event, hospital admission should be of short duration and the family invited into hospital to participate to the full. The implication of every obstetric event is clearer in terms of the family. Throughout obstetric practice all procedures should be framed to deal with it as a family experience. Healthy families can mobilize their strength to combat any complications and even in sick families the assets are not inconsiderable.

5

Conclusion

It is asserted here that childbirth and pregnancy are family experiences. The family is an organized system and any event within any part of that system affects the remainder. Childbirth is such an event affecting the whole family.

Childbirth is normally an unstressful experience. However, stresses particular to pregnancy can be precipitated by it. Some of these special stresses have been outlined. Stressful pregnancy affects the whole family, which is likely to show signs of it in all its dimensions. In obstetric practice these signs may first be noticed in an individual, especially in the mother. Equally, disability in other family members may be explained by the mother's pregnancy. Any disability at any point in the family should always lead to an exploration of the whole family. Treatment is only effective on a family basis. Furthermore, only in this way can one establish a stable family platform for the coming generations.

REFERENCES

1. BUCOVE, A. 1964. Post-partum psychoses in the male. *Bull. N.Y. Acad. Med.,* **40,** 961–971.

2. CURTIS, J. L. 1955. A psychiatric study of 55 expectant fathers, *U.S. Armed Forces med. J.,* **6,** 937.

3. FERREIRA, A. J. 1965. Emotional factors in prenatal environment. A review. *J. nerv. ment. Dis.,* **141,** 108–118.

4. FREEMAN, T. 1951. Pregnancy as a precipitant of mental illness in men. *Brit. J. med. Psychol.,* **24,** 49–54.

5. GREENACRE, P. 1960. Considerations regarding the parent-infant relationship. *Int. J. Psycho-Anal.,* **41,** 571–584.

6. HARTMAN, A. A. and NICOLAY, R. C. 1966. Sexually deviant behaviour in expectant fathers. *J. abnorm. Psychol.,* **71,** 232–234.

7. HARVEY, W. A. and SHERFEY, M. J. 1954. Vomiting in pregnancy: a psychiatric study. *Psychosom. Med.,* **16,** 1.

8. HOWELLS, J. G. 1968. *Theory and practice of family psychiatry.* Edinburgh: Oliver and Boyd.

9. HOWELLS, J. G. Unpublished Study.

10. KAPLAN, E. H. 1969. The husband's role in psychiatric illness associated with childbearing. *Psychiat. Quart.,* **43,** 396–409.

11. NEWTON, N. 1963. Emotions of pregnancy. *Clin. Obstet. Gynec.,* **6,** 639–668.

12. ROBERTSON, G. G. 1946. Nausea and vomiting of pregancy. *Lancet,* **251,** 336–341.

13. ROBIN, A. A. 1962. The psychological changes of normal parturition. *Psychiat. Quart.,* **36,** 129.

14. SONTAG, L. W. 1941. The significance of foetal environmental differences. *Amer. J. Obstet. Gynec.,* **42,** 996–1003.

15. SPELT, D. K. 1948. The conditioning of the human fetus *in utero. J. expl. Psychol.,* **38,** 338–346.

16. STOTT, D. H. 1969. The child's hazards *in utero.* In *Modern perspectives in international child psychiatry* (Howells, J. G., ed.). Edinburgh: Oliver and Boyd.

17. SZUREK, S. A. 1969. The child's needs for his emotional health. In *Modern perspectives in international child psychiatry* (Howells, J. G., ed.). Edinburgh: Oliver and Boyd.

18. TOWNE, R. D. and AFTERMAN, J. 1955. Psychosis in males related to parenthood. *Bull. Menninger Clin.,* **19,** 19.

19. TRAIN, G. J. 1965. Psychodynamics in obstetrics and gynecology. *Psychosomatics,* **6,** 21–25.

20. WEINER, A. and STEINHILBER, R. 1961. The post-partum psychoses. *J. int. Coll. Surg.,* **36,** 490.

21. WHITE, M. A., PROUT, C. T., FIXSEN, C. and FOUNDEUR, M. 1957. Obstetricians' role in post-partum mental illness. *J. Amer. med. Ass.,* **165,** 138–143.

22. WOLFF, P. H. 1969. Mother-infant relations at birth. In *Modern perspectives in international child psychiatry* (Howells, J. G., ed.). Edinburgh: Oliver and Boyd.

23. ZILBOORG, G. 1931. Depressive reactions related to parenthood. *Amer. J. Psychiat.* **10,** 927.

VIII

CHILDBIRTH IN CROSSCULTURAL PERSPECTIVE

NILES NEWTON
M.A., PH.D. (Columbia)
Associate Professor, Division of Psychology
Department of Psychiatry
Northwestern University Medical School, Chicago
U.S.A.

MICHAEL NEWTON
M.A. (Cambridge), M.B.B.CH. (Cambridge),
M.D. (Pennsylvania), F.A.C.O.G., F.A.C.S.
Clinical Professor, Department of Obstetrics and Gynecology
Pritzker School of Medicine, Division of Biological Sciences
University of Chicago
Chicago, U.S.A.

1

Introduction

All known human societies pattern the behavior of human beings involved in the process of reproduction.[65] Beliefs concerning appropriate behavior in pregnancy, during labor, and in the puerperium appear to be characteristic of all cultures. This review will concentrate on patterns of behavior during and surrounding birth. Special attention will be paid to the primitive and traditional cultures, but examples from modern industrial cultures will also be used. Major trends and contrasts in patterns will be emphasized, particularly in so far as they may have applicability to current clinical issues.

First, attitudes surrounding birth will be discussed: the importance placed on birth, privacy and sexual implications of birth, birth seen in terms of achievement or atonement, birth as dirty or defiling or close to the supernatural, and birth as a painful illness or a normal physiological process.

Then social variations in the management of labor will be discussed, particularly in regard to practices which differ markedly from one society to another, resulting in different types of birth experience for mother and baby. These variations include differences in biochemical management, rules about activity and relaxation, sensory stimulation, emotional support and companionship, and delivery position.

Finally, the effect of social attitudes and beliefs surrounding birth on birth behavior will be discussed, as well as other questions raised by the review.

Limitations on Available Information

Both medical and anthropological literature were searched for information on the patterns of culture in the area of birth. Particularly helpful were the Human Relations Area Files, which, at the time the search was made, contained 222 cultures coded in such a way that materials on childbirth could be located rapidly. Medical literature through the years has also concerned itself with certain aspects of patterns of childbirth and was therefore also searched.

Although both medical and anthropological literatures contain considerable information about certain patterns of obstetrical behavior, information is frequently lacking in regard to areas of behavior most relevant to this review. For example, Teit's[96] record of birth among the Nahane Indians of northern Canada devotes more than 450 words to describing the handling of the umbilical cord and to the beliefs concerning it and fewer than 150 words to the other behavior of the attendants and mother during labor. It was not until the 1920s, when the impact of psychoanalysis began to be felt, that ethnologists turned their attention to variations in emotion and personality and began to make more detailed records in this area.

One of the greatest handicaps in the recording of birth patterning among preliterate peoples is the fact that most primitive peoples exclude men from witnessing normal delivery. Although husbands are sometimes permitted to witness their children born, and medicine men may be called in in case of abnormality, other men are excluded from witnessing birth in many of the preliterature societies that have been studied.

Physicians contributing to medical literature are also handicapped, since they tend to see only the cases of extremely abnormal childbirth. Often modern medical advice is asked only when the primitive woman is on the verge of death. Normal childbirth as it takes place regularly in the tribal community is usually out of bounds for the physician as well as the anthropologist.

Implicit in most historical and anthropological writing and medical case reports is the assumption that relatively few observations of behavior in a culture can be generalized into statements about the whole. Due to the extreme paucity of studies done on broad samples collected with controls for observer bias, the limited data available have been used of necessity.

Nature of Conclusions

The nature of the data available at the present time makes it impossible to draw any precise conclusions. What the data can do is to suggest the many variations in the ways in which human beings handle birth. They can suggest certain aspects that have been muted in industrialized cultures and that are more fully developed in other cultures, thus opening new areas of understanding. They can also give perspective, by raising for question implicit assumptions held within our culture, and by exploring various ways in which behavioral issues in our culture are dealt with in other cultures.

A final word of caution is in order in regard to data gleaned from records of so-called primitive cultures. *The word "primitive" is used only in the anthropological sense, meaning peoples without written language.* It is likely that the *behavior of most peoples mentioned may often be different from that described in the text, due to rapid changes in culture occurring in most parts of the world.* The older accounts are often especially valuable for a study of this nature, since they may record relatively intact societies not yet overwhelmed by excessive contact with industrial culture. Despite the biased and fragmentary records produced by the early ethnographers and other early records, the scholarly world of today owes these men and women a deep debt of gratitude; for they recorded unique patterns of human behavior before they irretrievably disappeared.

2

Attitudes Surrounding Birth

Birth is an event that is treated with importance. Much cultural patterning surrounds birth as well as other aspects of reproduction. Despite widespread cultural interest in birth, the nature of attitudes toward birth vary greatly. For some it is an open sociable event, while others surround it with secrecy. The sexual implications of birth are developed in some cultures, and strictly taboo in others. Various peoples see birth in terms of pay or praise, dirt, defilement, and/or supernatural involvement; or as normal physiology, or painful illness.

Importance Placed on Birth

Among primitive groups and traditional village culture groups, as well as in modern industrial cultures, childbirth is an event of consequence that changes the behavior not only of the mother but of other people in the social group. In primitive culture, by far the most usual pattern is for the laboring woman to have two or more attendants for labor and delivery. Often special huts are built for delivery, and elaborate postnatal patterns have developed. Even among some primitive people, whose life depends on following the food supply, the group will stop migration if possible when delivery approaches, or leave a helper with the woman who must stay behind.

The intense interest in childbirth is reflected in the high degree of knowledge acquired. Thus some non-industrialized peoples have developed the use of oxytocic drugs,[7, 73, 99] cesarean sections,[105] and operations enlarging the birth passages.[37] Complex cultures have developed sophisticated systems of obstetrics. The medicine that developed in ancient India,[1, 80] Chinese medicine of the thirteenth century,[59] and Roman medicine of the early second century,[89] in some ways matches or surpasses the obstetrical knowledge of western Europe of only one hundred years ago.

Privacy Surrounding Birth

Although all cultures seem to emphasize in one way or the other the importance of childbirth, there are wide variations in specific aspects. One of these variations is in the area of secrecy with which they surround birth.

The frank open approach of some cultures to childbirth is indicated by the frequency with which they portray childbirth in their art. The Egyptian hieroglyphic for "to give birth to" depicts a squatting woman with the fetal head emerging from the perineum.[49] The ancient Mexican civilizations produced figures of women in the birth position with emerging infants.[99]

Many peoples pattern birth as a social event openly accepted by the community. Thus the Navaho of the south-western United States were reported to show "a great interest in birth. The hogan is open when a baby is being born. . . . Anyone who comes and lends moral support is invited to stay and partake of what food is available."[51]

In some cultures, the games of children reflect the frankness with which birth is regarded. For example, it is reported that a favorite game of Pukapuka preadolescents was to play at childbirth, immature coconuts being used to represent babies. "After a pretended cohabitation, the girl mother stuffed the coconut inside her dress and realistically gave birth to her child, imitating labor pains and letting the nut fall at the proper moment."[6]

In contrast to such open attitudes, other peoples feel extreme secrecy or the need for privacy about birth. Among the Cuna of Panama, children were kept in ignorance of birth as long as possible. They were not permitted to see dogs, cats, or pigs giving birth. Ideally they were not told until the last stage of the marriage ceremony about the existence of the sex act and childbirth.[94] Childbirth was called "to catch the deer": children were told that babies are found in the forest between deer horns or put on the beach by a dolphin.[44] The Chagga likewise surrounded birth with secrecy. Children were told that an animal brings babies or that they came from a beehive in the forest or steppe. In 1926 Gutmann reported: "In former years, the whole country was disgraced when a married man in conversation with minors replied to their questions as to the origin of man: *wandu veketsesau*—man happens to be born."[37]

In contemporary industrial cultures childbirth may also be cloaked with privacy. Seeing birth is often considered appropriate only for medical personnel. An illustration of this was the problem of an American obstetrician who bought a sculpture of a Mexican goddess in the act of giving birth. The fetus was half emerged. He tried putting it in his office, but his nurse and patients objected. He brought it home, but his wife felt it was improper to exhibit it in any part of the house.

Secrecy feelings may be so strong that they tend to persist despite administrative attempts to change them. For example, at St. Mary's Hospital in Evansville, Indiana, fathers are encouraged to participate in the child-bearing experience. Fathers attend prenatal classes with their wives and usually sit with them during the first stage of labor. Yet when asked whether fathers should be in the delivery room, 59·4% of 267 fathers said that they did not feel husbands belong there.[25]

However, a protest against the taboo on open childbirth may be developing in the United States. Not only is there a strong minority agitating for permission for husbands to be permitted to witness birth of their babies, but the hippies in communes of northern California are patterning birth as a social home event when it's nice to have one's friends around.[72]

Sexual Implications of Birth

Closely allied to feelings about secrecy are feelings about the sexual implications of birth. Niles Newton[77] has pointed out that there are similarities in the level of physiologically based behavior between undrugged childbirth as observed by Dick Read and the female sexual excitement documented by Kinsey et al.[46] The following aspects of behavior are similar: (1) type of breathing; (2) type of sounds made and facial expression during second stage labor and orgasm; (3) rhythmic contractions of the upper segment of the uterus; (4) periodic contractions of the abdominal muscles; (5) inhibitions and psychic blockages frequently relieved; (6) unusual muscular strength; (7) increased insensitivity to pain and restricted sensory perception at height of reaction; (8) sudden return of awareness at completion; (9) forceful emotional reaction of satisfaction at completion.

These physiological similarities between birth and sexual excitement are developed and recognized in some cultures and muted in others. A 1901 account of Laotian labor states that relatives, friends, or more often young men, hold the woman up and try to divert her with extremely licentious remarks. Some of the young men bring musical instruments and others bring phalli, to which they address such witty approaches that the patient, despite her pain, responds with an outburst of laughter.[83] A Lepcha man of the Himalayan States in Asia told of peeking at a woman in labor when he was eight or nine years old: "I only went because I was very interested to see how a baby was born and because I wanted to see what a woman's vulva was like. I could not now watch this sort of thing as it would have too exciting an effect on me."[75]

In contrast, other peoples have reacted to the sexual implications of birth by concern over modesty. The following remarks by Chippewa Indians of Ontario, Canada, illustrate this problem.[40]

Some of the full-bloods don't want men around, not even doctors. I, myself, think it is a disgrace the way women submit themselves to strangers today when their babies are born, especially to those doctors. . . . In the old days not even women looked at anyone more than necessary; a big piece of buckskin was placed over the mother to protect her modesty.

The current patterning of the second stage of labor in the United States is in keeping with the tendency to mute any recognition of the relationship between birth and other inter-personal reproductive acts. When delivery seems imminent, the American woman is transported from her bed, wheeled into a room with brilliant lights and medical instruments. She is then put on a special table that has equipment for tying her hands and her feet, and her buttocks are so adjusted that she pushes her baby out into space with no mattress to break its fall should the doctor fail to catch it. Labor is then quite usually artificially shortened by cutting the woman's perineum.[77]

Achievement and Atonement at Birth

In some cultures birth is patterned as representing achievement or an event to be paid for. However, there are marked variations as to who gets the credit and who does the paying. Atlee[2] has pointed out that modern women may derive very little prestige or satisfaction from childbirth. Instead, the feelings of achievement at birth may center around the actions of the obstetrician.

American parlance reflects this feeling. The obstetrician says, "I delivered Mrs. Jones," using the active voice. Mrs. Jones is likely to say, "Dr. Smith delivered me," using the passive voice. The husband and family are more likely to thank the obstetrician for the delivery of the baby than to thank the wife for giving birth.

In contrast to this, the Ila of Northern Rhodesia consider that birth is an achievement for the mother. "Women attending at birth were observed to shout praises of the woman who had had a baby. They all thanked her, saying, 'I give much thanks to you today that you have given birth to a child.'" After the birth, the Ila mother's husband may come in to see her and congratulate her. "Her male relations may also enter the hut, clasp their hand to hers and give her bracelets or leglets by way of congratulation."[88] This feeling of "personal achievement" about labor is so important to some South African tribes that the husband and father may refuse to get medical assistance for a woman in labor on the grounds that she would be better off dead than unable to bring forth a live child by herself.[56]

Perhaps allied with this feeling that birth is an achievement is the attitude that birth must be "paid for". Among the Goajiro of Colombia the father "pays" the relatives of the mother for the suffering and discomfort she experiences in childbirth.[11] The Araucanians of South America may feel that children should be made to "appreciate' their mothers' suffering. Said one informant, "I have often thought that when children grow up they need to be told how much their mothers suffered giving them birth."[41] However, the Laotians felt that the mother herself should "pay" for the birth. After delivery she underwent sitz baths and hot body effusions which are part of the custom known as "You Kam"—"to submit to penitence".[21]

Birth as Dirty or Defiling

Ordinary birth was frequently regarded as dirty or defiling. Among the Arapesh of New Guinea, "birth must take place over the edge of the village, which is situated on a hilltop, in the 'bad place' also reserved for excretion, menstrual huts, and foraging pigs."[62] Post-partum purification ceremonies were also reported from such widely scattered peoples as the Hottentots of South Africa,[42] the Jordan village peoples of the Middle East,[32] and the Caucasia region of Russia.[55] Hebrew-Christian tradition has firmly imbedded in it the feeling that birth is unclean. The ancient Hebrews felt so strongly about the defiling nature of birth that the whole of Leviticus Chapter 12 is devoted to the ritual purification of women following childbirth,[49] and even today the Catholic church has a special ritual for women after childbirth, although this is falling into disuse.

The "dirty" view of birth was especially strongly held in some parts of Asia. When labor started, the woman of Kadu Gollas of India was required to move into the jungle hut built for the purpose. She was considered impure for three months after delivery. Anyone touching her during labor "caught" the contamination and was isolated as well. Mother and child could not re-enter the house until they got permission from their deity.[92] Some women in India are reported to be considered unclean and "untouchable" during childbirth and for ten days thereafter.[93] The Vietnamese considered birth so contaminating that, although the village father did all he could during and after birth, he could not enter his wife's room but could speak to her only from the door. In order not to bring bad luck to others, Vietnamese mothers avoided going out for 30 to 100 days after delivery.[17]

Birth as Close to Supernatural

Many peoples see birth as a time of particular vulnerability, when death may be near and supernatural forces are at work. This was expressed very clearly in the Jordan village culture, where the midwife admonished: "The mother is in God's hands and she hovers between life and death. . . . Angels go up and down to record what happens . . . and the mother, after safe delivery of a boy, may be congratulated. 'God be thanked that thou hast risen unhurt'."[33] The seventeenth-century diary of Samuel Sewall suggests this same sense of vulnerability and closeness to God in colonial New England culture. A 1690 entry reads: "At last my wife bade me call Mrs. Ellis, then Mother Hull, and the Midwife, and throw the Goodness of God was brought to Bed of a Daughter between three and four o'clock."[87] The Moravian village people of Czechoslovakia of the last century are reported to have had strong feelings about vulnerability immediately after birth, when the lying-in woman was susceptible to demoniacal forces, which were particularly strong between sunset and 6 a.m. and again for three hours at mid-day. To avoid their influences, the lying-in woman was supposed to stay in bed and thus obtained some extra postpartum rest.[4]

Death of the laboring woman is widely looked upon as particularly horrifying. Posthumous removal of the fetus was a common pattern, occurring not only in the Pacific Islands[61] but also in Africa[13] and Burma.[58] In Samoa the child was cut out of the dead woman, since otherwise, it was believed, it would become an avenging ghost.[61] In some areas of West Africa it was considered a disgrace to die in labor. The body of the woman was "treated with contumely" and was burned, as was everything else belonging to her.[105] The deep fears stirred by death during pregnancy or labor were particularly prominent in the report of what happened among the Bambara of Africa. The entire female population of the village was upset, marking the event with an elaborate ceremony.[38]

Birth as Painful Illness or Normal Physiology

Is normal birth really a normal phenomenon or one to be treated as a painful illness? This basic question is viewed in different ways by different people. Many peoples in many parts of the world regard childbirth as a normal function. Du Bois,[23] observing the people of Alor, of the Lesser Sundas Islands, states: "One gathers the impression that birth is considered an easy and casual procedure. . . . This does not mean that difficulties never occur, but it does indicate that the society has not emphasized such difficulties." The Jarara woman of South America[36] gave birth in a passageway or shelter "in full view of everyone, even her small children. There was no concern at all over this matter; childbirth was considered a normal phenomenon." From the Pacific Islands it was reported: "Extremely realistic attitudes toward childbirth are held by the Pukapukans. No sense of mystery surrounds the event. It is considered of interest to the whole community as natural as any other fact of life."[5]

Indeed, the sensation of normal labor in some cultures may not be thought of as "pain". For instance, the Navaho have two words for labor—one means pain of labor and the other means labor alone.[60] Thus the vocabulary of the Navaho, which embodies the cultural expectation, encourages the Navaho woman to feel that it is possible to have labor sensations without interpreting them as painful. McCammon, after personally attending more than 400 Indian women who were delivered at the Navaho Medical Center, states: "Many appear to suffer severe pain for many hours. These women do not hesitate to request analgesics and anesthetics. . . . However, I am convinced that not a few go through labor and delivery without pain."[60]

One of the most detailed accounts of primitive labor is of the Aranda, an extremely primitive people of central Australia. The observer, de Vidas, reports that the Aranda recognize the onset of labor by strong contractions which are "painful".[20] However, during labor "little fuss" is made by the woman if the labor is normal.

Nor does excessive pain appear to be part of the usual pattern of the people of Alor of the Lesser Sundas Islands. Du Bois writes: "In the half-dozen births I witnessed, the mothers at no time showed signs of pain beyond acute discomfort. They groaned softly and perspired freely, but seemed on the whole to give birth with little difficulty."[23]

In other cultures pain may be quite definite, even among people who have had little contact with Western Industrial culture. For instance, de Lery[19] writes of the Tupinamba of the Brazilian coastal area he observed in 1557–1558, presumably before there was much contact with European culture. He and another Frenchman were lodging in a village, when about midnight they heard a great outcry from a woman. Thinking she had been surprised by a jaguar, they ran to her. They found her in labor with her husband acting as midwife. He caught the baby in his arms and cut the cord with his teeth. A Kurtatchi woman of the Solomon Islands described labor in her culture with these words: "Now it hurts, its mother cries out, now we cut some leaves, we make her drink. Now the child is about to be born. Now she is afraid because the child hurts her. She cries out because of the child."[9] Labor pain has puzzled the Ila of Northern Rhodesia so much that they have developed an elaborate theory concerning its origin as being the result of *mupuka* reluctant to let go of a woman.[90]

A number of primitive peoples do have cultural patterns of stoicism that prohibit women from showing the pain they may feel. In Samoa "convention dictates that mothers should neither writhe or cry out."[63] In some cultures, where the expectation of pain is intense the culture uses extreme fear to keep screaming under control. The Chagga are told from childhood that it is man's nature to groan like a goat, but women suffer silently like sheep.[81] Clitoridectomy scars may interfere with delivery and increase pain, yet the laboring woman believes she will kill her baby if she screams and that her husband may divorce her if, through lack of self control, "the child is killed".[81] She also knows that screams would shame her mother and make her mother-in-law critical of her. Thus most Chagga women are stoic during labor, suppressing loud cries.[81]

American culture has not developed such strong sanctions against expressing pain, but birth customs are patterned around the expectation of pain in labor. Uterine contractions of labor are called "pains" not "contractions", and instead of having separate birth attendants specializing in normal birth, the differences between normal and abnormal are so muted that it is considered desirable for a specialist in obstetrical disease to deliver every woman. Atlee[2] described the attitudes of his North American colleagues as follows:

"We obstetricians seem to think and act as if pregnancy and labor constitute a pathologic rather than a physiologic process. . . . Our entire basic medical education is so obsessed with pathology that it is practically impossible for us to think of any woman who comes to us as other than *sick*."

When there is belief that labor is extremely painful, there may be a kind of resignation about the pain and willingness to add to the inevitable; whereas, when pain is not considered "normal", extra care may be taken to avoid placing the parturient in extra discomfort. For instance, in U.S.S.R., where psychological methods of pain control are widely practised,[14] there is a belief that labor is not necessarily painful. Enemas, often used in American labor upon admission to the hospital, are avoided in U.S.S.R. as "painful stimuli".[67]

3

Obstetrical Techniques: a Crosscultural View

Since patterning of behavior may be particularly elaborated or particularly rigid when events have emotional impact, it is not surprising to find a large variety of well developed behavior patterns elicited by birth. Differences in management of labor occur in at least five different dimensions, including biochemical management, relaxation and activity, sensory stimulation, emotional support, and delivery position.

Biochemical Management

The culture largely determines the woman's biochemical status during labor. Not only does each society regulate the availability and type of medication, but also determines the availability and type of nutritional support during labor, which in turn influences the parturient's biochemical status.

Non-industrialized peoples have developed the same variety of patterns in regard to biochemical support in labor as have those of Western culture. Some years ago, the first act of the Ukranian midwife was to give the mother a generous dose of whisky to ease her pains.[47] The Amhara of Ethiopia[70] gave a drink of mashed linseed to "relax the birth tract" and to "lessen the pain". On the other side of the world, in Muskrat, North America, a Crow Indian midwife,[53] was reported to know of two plants that eased the suffering at birth. The Ojibwa[45] had also developed a pharmacological pattern. They had standard medicines for easing childbirth and others to be taken after normal delivery.

Nutritional regulation was also found frequently in primitive labor. For instance, the African Hottentots[86] fed soups to laboring women to "strengthen them". The Yumans[91] and the Pawnee,[22] both of North America, on the other hand, had developed a strong prohibition against drinking water in labor; it must cease with the first labor pain. Maternal death was ascribed to the breaking of this taboo. The Bahaya of Africa permitted drinking during labor but prohibited eating.[74]

Currently the nutritional approach to labor is so muted in the United States that the idea that food and beverage may play a role in labor may be startling to Americans. American patterns sometimes emphasize the fear that liquid and food given during labor will predispose to the aspiration of vomitus during anticipated anesthesia. A usual pattern is for all food and beverage, and often even water, intake to be prohibited during labor. If labor continues for many hours, dehydration and low blood sugar are combated with intravenous fluids containing glucose. At the same time, a variety of pharmacological supportive measures are administered. The great interest in the United States in the medicinal rather than the nutritional aspect of biochemical support is indicated by the fact that *Williams' Obstetrics*[24] cites 99 references in the chapter on "Analgesia and anesthesia", but only 27 references in the chapter on the "Conduct of normal labor", none of which deals specifically with the problem of nutritional support.

This is a relatively new American pattern. An early-nineteenth-century obstetrical text[69] urges nutritional supplementation in labor but warns against alcohol, an analgesic drug, as follows: "She should be supplied from time to time with mild bland nourishment in moderate quantities. Tea, coffee, gruel, barley water, milk and water, broths, etc., may safely be allowed. Beer, wine or spirits, undiluted or diluted, should be forbidden. . . ."

Current European medicine does not seem to mute the nutritional aspect of labor to the same extent as modern American. For instance, a recent British text[79] states: "The labouring woman requires a certain amount of nourishment . . . her own appetite should be a certain guide to what she wishes to eat or drink." The text goes on to suggest that a patient in "trial labour" who may later need a cesarean section be encouraged to eat and drink such foods as eggs, milk, and glucose drinks. In the late 1940s two papers appeared in the U.S.S.R. concerning the oxytocic and analgesic effects of Vitamin B1 in a series of labors. Europeans, whose cultural orientation included some interest in nutrition in labor, picked up the idea and papers were published in Germany, Italy, Hungary, Bulgaria, Yugoslavia, Austria, France and Greece.[66] Notably absent in a search of literature were American papers, in keeping with their general tendency to mute the nutritional aspects of birth management in this culture.

Relaxation and Activity Implementation

Many cultures feel the need for regulating activity during labor. Patterns involving restriction or augmentation of activity are common.

Preliterate peoples have tended to pattern types of desirable movement during labor, although from birth descriptions it is difficult to tell how far labor has progressed before regulations on movement are invoked. The inactive approach to labor, in which much movement is scarcely possible, is described by Schultze[86] in his study of the Hottentots: "Once I saw six women squatting around in one hut scarcely 3 meters in width. . . . It was difficult to recognize which woman was the cause of this gathering who lay on the floor in the background covered with skins."

Other peoples, however, felt that vigorous exercise was beneficial. Among the Tuareg, a nomadic tribe of the Sahara, the young mother followed the advice of her aunt or mother. She walked up and down small hills from the first labor pain onward, in order "to allow the infant to get well placed". She returned to the tent for delivery in the kneeling position.[10] In another group in the same cultural area women not only walked up and down but "pound grain in mortar to provoke the final labour pains."[29]

In the United States activity in labor is usually strictly patterned only after the parturient arrives at the hospital, regardless of the stage of labor. Upon admission, she is put in a wheelchair and pushed to the labor floor. There she is placed supine in bed. Frequently bedpans may be substituted for walks to the toilet. Labor-room attendants may tell the laboring woman to "relax", but only in hospitals where there is interest in psychological methods of pain control may actual coaching in methods of relaxation be given. Relaxation instruction may aim to relieve muscular tension, focus attention away from the pain, or put the patient in a more suggestible state, depending on theoretical orientations,[15] but in all cases inactivity of the major muscles is required.

Patterned *inactivity* is a relatively new development in American culture, contrasting with previous beliefs that exercise in labor was desirable. An 1816 obstetric text encourages movement:[69] ". . . During the first and second stages (the second stage was defined as terminating before delivery) . . . the patient may be allowed to sit, stand, kneel or walk out as her inclination may prompt her; if fatigued, she should repose occasionally upon the bed or couch, but it is not expedient during these two stages that she should remain very long at a time in a recumbent posture."

As late as 1894 an obstetrical text[54] warns: "The patient should be encouraged not to take to bed at the outset of labor. In the upright or sitting posture gravity aids in the fixation of the head and promotes passive hyperaemia and dilation of the cervix." However, by this time undressing and lying down are recommended as the end of the first stage approaches.

Sensory Stimulation

In quite a number of primitive cultures, sensory stimulation of many sorts plays a prominent part in the management of labor. Music in labor was used by widely separated groups: the Laotians in Indochina,[83] the Navaho of North America,[3] and the Cuna of Panama.[95] Conversation also involves an element of pure sound stimulation and was used by primitive groups who patterned labor as a social event.

Heat is sometimes applied to women in labor in various ways. The Tübatulabel[101] dug a trench inside or outside of the house, depending on the weather, in which a fire was built. The fire was covered with slabs of stone and layers of earth and tule mats were added. The laboring woman lay on top of all this. The North American Comanche[102] simplified the procedure by putting hot rocks on the back of the laboring woman. Farther south, the Tewa[84] fumigated the laboring woman by wrapping her in a blanket and had her stand over hot coals upon which medication was placed.

A common form of sensory stimulation is abdominal stimulation. A tedious labor among the Kurtatchi was treated by an older woman attendant who chewed special roots and vegetation:[9] "She spat the resulting red saliva on to her hand and rubbed Manev's abdomen with it, with a circular motion, all round the edge of the tumid belly. . . . Once in a while the woman kneeling behind moved her clasping hands from the top of the protuberant abdomen to the bottom and shook it violently."

This pattern of abdominal stimulation appears in other widely separated primitive peoples, suggesting independent invention of the technique. The Yahgan midwife of Tierra del Fuego, at the southern tip of South America, made circular strokes on the abdomen with the flat of her hand to stimulate birth.[35] The Navaho sprinkled pollen over the stomach area to make birth easy.[3] The Punjab midwife rubbed melted butter on the abdomen.[30]

Firm pressure applied to parts other than the abdomen was also used in primitive cultures. Among the Pukapuka, the *tangata wakawanau* (medicine man specializing in obstetrics) helped a woman in delivery by pushing with the heel or palm of the hand on the small of her back.[5] The Kurtatchi[9] and the Kazakhs of Kazakhstan in Asia[34] used knee pressure of the attendant holding the woman from the rear. The Punjab village midwife applied strong steady pressure with her feet on either side of the birth canal in the second stage of labor, a measure which was reported to feel "good".[30]

Many primitive peoples provide for skin stimulation by having the woman held in the labor position by others. The contact of body to body, skin to skin, may involve considerably more sensation than the support of an inanimate object. Ford[27] lists twenty-five primitive cultures in which women are supported from behind. Abdominal pressure is often applied as well.

Interest in sensory stimulation is muted in the management of labor in the United States today, except for occasional interest among groups that use psycho-physical methods of pain control. The woman using the Lamaze method of preparation for delivery is often instructed to stimulate her abdomen during labor in the manner similar to that used by various pre-literate people. A natural childbirth mother may have a warm water bottle placed on her lower abdomen and have her husband put firm pressure on her sore back. Music may be piped into the delivery room and television viewing may be encouraged during labor. However, this use of sensory stimulation in labor, as a diversionary technique to reduce the sensation of pain, is an atypical rather than a typical pattern.

Companionship and Emotional Support

Birth in most societies is patterned not as an unaided solo act but as a social one in which others help in some way. The emotional impact of the labor attendants is a key variable in the patterning of labor.

Curiously, there is a widespread belief that primitive labors are casual unattended affairs, but records indicate otherwise. Unattended birth does occur in many cultures, but it is a rare event to be gossiped about in the same manner as an American birth taking place in a taxi-cab. Granqvist[33] comments, after giving an account of an unusual unattended delivery: "The peasant women move about outside so carefree although they are already in the last stage of pregnancy . . . their hard life full of heavy work does not allow them to spare themselves. Considering this, it is rather surprising that cases of birth in the open air are not much more numerous." Hilger[41] tells of the resentment felt by the South American Araucanian mother who went into labor when no one except her little boy was at home, so that she could not send for help. In the mountains of Yugoslavia it was reported to be "not unusual" for women to give birth in a field or on the mountain,[98] and in a Bulgarian village[85] an "exceptional" woman was reported to prefer to deliver alone. But in neither case is this the "usual way". A most atypical account is that of the South American Talamanca which states: "When the time of parturition approaches, the father goes into the woods and builds a little shed at a safe distance from the house. To this the woman retires as soon as she feels the labor pain coming on. Here, alone and unassisted, she brings forth her young."[28] However, it is to be noted the father built the shed. This was not a "casual delivery", but one which involved considerable preparatory work by a family member.

Often the birth took place in the home of the mother's or the father's mother. Thus, the care of the heavily pregnant and newly delivered woman fell on the grandmother and her younger daughters. Frequently even when later births took place away from the original home, special efforts were made to return the primipara to her own mother for her first confinement. The Punjab girl left her husband and mother-in-law, with whom she still felt shy, and traveled to the home of her birth to be with her own mother and the village midwife, whom she had known for years.[30] Thousands of miles away, in Africa,[50] North America,[103] South America,[36] the Middle East,[33] and in the Pacific Islands,[9] the same return to mother's home for the first baby took place.

In primitive cultures all over the world, the elderly woman, rather than the skilled man, is the predominant attendant at normal labor. Ford[27] found elderly women assisting at birth in 58 cultures and not assisting in only two. In only four of his cultures was information lacking.

When social role differentiation has developed to such an extent that there is a person designated as a regular midwife, her personality and character are usually taken into account. Thus the Ojibwa felt that the midwife "should be a woman of mature years, preferably not under thirty-five. She should have had a few children of her own and be known to have had easy deliveries. She should be of calm temperament."[48] Among the Yahgan some women had the reputation of being good at delivery. "They get this reputation because of their frequent assistance and personal skill. . . . In general a woman will always be attended by the same midwife, because the latter has learned her physical characteristics from experience."[35]

Knowledge does not always come from personal experience, however.

Graybull's wife, a North American Crow Indian, gave a horse as payment to obtain her obstetrical knowledge from a visionary.[52] At Tau, in Samoa, barren women past childbearing age compensated for their barrenness by acting as midwives and were reputed to be very wise.[61]

In modern American culture there may be a tendency to mute the help available from older experienced women. Young couples often living many miles from their parents find the help of relatives at the time of child-bearing difficult to obtain. Among some families there is even a feeling that it is somehow better to try to manage alone without feeling "dependent" on the help and experience of the older generation. During labor in America, female relatives of the parturient are often excluded. Other women—practical nurses or registered nurses—do look after women in the hospital in the first stage of labor and post-partum, but these women are strangers, not friends or relatives. There is no requirement that a nurse have experienced childbearing herself. A registered nurse who has never had a baby is usually considered more desirable as a labor attendant in normal labor than the practical nurse who has experienced several labors and deliveries.

Although females all over the world attend women in labor, giving them emotional support by their presence as well as ministering to their simple needs, the role of males in labor is extremely variable.

The tendency to feel that birth is woman's business is so strong that men, other than husbands, are usually excluded from entering the same abode as the laboring woman. Even the male healer is frequently excluded. For example, in Africa, the Tuareg midwife, in case of abnormality, may ask for the help of a marabout (a Mohammedan hermit or saint), but he must stand outside the tent, for he may not go near the parturient woman.[50] The Cuna, who consider all labor a fearful ordeal, do call on the shaman for supervision regularly, but he must stay away from the laboring woman and depend on the female attendant's description.[58]

However, the feeling against males attending labor is by no means universal or absolute. In some industrial countries males command a much higher price for officiating at a delivery than does the midwife, and affluent women prefer to have such prestigious persons assist them even in normal deliveries, although the emotional support during labor is still usually left to women.

In preliterate cultures males may be called in under certain circumstances. Quite frequently, when labor is abnormal, male healers participate actively. When the Aranda woman had delayed labor, the male Mura took a hair girdle, and, violating the usual prohibition against men, went to her and tied the belt around her body.[90] The Sakai of Malaya have made the mid-wife role a hereditary one which both men and women inherit.[104] The Lepcha of the Himalayan mountain region appeared to have no sex preferences—the parents-in-law or anybody who knew how would help the woman in labor.[31] The pattern of the Araucanians of South America was changing at the time they were studied. In one area they had not yet developed a word for male obstetrician, but several middle-aged men were actually assisting at deliveries.[41] The Araucanian husbands also assisted their wives in dire necessity, such as when everyone else had gone to a fiesta or when they were too poor to hire a midwife.

The father very frequently had a patterned role to play, but not necessarily as an emotional supporter and companion to his wife. The Pacific Ocean Easter Islander father got a real sense of participation in birth by having his wife recline against him during labor and delivery.[71] The Kurtatchi father of the Pacific Islands was excluded from the labor, which took place in another hut, but the importance of his impending fatherhood was emphasized by the fact that he must stop work and remain in seclusion. On no account might he lift anything heavy or touch a sharp instrument.[9]

The custom of couvade* occurred in many parts of the world. Essentially it involved a period of activity restriction and "regulation" for the father as well as the mother for a time after birth. Ford's sample[27] of 64 cultures contains records of the customs of 18 tribes in this regard. Seventeen tribes from Asia, North America, Oceania, and South America involved the father in couvade after delivery. In only one group was it definitely recorded that there was no couvade. There may be real survival value in this custom, as it may particularly emphasize the father's role and responsibilities at the crucial time as each child is born. It may help him to identify with mother and baby.

Delivery Position

The most essential aspect of birth is the movement of the baby from the uterus to the outside. Thus the body mechanics of second-stage labor are fundamental to the whole problem of normal, spontaneous birth. One would perhaps expect that biological factors would determine the position and movements of the woman at this time. but even here ideas and cultural patterning or customs may overrule physiological and anatomical cues.

Delivery is possible in a great variety of positions.[26] A recent crosscultural survey of 76 non-European societies in the Human Relations Area Files found that 62 used upright positions.[76] Of these upright positions, the most common was kneeling, with 21 cultures represented. The next most common position was sitting, with 19 cultures using this method. Fifteen cultures used squatting, and 5 used standing positions.

Sometimes the culture patterns delivery in more than one way.[82] The Siriono woman lies in her hammock for the delivery of the baby but kneels for the delivery of the placenta.[43] The Sierra Tarascans[7] use both kneeling and flat deliveries, depending on "circumstances", according to a midwife. It is reported that the mother makes the choice for herself. A 1948 report indicated that the Goajiro woman had four different positions to choose from, for the sitting, kneeling, and squatting positions are all included in

---

* See also Chapter IV in this volume.

the traditional cultural pattern, and the supine position was also used occasionally.[36]

Among primitive peoples, the curved back is typical of most birth positions. In the sitting, squatting, and kneeling positions, the back automatically curves forward unless unusual effort is made. Bearing down in the standing position almost automatically forces some curving of the back. It is probable that many supine deliveries also involve a curve in the back. Thus the hammock deliveries[43, 57] may take place with backs curved forward. However, two peoples clearly have an opposite pattern. The Bambara woman[78] kneels with her hands thrown behind her while the midwives support the small of her back. The Jordan city woman sits on the side of her bed leaning backwards.[33]

Unfortunately, since most material dealing with primitive peoples does not indicate how far apart the legs were at the time of delivery, there is no way of knowing how much tension is usually put on the perineum at this time. The Laotians were reported to sit with legs folded and spread wide apart.[83] Blackwood[9] reports a Kurtatchi delivery with knees drawn up and wide apart. However, the birth description of the Hottentots, although not specific suggests that the legs may be together, since a hand is kept constantly between the legs of the woman to ascertain the progress of the child's head.[86]

Many primitive peoples used pushing, pulling, and bracing devices to help the parturient in her expulsive efforts. Ropes, which furnish firm resistance to pulling but are easily adjustable in regard to angle and height, are used by groups in Asia,[31] North Africa,[10] North America,[7] and South America.[41, 43] Poles and stakes are also used for grasping during delivery.[96, 102] In Manus houses, where labor takes place, an extra post or board will be fastened firmly to the leaf wall so that the laboring woman will have something to push her feet against.[64] The Yahgan woman squats, spreading her legs wide apart, and braces herself with hands and feet flat on the ground.[35]

Today in the United States the position for delivery is similar to that used for surgical operations. The body is flat and neck is straight without a pillow to support it, as is the custom on operating tables. Arms are tied so that they will not stray into the sterile field. The legs are mechanically spread wide apart with leg braces to allow the physician to have an unobstructed view of the operative area.

This rigid surgical structuring of position for normal delivery is quite new in American obstetrics. The 1913 edition of the DeLee textbook illustrates delivery with the woman lying on her side in the lateral Sims position, her back curved and her legs only a few inches apart.[18] Lusk[54] in 1894 expressed a permissive attitude toward the position of the woman for delivery: "During the second stage, the patient's posture should be left in general to her own volition. The physician should accustom himself to conduct labor with equal facility, no matter where the woman lies, upon her side or upon her back."

The problem of the body mechanics of labor is mentioned by earlier American obstetrical textbook writers. Adequate foot support to use for bracing during contractions is considered a matter of concern.[12, 54] As late as 1947, some thought was being given to labor as a muscular event. In that year Beck's[8] obstetrical textbook advocated "pullers" and snug abdominal binders to facilitate the body mechanics of delivery and to "retain the advantages of the squat position".

Recent American texts, however, do not appear to give much consideration or discussion to problems of efficient body position and bracing for effective expulsive effort. In a few hospitals a triangular pillow or backrest is occasionally used to help the women achieve a curved back position, but the need for the parturient to push or pull by bracing and holding is almost entirely muted in American hospital practice today.

4

Concluding Comments

In seeing the possibility of other ways of feeling and acting, one's own way is more clearly delineated. Basically, the questions raised can only be answered by each individual for himself. Questions similar to the following are pertinent. What are my personal attitudes toward birth? What are the attitudes of the majority of persons working with me? Are the attitudes of childbearing women different in my group from those of males and non-reproducing women?

To be sure obstetrical *behavior* is also noteworthy. In so far as it mutes or develops emotional support, sensory stimulation, body mechanics and biochemical manipulation, it can have a profound influence on the emotions of the parturient and those around her. However, emphasis on the varying patterns possible for birth behavior should not obscure the fact that behavior tends to reflect culturally determined attitudes.

An example of the force of attitudes in determining birth behavior is the fate of research studies which conflict with current obstetrical attitudes. For instance, considerable research on the problem of position in labor in relation to ease of delivery suggests that the flat, supine position for delivery may make spontaneous delivery more difficult. Mengert and Murphy,[68] in an extensive experimental study, recorded actual intra-abdominal pressure at the height of maximum straining effort in more than 1,000 observations with women placed in 7 postures. The researchers used sophisticated statistical techniques to analyse their data. They found that the greatest intra-abdominal pressure was exerted in the sitting position. This was due not only to major visceral weight but also to increased muscular efficiency. Vaughan presented X-rays and measurements which indicate that squatting alters the pelvic shape in a way that makes it advantageous for delivery. Had Mengert and Murphy[68] and Vaughan[100] advocated a new drug to speed labor, it is likely that culturally accepting attitudes would have resulted in adoption of their findings—even with far less scientifically controlled data. However, instead, the proposition of improving labor efficiency through sitting and squatting conflicted with the strongly held cultural attitude that birth is an event experienced lying down. This extensive research, instead of becoming part of the fundamental knowledge required of obstetricians, was ignored.

The importance of cultural attitudes in determining birth patterning can also be seen in the history of the "natural childbirth" program set up at Yale University under the leadership of Dr. Herbert Thoms. While Dr. Thoms continued work at Yale, published statistics indicated that 88% of the mothers had spontaneous deliveries and 29% had no anesthesia at birth.[97] Dr Thoms retired, and some others working closely with him left. The formal patterns of education for childbirth and support during labor continued, but they no longer appeared to influence patterning of birth. A follow-up study,[16] published just eight years after the previous study, indicated that the once deviant Yale practice had quickly changed in the direction of the norm of the surrounding culture. Now only 47% of the women had normal spontaneous deliveries, and less than 1% of the women received no anesthesia at birth, although all of these still received pre-natal training and support in labor.

Socially determined attitudes may also determine how the mother behaves in labor, even to the point of possibly regulating her uterine contractions. Heyns[39] presents statistics showing that Bantu women of South Africa, although their pelves are so small that Western women would require cesarean sections, deliver babies spontaneously. This seems to be accomplished by a moulding of the fetal head by extraordinarily forceful contractions. In extreme cases the baby may be born dead, but the mother's life may be saved through her ability to get rid of the products of conception.

Heyns[39] believes that psychological differences may account for the differences in uterine contractions. "It is submitted that in the European there is an unfavorable emotional background, which has an inhibitory effect on efficient uterine action. . . . Where in any individual parturient there is emotional stability supported by an unwavering resolution to push through with the task of spontaneous delivery, and where the realization that obstetric aid is readily available is not over-emphasized, the achievement of the Bantu woman may always be equalled. . . . Simple dystocia, due to contracted bony passages, can almost be eliminated by fostering the will in the parturient to deliver herself."

This illustration particularly shows the interaction of birth behavior and birth attitudes. The availability of forceps and cesarean sections depends on cultural attitudes which accept the idea of non-spontaneous birth. In turn, the widespread use of operative procedures may decrease the desire to push the baby out spontaneously.

The close interrelation of attitudes and behavior emphasizes that attempts to change obstetrical patterning may meet with unanticipated ramifications.

A broad view is required, which takes both attitudes and procedures into account. Perhaps the chief value of reviewing patterns of behavior surrounding birth is that it widens the perspective in the same way as historical knowledge increases understanding. In learning how others have done it, it is possible to get new insight into current patterns, their possible origin and interactions.

REFERENCES

1. ADALJA, K. V., 1940. Ayurvedic midwifery. *E. Afr. med. J.*, **17**, 142.
2. ATLEE, H. B. 1963. Fall of the Queen of Heaven. *Obstet. Gynec.*, **21**, 514.
3. BAILEY, F. L. 1950. Some sex beliefs and practices in a Navaho community. *Papers of the Peabody Museum of American Archaeology and Ethnology*, **40**, 2. Cambridge: Harvard University Press.
4. BARTOS, F. 1897. Volksleben der Slaven. In *Die Osterreichish-Ungarische Monarchie in Wort und Bild: Mähren und Schlesien*. Vienna: Kaiserlich-Koniglichen Staatsdruckerei.
5. BEAGLEHOLE, E. and BEAGLEHOLE, P. 1938. Ethnology of Pukapuka. *Bernice P. Bishop Museum Bulletin*, **150**. Honolulu.
6. BEAGLEHOLE, E. and BEAGLEHOLE, P. 1939. Brief Pukapukan case history. *J. Polynesian Soc.*, **48**, 135.
7. BEALS, R. L. 1946. *Cherán: a Sierra Tarascan village*. Pub. No. 2, Smithsonian Institute of Social Anthropology. Washington.
8. BECK, A. C. 1947 *Obstetrical practice*, 4th ed. Baltimore: Williams & Wilkins.
9. BLACKWOOD, B. 1935. *Both sides of Buka Passage*. Oxford: Clarendon Press.
10. BLANGUERON, C. 1955. *Le Hoggar*. Paris: Arthaud.
11. BOLINDER, G. 1957. *Indians on horseback*. London: Dennis Dobson.
12. BURNS, J. (with improvements and notes by JAMES, T. C.) 1831. *The Principles of midwifery: including the diseases of women and children*. New York: Clafton and Van Norden.
13. CANE, L. B. 1945. African birth customs. *St. Bartholomew's Hosp. J.*, **49**, 94.
14. CHERTOK, L. 1959. *Psychosomatic methods in painless childbirth*. New York: Pergamon Press.
15. CHERTOK, L. 1961. Relaxation and psychosomatic methods of preparation for childbirth, *Amer. J. Obstet. Gynec.*, **82**, 262.
16. DAVIS, C. D. and MORRONE, F. A. 1962. An objective evaluation of a prepared childbirth program. *Amer. J. Obstet. Gynec.*, **84**, 1196.
17. DÊ, T. D. 1951. Notes on birth and reproduction in Vietnam. Unpublished manuscript by Margaret Coughlin.
18. DELEE, J. B., 1913. *The Principles and practices of obstetrics*. Philadelphia: Saunders.
19. DE LERY, J. 1906. Extracts out of the Historie of John Lerius, a Frenchman, who lived in Brasill with Mons., Villagagnon, Ann. 1557 and 1558. In *Hakluvtus Posthumus of Purchas His Pilgrimes*, **16**, 518. Glasgow: MacLehose.
20. DE VIDAS, J. 1947. Childbirth among the Aranda, Central Australia. *Oceania*, **18**, 117.
21. DEYDIER, H. 1952. *Introduction à la connaisance du Laos*. Saigon: Imprimerie française d'Outre-Mer.
22. DORSEY, G. A. and MURIE, J. R. 1940. Notes on Skidi Pawnee society. *Field Museum of Natural History, Anthropology Series*, **27**, 2, 65. Chicago: Field Museum Press.
23. DU BOIS, C. 1944. *The people of Alor*. Minneapolis: University of Minnesota Press.

24. EASTMAN, N. J. and HELLMAN, L. M. 1961. *Williams' Obstetrics*, 12th edn. New York: Appleton-Century-Crofts.
25. ENGEL, E. L. 1963. Family-centred hospital maternity care. *Amer. J. Obstet. Gynec.*, **85,** 260.
26. ENGLEMANN, G. J. 1883. *Labor among primitive peoples*, 2nd edn. St. Louis: Chambers.
27. FORD, C. S. 1945. *A comparative study of human reproduction.* Yale University Publications in Anthropology, No. 32: New Haven.
28. GABB, W. M. 1876. On the Indian tribes and languages of Costa Rica. *Proc. Amer. Philosoph. Soc.,* **14,** 483.
29. GAMBLE, D. P. 1957. *The Wolof of Senegambia.* London: International African Institute.
30. GIDEON, H. 1962. A baby is born in the Punjab. *Amer. Anthropol.,* **64,** 1220.
31. GORER, G. 1938. *Himalayan village: an account of the Lepchas of Sikkim.* London: Michael Joseph.
32. GRANQVIST, H. 1935. Marriage conditions in a Palestinian village. *Commentationes humanarum litterarum,* **6,** No. 8.
33. GRANQVIST, H. 1947. *Birth and childhood among the Arabs: Studies in a Muhammadan village in Palestine.* Helsingfors: Söderström.
34. GRODEKOV, N. I. 1889. *Kirgizy i Karakirgizy Syr-Dar'inskoi Oblasti,* Vol. I. Tashkent: The Typolithography of S. I. Lakhtin.
35. GUSINDE, M. 1937. *Die Yamana: vom Leben und Denken der Wassernomaden am Kap Hoorns,* Vol. II. Mudling, near Vienna: Anthropos-Bibliothek.
36. GUTIERREZ DE PINEDA, V. 1948. Organizacion social en la Guajira. *Rev. Inst. Etnolog. Nac. (Bogota),* **3.**
37. GUTMANN, B. 1926. *Das Recht der Dschagga.* Munich: C. H. Beck.
38. HENRY, J. 1910. L'aime d'un peuple Africain. *Bibliotheque-Anthropos,* **1,** No. 2.
39. HEYNS, O. S. 1946. The superiority of the South African negro or Bantu as a parturient. *J. Obstet. Gynaec. Brit. Emp.* **53,** 405.
40. HILGER, M. I. 1951. *Chippewa child life and its cultural background.* Washington: Bulletin 146, Bureau of American Ethnology, Smithsonian Institution.
41. HILGER, M. I. 1957. *Araucanian child life and its cultural background.* Washington: Smithsonian Miscellaneous Collection, Vol. 133, Smithsonian Institution.
42. HOERNLÉ, A. W. 1923. The expression of the social value of water among the Naman of South-West Africa. *S. Afr. J. Sci.,* **20,** 514.
43. HOLMBERG, A. R. 1950. *Nomads of the Long Bow: the Siriono of Eastern Bolivia.* Washington: Publication No. 10, Smithsonian Institute. Institute of Social Anthropology.
44. JELLIFFE, D. B., JELLIFFE, E. F. P., GARCIA, L. and DE BARRIOS, G. 1961. The children of the San Blas Indians of Panama. *J. Pediat.,* **59,** 271.
45. KINIETZ, W. V., 1947. *Chippewa village: The story of Katikitegon.* Bloomfield Hills: Cranbrook Press.
46. KINSEY, A. C., POMEROY, W. B., MARTIN, C. E. and GEBHARD, P. H. 1953. *Sexual behavior in the human female.* Philadelphia: Saunders.
47. KOENIG, S. 1939. Beliefs and practices relating to birth and childhood among the Galician Ukranians, *Folk-lore,* **50,** 272.
48. LANDES, R. 1937. *Ojibwa Society.* New York: Columbia University Press.
49. LEVIN, S. 1960. Obstetrics in the Bible, *J. Obstet. Gynaec. Brit. Emp.,* **67,** 490.
50. LHOTE, H. 1944. *Les Touaregs du Hoggar.* Paris: Payot.
51. LOCKETT, C. 1939. Midwives and childbirth among the Navajo. *Plateau,* **12,** 15.
52. LOWIE, R. H. 1922. The religion of the Crow Indians, *Anthropological Papers of the American Museum of Natural History,* **25,** 309.
53. LOWIE, R. H. 1935. *The Crow Indians.* New York: Farrar and Rinehart.
54. LUSK, W. T. 1894. *The science and art of midwifery.* New York: Appleton.

55. LUZBETAK, L. J. 1951. *Marriage and the family in Caucasia: a contribution to the study of North Caucasian ethnology and customary law.* Vienna-Modling: St. Gabriel's Mission Press.

56. MARCHAND, L. 1932. Obstetrics among South African natives, *S. Afr. Med., J.,* **6,** 329.

57. MARSHALL, D. S. 1950. Cuna Folk. A Conceptual Scheme Involving the Dynamic Factors of Culture, as Applied to the Cuna Indians of Darien. Unpublished manuscript, Department of Anthropology, Harvard University.

58. MARSHALL, H. I. 1922. The Karen people of Burma: a study in anthropology and ethnology. *Ohio State University Bulletin,* **26,** No. 13.

59. MAXWELL, P. 1927. Obstetrics in China in the 13th century. *J. Obstet. Gynaec. Brit. Emp.,* **34,** 481.

60. McCAMMON, C. S. 1937. Study of four hundred seventy-five pregnancies in American Indian women. *Amer. J. Obstet. Gynec.,* **61,** 1159.

61. MEAD, M. 1928. *Coming of age in Samoa.* New York: William Morrow.

62. MEAD, M. 1935. *Sex and temperament in three primitive societies.* New York: William Morrow.

63. MEAD, M. 1939. *From the South Seas.* New York: Morrow.

64. MEAD, M. 1956. *New Lives for Old.* New York: Morrow.

65. MEAD, M. and NEWTON, N. 1965. Conception, pregnancy, labor and the Puerperium in cultural perspective. In *First International Congress of Psychosomatic Medicine and Childbirth,* p. 51. Paris: Gauthier-Villars.

66. MEAD, M. and NEWTON, N. 1967. Cultural patterning of perinatal behavior. In *Childbearing—its social and psychological aspects,* edited by S. A. Richardson and A. F. Guttmacher. Baltimore: Williams and Wilkins.

67. Medical Exchange Mission to the U.S.S.R. 1960. Maternal and Child Care. *Public Health Service Publication,* **954.** U.S. Government Printing Office.

68. MENGERT, W. F. and MURPHY, D. P. 1933. Intra-abdominal pressures created by voluntary muscular effort. *Surg. Gynec. Obstet.,* **57,** 745.

69. MERRIMAN, S. (with notes and additions by JAMES, T. C.). 1816. *A Synopsis of the various kinds of difficult parturition, with practical remarks on the management of labours.* Philadelphia: Stone House.

70. MESSING, S. D. 1957. The Highland-plateau Amhara of Ethiopia. Philadelphia: Doctoral (anthropology) dissertation, University of Pennsylvania.

71. MÉTRAUX, A. 1940. Ethnology of Easter Island. Honolulu: *Bernice P. Bishop Museum Bulletin,* **160,**

72. MILLER, J. S. 1970. The role of the physician. Unpublished paper given April 30 at Jefferson Medical College: Continuing Medical Education Symposium on Safety and Satisfaction in Childbearing.

73. MOLLER, M. S. G. 1958. Bahaya customs and beliefs in connection with pregnancy and childbirth. *Tanganyika Notes, Records,* **50,** 112.

74. MOLLER, M. S. G. 1961. Custom, pregnancy and child rearing in Tanganyika. *J. Trop. Pediat.,* **7,** 66.

75. MORRIS, J. 1938. *Living with Lepchas: a book about the Sikkim Himalayas.* London: Heinemann.

76. NAROLL, F., NAROLL, R. and HOWARD, F. H. 1961. Position of women in childbirth. *Amer. J. Obstet. Gynec.,* **82,** 943.

77. NEWTON. N. 1955. *Maternal emotions.* New York: Hoeber.

78. PAQUES, V. 1954. *Les Bambara.* Paris: Presses Universitaires de France.

79. PHILIPP, E. E. 1962. *Obstetrics and gynaecology combined for students.* London: Lewis.

80. RAO, K. 1952. Obstetrics in ancient India. *J. Indian Med. Ass.,* **21,** 210.

81. RAUM, O. F. 1940. *Chaga childhood.* London: Oxford University Press.

82. RAYNALDE, T. 1626. *The Byrthe of mankynde.* London: Boler.

83. REINACH, L. DE. 1901. *Le Laos*. Paris: Charles.

84. ROBBINS, W. W., HARRINGTON, J. P. and FREIRE-MARRECO, B. 1916. *Ethnobotany of the Tewa Indians*. Washington: Smithsonian Institution.

85. SANDERS, I. T. 1949. *Balkan village*. Lexington: University of Kentucky Press.

86. SCHULTZE, J. 1907. *Aus Nanaland und Kalahari*. Jena: Fischer.

87. SEWALL, S. 1878. *The diary of Samuel Sewall, 1674–1729*. Boston: Massachusetts Historical Society.

88. SMITH, E. W. and DALE, A. M. 1920. *The Ila-speaking peoples of Northern Rhodesia*. London: Macmillan.

89. SORANUS: *Gynecology*, translated by O. Temkin. 1956. Baltimore: John Hopkins Press.

90. SPENCER, W. B. and GILLEN, F. J. 1927. *The Arunta: a study of a Stone Age people*. London: Macmillan.

91. SPIER, L. 1933. *Yuman tribes of the Gila River*. Chicago: University of Chicago Press.

92. SRINIVAS, M. N. 1942. *Marriage and family in Mysore*. Bombay: New Book.

93. STONE, A. 1953. Fertility problems in India. *Fertil. Steril.*, **4**, 210.

94. STOUT, D. B. 1947. *San Blas Cuna acculturation: an introduction*. New York: Viking Fund Publications.

95. STOUT, D. B. 1948. The Cuna. *Handbook of South American Indians*, **4**, 257. Bureau of American Ethnology Bulletin 143, edited by Julian H. Steward. Washington: Smithsonian Institution.

96. TEIT, J. A. 1956. *Field notes on the Tahltan and Kaska Indians, 1912–15*. Ottawa: The Research Center for Amerindian Anthropology.

97. THOMS, H. and KARLOVSKY, E. D. 1954. Two thousand deliveries under training for childbirth program: a statistical survey and commentary. *Amer. J. Obstet. Gynec.*, **68**, 279.

98. TOMASIC. D. 1948. *Personality and culture in eastern European politics*. New York: Stewart.

99. VAN PATTEN, N. 1932. Obstetrics in Mexico prior to 1600. *Ann. med. History*, 2d series, **4**, 203–12.

100. VAUGHAN, K. O. 1937. *Safe childbirth: the three essentials*. London: Baillière, Tindall and Cassell.

101. VOEGELIN, E. W. 1938. *Tübatulabal ethnography*. University of California Anthropological Records. **2**, 1–90. Berkeley: University of California.

102. WALLACE, E. and HOEBEL, E. A. 1952. *The Comanches: lords of the South Plains*. Norman: University of Oklahoma Press.

103. WHITMAN, W. 1947. *The Pueblo Indians of San Ildefonso*. New York: Columbia University Press.

104. WILLIAMS-HUNT, P. D. R. 1952. *An introduction to the Malayan aborigines*. Kuala Lumpur: Government Press.

105. WRIGHT, J. 1921. Collective review—the view of primitive peoples concerning the process of labor. *Amer. J. Obstet. Gynec.*, **2**, 206.

PART TWO

CLINICAL

Pre-Natal

IX

THE CONTROL OF CONCEPTION

ELEANOR MEARS

M.B., CH.B.

London
England

1

Introduction

Attempts at conception control have been documented even among the earliest civilizations. Yet until the middle of the last century they had little or no influence on the course of events; the forces of nature were in command and high birth rates, low survival rates and a short life span were the rule. Indeed it took from the beginning of time until 1850 for the human race to reach a billion. But since then, scientific and medical measures have so improved health and reduced death rates that the balance of nature has been thoroughly upset and world population has now grown to three billion.

In Western countries death control has been balanced by birth control as people gradually found the economic advantages of smaller families. People marry earlier, live longer, regulate their fertility and, free from the primitive struggle for survival, have achieved an extraordinary increase in the standard of living. An average of less than 2·5 children per family is enough to keep the population stable under present conditions, so that family planning is an accepted practice in some form or other for all but sub-fertile couples.

In other countries, however, despite the control of disease and the consequent reduction in death rates and the longer life span, birth rates continue to be high, giving rise to a terrifying increase in world population of 65 million every year. If present trends continue, world population is expected to double before the end of the century. This serves only to worsen the problems of hunger and malnutrition at all ages in these countries, and makes it impossible to increase the medical care and education, already pitifully inadequate, of children, who now form an ever growing percentage of such populations. As a result, the gap between the developed and the developing countries grows wider and it has become a necessity for nations as well as individual families to control fertility.

2

The Importance of Methods

The reduction in birth rates in the West prior to 1930 was effected by coitus interruptus, abstinence, late marriage, self-induced abortion and to a lesser extent by the use of condoms and chemical contraceptives—all methods which had been used in various forms over the centuries. Thus the reduced birth rate was due not to the introduction of new family planning methods but to the use of already existing ones showing that motivation came first. In other words, couples who were anxious enough to limit their families always found ways of doing so. It is interesting, however, that the methods used vary from one country and one culture to another, e.g. female methods were preferred in the U.S.A., male methods in the U.K., the rhythm method, coitus interruptus and sexual play without penetration in Roman Catholic countries.

A more scientific attitude was adopted about 1930, when the safe period became scientifically based and was accepted by the Roman Catholic Church, testing procedures for available contraceptives were initiated, and the diaphragm method (a more sophisticated form of the ancient vaginal plug) was used more widely and associated particularly with the growth of feminism and the family planning movement; the condom was improved through the use of latex, and became relatively cheap and widely available. In sophisticated countries these methods gradually began to replace the old; but on a worldwide scale abortion and coitus interruptus were still the dominant methods. Doctors, who have a long history of indifference and antipathy to becoming involved in this field, were reluctant to accept the responsibility, and therefore slow to equip themselves to give contraceptive advice to their patients as part of medical care. The advent of the Pill and the I.U.D. in the 1960s however, caused a revolution in methods; for they brought increased efficiency and acceptability, and a bigger choice to the individual couple. These new methods had little effect on the relatively stable birth rates in the West, but they did transform overnight attitudes to birth control in the U.K. where lingering Victorian attitudes to birth control were finally abandoned. The Church quickly followed, recognizing that procreation can no longer be considered the primary purpose of marriage. Members of the medical profession, hustled by the changing attitudes and demands of their patients, and encouraged by the more medical type of methods into overcoming their antagonism and prejudices, began to accept birth-control advice as an important element in preventive medicine.

These new methods had an even greater effect in the developing countries. It was very quickly realized that the old conventional methods by which people in the West learned to plan their families were quite unacceptable to the majority of people new to family planning. Early attempts to introduce these methods, e.g. in India and Turkey, proved quite useless. The Pill became the first of the magic new methods to be found acceptable to people (and this includes the problem families in our own country) who would not, or could not, use previous methods.

3

Population Planning

The population explosion in the under-developed countries of the world is one of the most pressing problems of our day, particularly where economic growth is largely or entirely cancelled out by the increase in population. Apart from the continuing high birth rates, other factors add to the complexities of the problem. Their people now live longer and marry earlier than in the West; age-old cultural attitudes persist which encourage large families and they are rural communities with no middle-class incentives for family planning and already they suffer deficient standards of living, of education, of medical care and nutrition. Religious opposition is not as often a problem as it is often thought to be, with the exception of the Roman Catholic Church in European countries; its doctrine prohibiting birth control except by the rhythm method, has been promoted aggressively throughout the Christian world, until very recently hindering family-planning efforts and preventing governments and world agencies such as W.H.O. from tackling world population problems. Fortunately, Catholic countries as far removed from Rome as Latin America have few inhibitions over promoting government family-planning programmes without waiting for Papal approval recognizing the absolute necessity of so doing.

Of course, people with a rising standard of living gradually want to plan their families, but we cannot afford to wait for the two or three generations it takes for this to happen spontaneously. Food production must be increased, but that increase does not provide an adequate solution; for already one-third of the people in the world are underfed, and food supplies lag behind population growth. Increasing the economic prosperity of a country is useful and necessary, but that again does not solve the problem because of the increased population which it has to feed. The solution can only come about if these measures are combined with reducing the birth rates, preferably by Government intervention. Only Governments can provide the organization to deal effectively with the problem, and a strong lead from their own Government has more effect in motivating people in any country than exhortations from Western countries, where there are no population policies and populations are relatively stable more by chance than otherwise.

Until recently most efforts have been due to individuals and a few privately sponsored organizations, but fortunately in the last few years Governments have become increasingly involved. Japan shows the outstanding example of what a country can achieve with a Government-sponsored programme, for the Japanese succeeded in halving their birth rate in fifteen years. This was achieved mainly by a combination of sterilization and abortion (legalized in 1949), with birth-control methods playing only a very small part. India was one of the earliest countries to have a population policy, but this was devoted only to promoting western methods and had no practical impact whatsoever on the population. Yet the Government has been resistant to using the newer methods, particularly the Pill; and the only method which has so far made any impression has been voluntary sterilization, with a small cash payment to volunteers.

One method only is universal—*abortion*. The high abortion rates in countries where family-planning methods are illegal or taboo for religious reasons, or even where neither of these holds but there is apathy and reluctance and lack of motivation for family planning, show that individuals do want to restrict the number of children they have, even where the risks of attempting abortion under primitive conditions are very high indeed. It is important to recognize, even if we do not approve of abortion as a method of population control, that it is important as a first sign of motivation among people, even if it has to be replaced with preventive methods which are acceptable to them. No conventional contraceptive seemed to be acceptable until the advent of the Pill and the I.U.D. which, together with abortion and sterilization, are the best we can offer at present.

The *I.U.D.* (Intra Uterine Device) is proving a particularly useful method, as it calls for only one visit to have the device inserted and if complications occur they do bring the woman (who is normally a poor attender for routine examination) back to the clinic. It has proved possible to train nurses and midwives to insert these satisfactorily; and after all, why not? Surely it is similar to our practice of leaving midwives to deliver babies and training them to call in the doctor if anything goes wrong. I.U.D's are often unacceptable medically, however, e.g. to a woman already anaemic, as menorrhagia is a common complication; to women in every country who dislike having foreign bodies in the uterus; and to Moslem women who may not co-habit with their husbands or pray during menstrual bleeding, and are made distressed and anxious by the more prolonged bleeding which this method so often causes. As this seemed the ideal method, I.U.D's were introduced in some countries, e.g. in South Korea and Taiwan, as the sole recommended method of fertility control, but drop out rates were so high (40% at the end of one year) that oral contraceptives have since been introduced as an alternative.

Oral Contraception certainly requires more conscientiousness on the part of the individual woman but its complete effectiveness, when taken properly, gives security, the reduced and regular menstrual bleedings improve general health, and its regular administration without any relation to intercourse and the absence of any genital manipulation are some of the factors which seem to make it one of the most acceptable methods. However, the need to take it regularly makes it difficult for some, while the anxiety over interfering with nature often make it unsuitable and unacceptable.

Obviously, methods which require no kind of medical supervision would be cheaper and simpler in developing countries, but since present methods which come into this category are just not acceptable, we have to allow the introduction of these with paramedical personnel. They are much easier to introduce of course where there is already some kind of public health service, e.g. Maternity and Child Welfare services as in South Korea; whereas in Turkey they are much more difficult, as there are hardly any medical services outside the main towns.

Our role as doctors in this field is limited: we can only develop new methods and train doctors and paramedical workers to advise on these. Education to promote preventive family planning depends on newspapers, radio, television and other mass media; and politicians and religious leaders have far more influence than doctors.

4

Effectiveness and Acceptability of Contraceptive Methods

Failures with any contraceptive method may be due to the method itself or to its misuse (patient failure). It is generally agreed that the failure rate of any contraceptive method must include the accidental pregnancies whether these are due to patient or method failure, because it is impossible to be sure of distinguishing between these and the failures in the months when the method has been used inconsistently as well as when used consistently. This means, of course, that the effectiveness is not so high when motivation for family planning is poor and the methods offered are not acceptable. It means too that acceptability is probably the most critical factor in the effectiveness of any contraceptive method and that individual couples will use a method conscientiously and therefore effectively, only if they like it.

The acceptability of any method to any couple depends upon a great many factors, many of which are irrational and emotional. It may be affected by governmental attitudes, as in India, where there is a reluctance to introduce oral contraceptives, by social factors, as in U.K. where couples in the lower social brackets resort only later or not at all to birth control and use withdrawal more than any other method, whereas in social classes 1, 2 and 3 they mostly start attempting straight away to regulate their fertility, and the majority seek premarital advice. It is affected by cultural and racial mores and prejudices towards birth control in general or any method in particular, e.g. a distinction between the so-called artificial and natural methods by Catholics, and the greater extent of the use of female methods in the U.S.A. compared with U.K., where male methods predominate. It is affected by religious views and practices, by educational level, by emotional attitudes—many of them unconscious—by the opinion of family and friends and, indeed, by the prejudices of the doctor or other professional adviser.

In India, where the views of grandmother are influential, education must be aimed also at her. In the U.S.A. fashions change quickly, and any new method tends to predominate, or in the absence of such, any new gadget attached to an old method. In Australia and New Zealand doctors are paid per item of service to patients; they have more readily accepted the new methods, and oral contraceptives are used more often per head of population than any other country. In Turkey, few men allow their wives to use birth control in case they should be unfaithful.

Since we live in a time of changing climate of opinion and of newer methods and re-assessment of the old, patterns of acceptability are likely to alter markedly. It seems that doctors should do their best to overcome their own emotional prejudices and help their patients to find what is acceptable to them, bearing in mind that people with little or no experience of birth control are likely to want to try more than one method before deciding what suits them best.

5

Contraceptive Methods Requiring No Medical Supervision

The Condom

The condom is one of the oldest, most effective, most widely used and acceptable of all methods, first introduced as a linen sheath to be used as a protection against venereal infection. Condoms are still often called protectives, and are the only birth-control method to give some protection against venereal disease. When first used as contraceptives, probably in the eighteenth century, they were made of animal membrane and consequently expensive. In the middle of the nineteenth century, vulcanization of rubber was applied to their manufacture, making them available more cheaply at a time when birth control methods were being popularized. The latex process, developed about 1930, significantly improved condoms making them finer, stronger and longer-lasting.

The condom acts as a barrier to prevent the direct insemination of the cervix. For maximum efficiency, condoms have to be applied before any genital contact takes place and care must be taken in removing them not to spill any of the semen in the vagina.

Used carefully and conscientiously, this is a highly efficient method. Any pregnancies which occur may be due to the escape of spermatozoa into the vagina if the condom leaks or ruptures; so it is still more efficient if the wife uses a spermicidal pessary or cream inserted to the top of the vagina before intercourse to act as a chemical barrier if the mechanical one fails. This is not necessary with the thicker washable sheath, which is strong enough to be used over and over again. Both types are made in plain or teat end, the latter designed to contain the ejaculate; where the plain one is used, half an inch should be left for this purpose at the end as it is being unrolled over the erect penis. Condoms are available in a great variety of colours, and packs and prices (recently the pre-lubricated type has become very popular), and are easily obtainable from most chemists and barbers, and from a multitude of mail order firms; and, of course, they require no medical supervision. They are particularly suitable if the husband prefers to take charge of the birth-control method or if the use of female methods is unacceptable to the wife; they are also suitable where vaginal infections occur and for reducing sensitivity where premature ejaculation is caused by this. The condom is also useful as an interim method after the birth of a baby, or as a method to alternate with female methods such as the cap for couples who like to ring the changes. It is particularly useful too where acts of intercourse are occasional or unpredictable, as in the case of the unmarried. Some couples like the protective effect as it provides a barrier to prevent too close contact or mess in the vagina; other couples find that such a barrier interferes with pleasure and that the method interferes with spontaneity.

Coitus Interruptus

The use of coitus interruptus, i.e. withdrawal, is widespread and common. It is often described by the patient as "being careful", as it involves withdrawal before ejaculation. Some failures do occur because in some men sperms may be present in the erect penis before ejaculation, or because withdrawal is mistimed. When a husband has difficulty in controlling ejaculation, this method can cause anxiety in either or both partners. For some couples, the restraint imposed by the method spoils the element of relaxation essential to satisfactory intercourse. Prolonged use of the method is sometimes said to cause nervous strain in some couples, though its widespread use suggests that this is really quite rare. The absence of cost and the need to be prepared in advance for coitus are obvious advantages for this method and explain why it is used more often by manual workers. The trend in recent years among the social classes 1, 2, and 3, is away from this towards more sophisticated and more expensive methods. As with all methods, there are geographical differences, e.g. about half of all couples in U.K. have tried this method at some time, while only a small percentage of couples in U.S.A. have ever done so. The fact that it is entirely in the husband's control may be an important factor in choosing this method, though it must often be used simply because nothing else is available where intercourse is not premeditated.

Rhythm Method

The rhythm method—or safe period—is also widely used, either alone or in conjunction with other methods. It is important as the only method, apart from abstinence, permitted so far by the Roman Catholic Church. It is based on the idea of avoiding intercourse at the time of ovulation when conception is most likely to occur; its success, therefore, depends on the accurate assessment of the time of ovulation. In most women ovulation occurs fourteen days before the onset of the next menstrual period, so that it can only be reliable in women with a reasonably regular menstrual cycle. Spermatozoa can remain viable in the female genital tract for up to five days, though they are probably capable of fertilizing for only two or three days. The ovum is only capable of being fertilized for twelve to twenty-four hours after it is shed. To be reasonably safe, therefore, it is advisable for intercourse to be avoided for five days before ovulation and two days afterwards. The difficulty of course lies in working out the date of ovulation with sufficient accuracy. It should be calculated with reference to several of the patient's previous menstrual cycles and should take account of the shortest and the longest cycle over at least six months. It is, therefore, not reliable before the cycle is re-established after a pregnancy or for a woman with irregular cycles, or for women over forty, at which age cycles may begin to be irregular.

Ovulation can occur at any time in the cycle, and possibly more than once in a cycle in some women, as a direct response to the stimulation of intercourse; such factors obviously increase the failure rates.

There are several expensive gadgets for calculating the safe period on the market but it is just as easy to calculate without them. The calculation is made as follows:

Once the shortest and longest cycles over at least six months are known, deduct 18 from the number of days in the shortest cycle, to find the first fertile or unsafe day.
Deduct 10 from the number of days in the longest cycle to find the last of the fertile or unsafe days, e.g. if the cycle varies from 25 to 31 days, conception is possible from cycle-day 7 up to and including cycle-day 21: thus the safe days, when fertilization is unlikely, are cycle days 1 to 6 and from day 22 onwards to the end of the cycle.

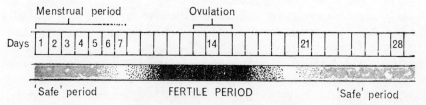

Fig. 1. The typical female cycle.

The use of a basal temperature chart can increase the efficiency as it will show when ovulation is safely over, though it cannot predict ovulation. The temperature should be taken first thing on waking, the thermometer being left under the tongue for a full four minutes. The temperature rises after ovulation, as the production of progesterone by the corpus luteum increases metabolism and causes the temperature to rise to a higher level, where it remains until just before menstrual bleeding starts. It can be assumed that ovulation is over when the temperature remains at the high level for two or three days.

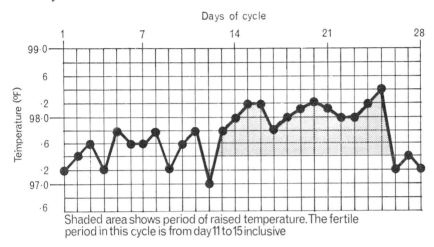

Shaded area shows period of raised temperature. The fertile period in this cycle is from day 11 to 15 inclusive

Fig. 2. Typical normal temperature range. Note how it is consistently higher after ovulation until just before the next menstrual period.

Failures occurring with this method are due to the obvious difficulties in working out the time of ovulation and in avoiding intercourse over the fertile phase. Women with an increased desire for intercourse at the time of ovulation will find this method frustrating; and not all men find it easy or possible to have intercourse only according to the calendar. For success the method requires a strong sense of motivation on the part of both partners. Since this method is approved by the Roman Catholic Church, it is very important to some couples, many of whom have the necessary motivation.

Some couples conveniently combine it with other methods; for example they use some other form of contraceptive over the fertile phase and none at the safe period. Where the woman has reasonably regular cycles, such a combination can be good. This is probably one of the methods used by many couples in the early days of marriage, but likely to be given up because of failure. Where it is the only permissible method and the menstrual cycles are irregular, it can be a constant source of unwanted pregnancies and anxiety.

Spermicides

Vaginal contraceptives or spermicides are available in the form of pessaries, gels, foaming tablets and, more recently, aerosol foams. These products are readily available without prescription at most chemists. They require insertion to the top of the woman's vagina just before intercourse, and they provide a physical barrier to the penetration of the cervix by sperms as well as exerting a contraceptive action.

Insertion is by means of the finger for soluble pessaries and foaming tablets, by means of an applicator for the creams, jellies and aerosols. They must be inserted a few minutes before intercourse—long enough for body heat to melt and spread the contents, but not long enough for it to leak out of the vagina.

Failures occur, as the cervix is not always covered or the amount is insufficient to kill off all the sperms; and fertile couples should use these preparations along with a mechanical device, though less fertile couples might find them adequate when used alone. The more recent aerosol foams are more efficient than the others for use on their own but should not be recommended for the fertile multiparous woman.

The advantages of spermicides are the wide availability and easy insertion; the disadvantages are the inconvenience and messiness, and some couples find it unpleasant to have to use anything at the time of intercourse. Occasionally a patient or her husband may be allergic to one spermicidal preparation; this allergy is usually manifested by local irritation and possibly swelling. A change should be made to another product containing a different spermicide and different base.

Douches and Sponges

Douching to wash the sperms out of the vagina immediately after intercourse is used by some women as a method of contraception. It is probably the most inefficient of methods, for even if douching is carried out as soon as possible after intercourse, it may be too late to prevent some sperms entering the cervix. Some women choose this method because they like to make themselves clean after intercourse. A vaginal douche apparatus is required but there is no particular virtue in using any chemical in the douche; time is all-important, and removal of the sperms is more efficient than trying to kill them by chemical means.

Home-made sponges soaked in oil, vinegar or spermicide and inserted high into the vagina have been used for years where more sophisticated methods have not been available.

6

Methods Requiring Medical Supervision

Cap and Chemical

Devices to cover the cervix and prevent the access of sperms are not new; for all kinds of sponges, leaves, fruit, e.g. half a lemon, have been used throughout the ages. Rubber caps to form a mechanical barrier gradually replaced these and became all important in the birth-control clinics. They are usually used with a spermicidal cream or jelly, which facilitates insertion and provides an added safety factor, and properly used they are one of the most efficient methods, though some pregnancies do occur. Caps have to be the right shape and size for the woman's vagina so that individual fitting and teaching is required.

They are made in various shapes. The most commonly used is the diaphragm which has a spring rim and a soft rubber dome and lies diagonally across the vagina, separating the cervix and upper part of the vagina from the vaginal opening and cavity.

This is the simplest type for most patients to insert and the most suitable where there is good vaginal muscle tone, because the cap is kept in position by a combination of its own spring and the vaginal muscles. The flat spring is more rigid than the spring rim and usually easier to manage. For the woman with poor vaginal muscle tone or a retroverted uterus, and for some awkward shapes of vagina, other types of cap are available, mainly the vault, vimule and the cervical.

With all of these the cap, with about a teaspoonful of spermicide in the bowl, is inserted into the vagina to cover the cervix at any convenient time before intercourse, and is left in place for at least six hours afterwards. The most satisfactory way is for the woman to insert her cap regularly each night. When removed next morning it should be washed in warm soapy water, dried well and powdered.

Diaphragms are available in sizes from 45 mm up to 105 mm with $2\frac{1}{2}$ or 5 mm difference between one size and the next, depending on the make— the vault and cervical types of cap in five sizes, the vimule type in three. It is important that the woman be fitted with the right type and size to suit her, that she be instructed how to insert and remove it, and that she attends for a second visit wearing the cap to ensure that she is using it properly and that the right size has been chosen (at a first examination many women have tense vaginal muscles and, therefore, appear to be smaller than they are). She should be taught to determine whether the cap is covering the cervix each time that she inserts it.

Cap and chemical, like the other methods already considered, produce no side effects. It is usually easy to insert them once the patient has learnt to do so. It is a comparatively cheap method, although it does involve a visit to a doctor or clinic; and they can be inserted routinely before going to bed, rather than calling for genital manipulation at the time of intercourse. The disadvantages are that some women find the vaginal manipulation involved in inserting the cap distasteful; regular check-ups are required at intervals for size—more often in early marriage, after childbirth, and if the patient has any gross weight change—and a few pregnancies do occur even with conscientious and careful use. The method requires, moreover, a fairly reasonable level of intelligence and even more motivation on the part of the user.

This method leaves the control of pregnancy entirely in the hands of the woman, which probably explains its much more frequent use in U.S.A.

than in U.K. where it has never been used by more than about 12% of couples. Some women inevitably use the cap to get their own way as to when intercourse happens, or otherwise to control the sexual situation. It is still a most useful alternative method for some couples.

Intra-uterine Contraceptive Devices

Intra-uterine devices, or I.U.D's, have been revived as a useful method. Earlier this century, being made of metal, e.g. the Grafenberg ring, they fell into disrepute in most countries, largely because of side effects such as pelvic inflammation, endometrial reaction and sometimes even perforation of the

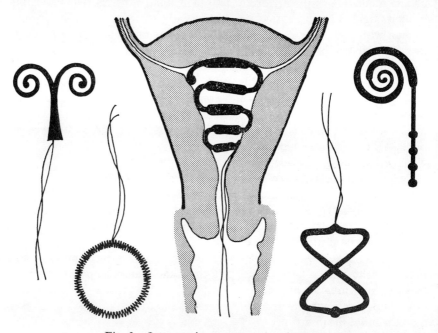

Fig. 3.   Intra-uterine contraceptive devices.

uterus when follow-up had not been adequate. Recently, first in Japan and later in U.S.A. and Israel, investigators began to experiment with new materials and new designs. Plastics, which were known not to cause foreign body reaction in other human tissues, impregnated with a barium salt to make them radiopaque, were made into shapes which could be stretched for insertion into the uterus through an introducer, and resumed their moulded shape after introduction into the uterine cavity. By now these have proved so useful that a great variety of shapes are available. It appears that any foreign body in the uterus will have some contraceptive action, although indications are that a comfortable fit, i.e. not distorted and big enough to touch at all points, gives best results, both from the point of view of efficiency and side effects.

World-wide trials of the earliest of these plastic intra-uterine devices, using in the first place a spiral, a loop and a bow, have been carried out under the auspices of the Population Council, thus giving a speedier and more valid assessment of the advantages and disadvantages of each than would otherwise have been possible.

Efficiency and Acceptability. These are one of the most efficient of available contraceptive methods. The pregnancy rate averages about 3 per 100 women-years and is, therefore, roughly similar to the failure rate with condom or cap and chemical method, conscientiously used. Only oral contraceptives are more effective. Half of these pregnancies occur with the device still in place, the other half when the device has been expelled without the patient noticing it.

The most important reason for the effectiveness of this method is that it virtually does away with the possibility of patient failure; the device is inserted by the doctor and the patient has no further responsibility in the matter apart from reporting for check-ups, as and when required to do so. It is, therefore, particularly useful for people with poor motivation for family planning or those who dislike conventional methods. It is also acceptable to doctors who like more "medical" methods, and obviously it appeals to the woman who is tired of taking contraceptive precautions and likes to hand over the responsibility to her doctor.

Disadvantages and Side Effects. Other women dislike a method over which they have no control, or dislike the idea of a foreign body in the uterus. A considerable proportion of women have menorrhagia, inter-menstrual bleeding or pre-menstrual spotting, particularly in the first three cycles. A small number continue to have heavier periods beyond six months, and indeed as long as they have the device in situ. Many of these women, however, regard this as a small price to pay for such a satisfactory method. It is always advisable to warn patients to expect an alteration in their menstrual flow. Pelvic inflammatory disease has been reported in a small proportion of cases—probably a reactivation of a previous infection.

In some 5 to 10% of cases, the device is spontaneously expelled. This usually happens in the first one or two cycles, particularly at the time of menstruation and is usually preceded by some uterine colic; occasionally, however, the device is expelled without the patient noticing it. Where conception does happen with the device in situ, no ill effect on the pregnancy or foetus has been reported and the device is usually expelled at the time of confinement. There is, therefore, no need to remove it when pregnancy occurs.

A few women complain of discomfort for a few days after insertion and sometimes get dysmenorrhoea—both are particularly common with the nulliparous woman. On the other hand, occasionally a woman finds that the presence of a device relieves her previous dysmenorrhoea.

Selection of Cases. A careful medical history and pelvic examination should be carried out before considering this as a method. It may be unsatisfactory with an acutely flexed uterus, a fixed retroversion or fibroids, particularly if near the cavity, and for patients with heavy periods and those with a history of recent pelvic infection (the possibility of sterility following pelvic inflammation after the insertion of an I.U.D., although slight, suggests that it might be wiser to discourage their use in nulliparous women).

An I.U.D. must, of course, be inserted under sterile conditions. The plastic introducers may be sterilized by boiling; but the devices themselves must never be boiled. They are best stored in screw-top glass jars, in an antiseptic solution, e.g. benzalkonium chloride, for a minimum of twenty-four hours; or they may be covered with an alcohol, e.g. isoproponal for five minutes before use. They can also be obtained in individual packs sterilized by gamma radiation, sometimes packed with disposable introducers and correspondingly more expensive. These are particularly useful for the physician inserting an occasional one only.

Mode of Insertion. A routine pelvic examination is carried out to determine the position of the uterus and ensure that everything is normal; and the cervix is exposed with a speculum, mopped with sterile gauze or cleansed with an antiseptic and a sound introduced gently to find the angle and length of the uterus and cervical canal. The type of device to be used is decided upon and prepared. With the Lippes loop (which is overall the most satisfactory), the loop is loaded into the inserter with a no-touch technique, and the inserter introduced half an inch or so beyond the internal os. This is then rotated 90° to bring it into the plane of the uterine cavity and the device expelled by pushing the plunger, which should then be removed before gently pulling out the introducer. The devices must be loaded immediately prior to use or they tend to lose their shape. Occasionally a volsellum is required, particularly if the uterus is acutely ante- or retroflexed. Force should never be used at the time of insertion.

Most devices have a nylon thread which is left protruding from the cervix and the woman should be taught to feel this from time to time to ensure that it is still present, particularly in the earlier months. Ideally, a check up at two and three months is advised and yearly thereafter. So far as is known at present, these devices may be left in place indefinitely unless any complications arise.

The majority of women, if relaxed and at ease, are unaware of the insertion of the device; a small number, and particularly those who are tense and anxious, experience discomfort of varying degrees; an occasional woman becomes shocked and unconscious but recovers quickly, whether the device is removed or not.

Expulsion is more likely to happen if the device is not completely within the cavity—if the open end is left in the cervical canal, it will almost certainly cause discomfort and become expelled. Where spontaneous expulsion does happen, it is worthwhile trying a second time—and it seems a good idea to try a different shape of device and different plastic.

The uterus is occasionally perforated—presumably at the time of insertion—although this is not usually recognized, as it is symptomless. If discovered, there is no hurry to operate with an open ended device though a closed one is better removed for fear of causing strangulation of the bowel.

Management of Bleeding. Any abnormal bleeding in the first two or three cycles after insertion may be ignored as it is likely to settle spontaneously. Some devices do have to be removed after a number of months because of the persistence of irregular bleeding. Intermenstrual bleeding or menorrhagia may be due to the device having been distorted at the time of insertion or subsequently due to uterine contractions, or it may be covered with calcium salts. Removal and insertion of a new device would help in such instances. Persistent menorrhagia may be treated, if required, in the usual manner, though it is doubtful if anything other than three months cyclic treatment with a strongly progestagenic oral contraceptive makes any difference. Where bleeding has been regular and months after insertion inter-menstrual bleeding or menorrhagia begin, this may indicate inflammation or congestion.

There is a wide variation in the pregnancy rate and the complication rates —which is hardly surprising, considering the number of different types and shapes of I.U.D's and the many different countries in which they are being used. One important factor is the experience of the doctor or paramedical personnel inserting the device, for a relaxed patient in competent hands is likely to have a more comfortable insertion with fewer complications. On the other hand, there is no doubt that in nine out of ten cases the simpler types of device may be inserted satisfactorily by a suitably trained midwife or health visitor.

Legal Implications. In U.K. doctors should note that it is advisable to have the consent of the husband before inserting one of these devices, as under English law the husband has the right to a say in the matter.

Oral Contraceptives

The oral contraceptive—"the Pill"—is the most efficient method ever known. It is the first new method resulting from scientific research and it has revolutionized birth-control practice all over the world. Not only has it given security to highly fertile couples who had failures with other methods and to couples to whom it is important or imperative that conception should not occur, but it has also proved acceptable to those who need family planning most but failed miserably with other methods because they did not accept them.

There are by now some thirty brands of the Pill produced by different drug firms and containing all kinds of combinations of the two female hormones progestagen and oestrogen. The majority are of the *combination* type, i.e. every pill contains both of these hormones. Pills of this type are the most efficient of all because not only do they inhibit ovulation but administration of even a small amount of progestagen from early in the cycle renders the cervical mucus hostile to sperms and prevents the oestrogen-induced proliferative changes in the endometrium which are essential for implantation. The patient who takes the combined oral contraceptive regularly as instructed ought not to get pregnant. The more recent *sequential* type of pill involves giving oestrogen only for the first part of the cycle and adding the progestagen in the last few pills, so that its effectiveness largely depends on inhibition of ovulation. As ovulation occurs occasionally during oral contraceptive treatment, pregnancy can and does occur with patients on the sequential type of pill.

Mode of Action. The consensus of present opinion is that the combined O.Cs. act by suppressing the mid-cycle peak of L.H. secretion while total gonadotrophins remain unaffected, whereas sequential preparations mainly reduce F.S.H. output. The ovulatory cycle in a woman arises from a complex interplay between the ovary and its two hormones, the pituitary and its three gonadotrophic hormones, the hypothalamus which controls pituitary hormones through its releasing factors, and various nervous factors located above the hypothalamus. Not only are oestrogen and progesterone secreted by the ovary in response to pituitary gonadotrophin stimulation, but they both have a feed-back action on the hypothalamic releasing factors; and this may be the most important mode of action of the O.C's.

Side Effects. The majority of side effects which trouble the woman in the early cycles of medication are related to the oestrogen/progestagen balance of the product, and are similar to those in pregnancy or the normal menstrual cycle or menopause. The commonest ones are gastric disturbances including increased appetite, breast tenderness, abdominal and leg cramp, fluid retention, weight increase, changes in libido, in the condition of skin and hair, and in the amount and type of vaginal discharge. Most of these disappear spontaneously after the first three or four cycles. But it is also true that many women lose their pre-existing complaints such as premenstrual tension, dysmenorrhoea, breast discomfort, nervousness and irritability, and the majority of women have much more regular cycles with a reduced menstrual loss, so that overall they alleviate more menstrual complaints than they cause. Many women have a sense of well-being and enjoy intercourse more, not only because of the freedom from anxiety over pregnancy but because of the anabolic effect of the product.

Weight gain, loss of libido, mood changes and headache may be troublesome in a small proportion of long-term cases.

Endocrine and Metabolic Effects. Of more importance is the effect on endocrine and biochemical functions of the continued administration of these hormones. In this respect we have to consider not only what changes are produced by medication but also the clinical significance of these. As oral contraceptives are steroids and act systemically, they effect many changes in other organs and, since they are taken regularly over a long period of time by normal women, they raise anxieties over the possibility of long-term effects and/or upsetting the mechanism of endocrine interrelationships. Some of the changes, however, are physiological, are reversible, and maybe no more harmful than the increase in gastric secretion which follows eating.

Thyroid. Oral contraceptives have no apparent effect on the normal thyroid, but they do affect some laboratory tests of thyroid function. They cause an increase in thyroxin-binding globulin and consequently an increase in protein bound iodine (P.B.I.). These changes are due to the oestrogen and are reversible when medication is discontinued.

Adrenal Cortex. The oestrogen component causes an increase in corticosteroid-binding globulin in the plasma and an increase in the total plasma cortisol level and consequently a raised total aldosterone. Water and salt retention and oedema sometimes occur, due to the oestrogen; and care should be taken in prescribing these for patients with a history of renal damage or cardiac trouble.

Carbohydrate Metabolism. Impairment of glucose tolerance has been found in some women on oral contraceptives—usually in women who are pre-diabetic or have a family history of diabetes; this risk is probably less than in pregnancy. They do not appear to alter the severity of the diabetes. This change is probably due to the oestrogen.

Recently alterations have been found in the cholesterol, lipo-proteins and in serum triglyceride—which are all raised—but the significance of this is not yet understood.

Liver. Since the liver conjugates and metabolizes steroids, it is not surprising that changes are found. Oral contraceptives (probably the oestrogen) apparently interfere with B.S.P. metabolism and hepatic cell excretory function; but these changes are reversible, are often transient, and may disappear spontaneously with continued medication. The changes are similar to, but less than, those found in normal pregnancy, and are probably due to physiological adaptation.

Women in Scandinavia and Chile occasionally have jaundice on oral contraceptives but there have been no cases of hepatic abnormality clinically in other countries. These raised values therefore do not appear to indicate hepatic dysfunction presumably because the hepatoxic dose is higher than the clinical one.

Cervix and Endometrium. There is no evidence of any carcinogenic effect on the cervix or the endometrium, though it is too early to define final long-term effects.

Blood Clotting and Venous Thrombosis. O.Cs. do produce changes in the blood clotting mechanism (the mean prothrombin time decreases and fibrinogen, fibrinolytic activity and factor *vii* and factor *viii* increase). These are similar to the changes in pregnancy when there is no increased incidence of thrombo-embolic phenomena: the increase is in the puerperium, usually days after the blood clotting factors have returned to pre-pregnancy levels, and is believed to be due to trauma and local alterations in blood circulation. The significance of these changes, then, is not understood: venous thrombosis and thromboembolic phenomena are in any case common, with an incidence of 1 to 3 per thousand woman of child-bearing age every year, and in the post-partum period 3 to 10 cases per thousand deliveries. However, prospective statistical studies carried out by the Medical Research Council confirm the increased risk of thrombosis for a woman on oral contraceptives. The chances of a fatal episode for Pill users aged 20–34 is one in 60,000 and aged 35–44 one in 20,000, and there is an increased risk of hospitalization with venous embolism to the extent that one in every 2,000 pill takers will be admitted to hospital yearly. To put this risk into perspective, however, it must be stated that the risk to women of the younger age group is only 1/6th of the risk in pregnancy and is considerably less than the risk of death from a road accident or an accident in the home, or from smoking one or two cigarettes daily.

It is now known that this is due to the oestrogen and is dose related (oestrogen given for other purposes, e.g. to inhibit lactation, also increases the incidence of thrombosis); so a preference should be given to those products with a low oestrogen content (see Table II). Indeed a recent recommendation to doctors in the U.K., based on as yet unpublished evidence, apparently shows an increased incidence of thrombosis among women on oral contraceptives containing 0·75 mgm of oestrogen or over compared with the low dose, i.e. 0·05 mgm of either oestrogen.

The woman with a history of previous thromboembolic phenomena is more likely to develop such a complication on oral contraception; but such a previous history also predisposes to puerperal complications, which is the greater risk, so that where no other contraceptive is efficient enough, oral contraceptives are clearly the lesser risk.

Lactation. The effect of oestrogens and progestagens on lactation is improperly understood. The amount of breast milk is decreased in some women on oral contraceptives: as this is a dose-response, low doses are to be preferred when a woman wishes to continue breast feeding.

Subsequent Fertility. Overall, there is no evidence that fertility is either increased or decreased following the use of oral contraceptives. The first spontaneous menstruation after stopping oral contraceptives is usually delayed by anything from a few days to three or four weeks, and a woman attempting pregnancy should be warned that such a delay might not mean that she is pregnant. Persistent amenorrhoea after stopping hormonal steroids has been reported, but as yet inadequately studied: in any case incidence in women who have not been on oral contraceptives is not known. There is no evidence that babies subsequently conceived have any increased incidents of congenital defects, foetal wastage, or perinatal mortality.

After a pregnancy oral contraceptives can be started in the usual way after the first spontaneous menstruation; however, for patients who cannot be relied upon to use other measures until then, they may be given at any time before six weeks without waiting for menstruation, as ovulation does not occur before then.

The Menopause. The menopause appears to be neither prolonged nor postponed by oral contraceptive therapy, although it hides menopausal irregularities and symptoms, so that at some stage, say at age 50, a woman has to stop to see whether she is still menstruating. It is a particularly good method of birth control at this age, where menstrual irregularities cause anxiety, where functional menorrhagia is debilitating, or where side effects call for hormonal medication.

Prescribing the Pill

Pre-medication Examination. Routine examination of any woman before prescribing the Pill should include a careful history of obstetric and gynaecological complaints, menstrual pattern and symptoms, and vaginal examination to exclude pelvic disease; a cervical smear for the early detection of cancer of the cervix; breast examination to eliminate pre-existing breast cancer, and a blood pressure recording, particularly if she gives a history of toxaemia in pregnancy or renal disease since the blood pressure may rise during medication in such cases; and her weight since she may gain weight while taking oral contraceptives. A comprehensive medical and family history should also be taken, for careful medical supervision is required where there is a history of jaundice, embolism, thrombosis, malignant disease, hypertension, obesity, epilepsy, migraine, steroid therapy, diabetes or allergic disorders.

Instruction to Patient. With all oral contraceptives it is important that the tablets should be taken each day as directed. Counting the first day of menstrual bleeding as Day 1 the first tablet should be taken on Day 5, whether the bleeding has finished or not. One tablet should be taken daily until the package is finished (usually 20 or 21 days). If a tablet is ever forgotten, it should be taken as soon as remembered even if this means taking two tablets next day. After seven days without tablets (during which menstruation should occur) the next packet should be started regardless of whether bleeding has started, finished, or is in progress. Most of the brands are now made in 21-day packages labelled for each day so that it is impossible to miss one without knowing; the gap without pills is always seven days, and the woman begins the Pill always on the same day of the week. Some packets are made up with dummy pills to be taken during the seven day gap, so that the patient continues to take one Pill every day.

When taken properly they work from the first Pill; the woman who has a very short cycle should be advised to start on Day 3 instead of Day 5.

Spotting and Breakthrough Bleeding. If slight bleeding or spotting occurs in the middle of any medication cycle the woman should ignore it and continue to take the tablets as directed. If, however, bleeding as heavy as a normal menstrual period begins in the middle of the cycle, she should stop taking the tablets and resume with a new packet to take a full course five days later. This is more likely to happen in the early cycles but if it persists beyond the 3rd or 4th a change to another product is advisable (see page 196).

Choice of Product. In choosing a suitable product it is useful first of all to assess the woman's own hormone balance, whether it is predominantly oestrogenic or progestagenic, from her obstetric and menstrual history and symptoms and from gynaecological examination, as follows:

TABLE I

Oestrogenic effects	Progestagenic effects
Fluid retention and oedema	Pre-menstrual depression
Premenstrual tension, irritability and increase in weight	Leucorrhoea, dry vagina
	Acne, greasy hair
Nausea and vomiting	Appetite increase with weight gain
Headache	Breast discomfort
Mucorrhoea, cervical erosion	Menses which are regular and not heavy
Menorrhagia	Leg and abdominal cramps
Excessive tiredness	Decreased libido
Vein complaints	

The overall hormone balance of oral contraceptives varies from predominantly oestrogenic to predominantly progestagenic in effect, and it seems that selection of a suitable Pill gives fewer side effects and by adjusting her hormone balance, relieves the woman of any pre-existing menstrual complaints. Thus, where oestrogen effects predominate, an oral contraceptive which is predominantly progestational should relieve these and vice versa. A clinical assessment of the woman's own hormone balance should be adequate and elaborate endocrine investigations unnecessary.

Classification of available oral contraceptives is complicated by the fact that although the two oestrogens are similar in potency, mgm for mgm, this is not true of the progestagens, which cannot be classified as strongly or weakly progestagenic according to the mgm dose. The *oestrogenic effect* of a formulation depends not only on the actual dose of oestrogen but also on the particular progestagen in the tablet, as some progestagens are metabolized to oestrogen, thus increasing the overall effect. On the other hand, most progestagens oppose or lessen the effect of oestrogen to a varying extent. Also endogenous oestrogens are much reduced by oral contraceptive medication while, since no corpus luteum is formed, the endogenous progesterone is limited to the small amounts produced by the adrenal and the ovarian stroma.

Because the oestrogen component is responsible for most of the untoward effects of oral contraceptives, it is important to keep the dose of oestrogen as low as possible and Table II provides a classification of oral contraceptives grouped according to their oestrogen content. The oestrogen is either ethynyl-oestradiol (EE) or mestranol (M). Since the dose of progestagen in the formulation gives no clue to the potency, this is indicated (P=strongly progestational, p = weakly progestational).

The efficiency should also be taken into account in prescribing a suitable Pill, that is whether a slight risk of pregnancy is acceptable to the couple or whether the need is for 100% efficiency. Combined oral contraceptives should always be given where maximum efficiency is required, remembering that the safety margin is higher with the strongly progestational compounds if the patient is liable to miss tablets or is overweight. The sequential formulations have always been less effective giving an occasional pregnancy even when properly taken and they all contain more than the recommended dose of oestrogen so that their use is rarely indicated.

TABLE II

Oral Contraceptives (I.Cs) classified according to oestrogen content

O.Cs containing 0·05mgm of oestrogen (low dose) Recommended dose		O.Cs containing 0·075 or 0·08mgm oestrogen (intermediate dose) Combined		O.Cs containing 0·1mgm oestrogen (high dose) Not recommended Combined	
P. Anovlar	EE	Conovid	M	Conovid E	M
Gynovlar	EE	Lyndiol 2·5	M	Demulen	M
Minilyn	EE	Ortho Novin 1/80	M	Nuvacon	EE
Norlestrin	EE			Ortho Novin 2mgm	M
Volidan	EE			Ortho Novin 0·5	M
p. Demulen 50	EE			Ovulen	M
Minovlar	EE			*Sequential*	
Norinyl 1	M			C-Quens 21	M
Ortho Novin 1/50	M	*Sequential*		Feminor 21	M
Orlest 28	EE	Ovanon	M	Ortho Novin SQ	M
Ovulen 50	EE	Sequens	M	Serial 28	EE

Indications and Contra-indications. This, the most efficient of all contraceptive methods, is particularly suitable for highly fertile couples with anxieties over fertility control, for those with irregular cycles, dysmenorrhoea, frequent or heavy menstruation and other gynaecological disorders, and for those with urgent medical or personal reasons why pregnancy should be avoided. For couples who have been unable or unwilling to persist with other contraceptive measures, it is well worth trying, because it often proves to be much more acceptable, presumably because of the absence of genital manipulation and of measures taken at the time of intercourse.

There are few contra-indications in normal women. Hormonal steroids should not be used in pre-menopausal women with an existing breast cancer, though it is not yet known whether the same restriction should apply to cases of genital tract carcinoma where this does not impair fertility. They should not be used in women with a previous history of cholestatic jaundice of pregnancy or certain other forms of hepatic excretory impairment. In considering whether to give this method to patients with endocrine disorders, other liver disorders including recent catarrhal jaundice, and venous thrombotic conditions it should be remembered that, apart from sterilization, this is the most effective method: possible side effects from medication should be assessed in relation to whether pregnancy may represent danger to the life and health of the mother. In patients who suffer from such illnesses as diabetes, tuberculosis, cardiovascular disorders, allergy, epilepsy, migraine, etc., oral contraceptive pills, in common with some other medicaments, are occasionally responsible for aggravating these disorders particularly those with an allergic basis; but it is well worth giving them a trial, as there is a good chance that the condition will be improved and even if aggravated it would return to normal as soon as medication is stopped.

Changing to another Pill. Severe sensitivity reactions will of course require a change of product at an early stage; such side effects may be due to a sensitivity reaction to the particular oestrogen or progestagen in the formulation. These include headache and migraine, allergic rhinitis, eczema, epilepsy, severe nausea and vomiting, nervousness and mood changes, vertigo, flushing and possibly some metabolic effect. If any of these is severe, a change should be made to a product with a different oestrogen and progestagen to avoid any risk of making the condition worse; where it is only slight, the responsible factor might be found by changing one of the constituents only.

Other side effects encountered are hormonal in nature; and if mild, patients should be encouraged to continue until the third cycle as they so often settle spontaneously by then, but if not, this is a convenient time to assess whether a suitable product has been chosen. Such side effects as do persist should be assessed as oestrogenic or progestagenic as in Table I and a change made to give the desired balance, e.g. if a woman complains of one or more of the following symptoms, fluid retention, tiredness, irregular bleeding and increased varicosities, which are oestrogenic effects, a change should be made to a more progestagenic one.

In changing from one oral contraceptive to another, the progestational potency may be increased either by increasing the dose of progestagen, or increasing the amount of oestrogen, or both; while the oestrogenic potency can be increased by reducing the dose of progestagen or both.

The following may call for a change of product:

Amenorrhoea (or scanty flow) can be ignored unless it makes the woman anxious, when a more oestrogenic preparation could be given.

Nausea is due to oestrogen; so change to the other one and as low a dose as possible.

Breast fullness may be part of general fluid retention, in which case it is an oestrogenic effect, whereas painful breasts are a progestagenic effect.

Breakthrough bleeding usually calls for a more strongly progestagenic product; if however, B.T.B. occurs—as it occasionally does with a strongly progestagenic compound—give more oestrogen (i.e. strong progestagen plus strong oestrogen) without reducing the progestagen.

Decreased libido is probably a progestagenic effect; so try a more oestrogenic formulation.

Headache. Oral contraceptives may relieve pre-existing headaches or may precipitate migraine or headache in the gap between courses.

Headaches at the beginning of medication are likely to be a sensitivity reaction—sometimes they develop after months or years when a change of product may be tried or a rest from medication.

Low dose "progestagen-only" pills. This is the most recent development in the oral contraceptive field with advantages in the low cost, one pill every day administration which makes it easier to remember, and an absence of oestrogen which is thought to be responsible for most of the troublesome side effects of the combined oral contraceptive pills. There are disadvantages in the unpredictability of bleeding and the possibility of pregnancy when amenorrhoea occurs; and, of course, it still requires continued motivation. It is undoubtedly a most useful addition to available methods as a pill a day for women who do not mind the lesser efficiency (pregnancy rates vary from 2–12 per 100 women years), but it might prove to be even more useful if it proves possible to give it in the form of a slow-release plastic silicone capsule small enough to be injected intramuscularly. There are still problems, however, as to whether the rate of absorption would be sufficiently regular, over individual dosage, and whether the capsule could be removed or would be harmless if left. If found practicable, this would provide a cheap method requiring minimum attention and only occasional motivation, and perhaps it could be tailored to suit the individual woman—a yearly dose for the woman planning her family, and a twenty-year dose for the woman who intends no more.

7

Sterilization

When a couple decide that they will never want another child, a sterilization operation can be considered for either the husband or the wife. For a woman this usually entails a general anaesthetic, an abdominal operation and a stay in hospital. For a man vasectomy is usually carried out with a local anaesthetic as an out-patient, and usually only involves a day or two off work. He should be kept at rest, however, for two or three hours and should not be allowed to drive himself home. Occasionally the development of a haematoma delays recovery.

Both of these operations involve cutting and tying of the tubes, in the case of the woman the fallopian tubes and in the man the vas deferens. Neither operation, of course, involves removal of the sex organs. Although some surgeons claim that a vasectomy is sometimes reversible, i.e. that the tubes can be re-opened, nobody should count on this being possible.

The sterilization operation on the woman is effective immediately, but it is important to understand that sperms are still present in a man's ejaculate for at least eight weeks after vasectomy so that other contraceptive precautions should be taken until two negative sperm counts have been taken after that time.

Until recently, attitudes towards sterilization as a contraceptive measure in men have been rather cautious, partly for legal reasons and doubts, now largely resolved, although it is often carried out in women, being justified on medical grounds. In 1966 the Council of the Medical Defence Union in the United Kingdom was advised that an operation for sterilization is lawful when it is performed on therapeutic or eugenic grounds or for any other reason, provided there is full and valid consent to the operation by the patient concerned. Thus written consent by both the applicant and his wife should always be obtained.

As long as there is no chance of a couple ever wanting to have another child—because there is no guarantee that the operation is reversible—sterilization as a once-and-for-all method has much to commend it, particularly where mental illness, hereditary defects or other eugenic considerations apply. In practice, it is found that men are much more resistant on the whole to having this operation carried out than their wives, probably because they are afraid of a possible effect on their libido resulting from interference with their fertility. There is of course no substance in this, but it is a deep-seated fear which cannot always be dissolved by rational explanation. That it can be overcome, however, is clear from the progress in India of the Government-sponsored sterilization programme, there. Although men were slow to come forward for this in the beginning, there are now 2 million operations per year, and this is at last having an effect on the birth rate.

8

Newer Methods

It would be wrong to await the development of newer methods to solve the population problem, for it must always be remembered that motivation is more important than method, and we have to press on and educate people to use what is available now. However, the increased acceptability of recent methods does emphasize the importance of continuing research to find simpler and cheaper methods. As feeling, attitudes, and prejudices all affect a couple's choice of method, it seems highly unlikely there will ever be one perfect method which meets every couple's needs, so that increased choice of methods is likely to help solve the problem.

Male Methods

The control of spermatogenesis is possible either by chemical means or by hormonal suppression of gonadotrophins. Many scientific workers, notably Nelson and MacLeod in the U.S.A., have been investigating chemicals which are anti-spermatogenic in the human male, but so far no compound has been found to be effective without unfortunate side effects. The nitro-furans are not tolerated in the human in the dosage required; the bis(dichloracetyl) diamines cannot be taken with alcohol because of an antabuse effect; the dinitrophenols are toxic in dogs and monkeys and do not seem very promising. These all have the same type of effect and function at the stage of primary spermatocytes; recovery is prompt after medication is stopped; no mutagenic effect has been shown to occur, and there is appar-ently no suppression of gonadotrophic hormone, so that some compound may emerge which proves possible for regular use. One of the big dis-advantages of these compounds, however, is that they take some fifty days to be fully effective after treatment is started and a similar time after stop-ping treatment for normal fertility to be restored.

It would also be possible to inhibit spermatogenesis indirectly through suppression of gonadotrophins by a variety of steroidal agents, all of which would have a more immediate effect on sterility; but much basic research is required before these will be ready for even preliminary clinical trial.

It must be obvious, therefore, that despite frequent newspaper publicity to the contrary, there is no male pill yet ready for clinical evaluation.

Immunological Methods

Interest in this field was aroused by finding that antibodies against sperms are a factor in causing infertility in human males and females. However, much more research is needed before experimental work on humans can be undertaken, or before we know whether it will be possible to develop this as a method of fertility control.

Hormonal Methods

Until recently, it was thought that hormonal control of fertility would soon be superseded by non-hormonal methods, but it becomes clear that the emerging methods which hold some promise for the immediate future are still hormonal.

Injectable Steroids

Injections of long-acting progestagens can be given in large doses with or without oestrogen, e.g. 150 mgm Medroxy Progesterone Acetate every three months, or 250 mgm each six months. Contraception by an occasional physician-administered injection will clearly appeal to some women and it is undoubtedly a most efficient method. It is liable, however, to disrupt the menstrual cycle completely, and not many women are good at tolerating irregular bleeding. It is possible to administer oestrogens at regular intervals (e.g. 0·1 mgm Etheinyl Oestradiol daily for seven days in the month), to produce a reasonably regular withdrawal bleeding, but this seems to destroy the advantages of an occasional injection. Other disadvantages are that menorrhagia is sometimes uncontrollable, that amenorrhoea is frequent, and that resumption of ovulation is very variable and may be delayed as long as fourteen months after a single injection. It seems better, therefore, until more is known of the mode of action and ultimate effect of giving such a large dose, that this should be given only to women who have finished child-bearing.

It is also possible to give a once-a-month slow release injection containing both oestrogen and progestagen and given approximately every 28 days so as to maintain the menstrual cycle. Such an injection is usually given on the eighth day of the woman's cycle. Monthly injections would inevitably cost more, though it might be easier for some women to remember to have them than to remember to return at much lengthier intervals for medication.

Once-a-month Pills

In the same way a single dose by means of a pill given about the same stage in the cycle containing both a long-acting oestrogen and progestagen would give anti-fertility cover until ovulation and the production of endogenous progesterone. The timing would obviously be important, and once a month might prove more difficult to remember than once per day. This is unlikely to be suitable for over-populated countries but it might be a useful alternative for the woman with continued motivation who prefers self-medication at a reasonable cost.

Post-coital and Post-ovulatory Pills

While low doses of oestrogens have been known for a long time to prevent pregnancy in laboratory animals, there has never been any evidence that these results could be extrapolated to women until recently when McLean Morris[1] used large doses of 1 and 2 mgm Ethynyl-oestradiol. These are toxic doses and would have to be 100% efficient or free of teratogenic effect if they were less so, and large-scale study is required in a country where abortion is permissible should medication fail. Even if the drug is efficient, there are still problems concerning the timing of medication for the post-ovulatory dose; so it is unlikely to be useful on a large scale among illiterate women. Such a drug, if effective and harmless, would be useful as a post-coital contraceptive in isolated incidences of exposure or occasional intercourse, but it would require something much less toxic if it were to be used regularly as a contraceptive. Compounds which have an anti-zygotic effect or prevent implantation are being studied in laboratory animals, and the same reservations and comments apply to them.

Abortifacients

We have seen that the motivation of people new to family planning does not grow overnight, and it is clear that before a woman is ready to take premeditated action to avoid pregnancy she may be distressed enough by an unwanted pregnancy to find a means, however dangerous and despite her religion or her culture, to put an end to this. It is indeed frightening to realize that abortion is still the most common method of birth control on a world-wide scale, despite all the risks involved. It is my belief that side by side with all possible measures to educate couples in family planning by the use of present methods, what we urgently need is to make available a pill or injection to precipitate menstruation for any woman whose period is over-due; for this is the stage when a woman, new to family planning, seeks advice. Of course, such medication would have to be 100% efficient or completely free from teratogenic effects, but the problem is so urgent that I believe if such a pill could be found, it would rapidly gain world-wide acceptance. We have already seen how the advent of the pill changed atti-tudes overnight in so many countries and precipitated an agonizing re-appraisal in the Catholic church of the theological basis of its doctrine and indeed of Papal authority. The taboo on sterilization, except for medical purposes, has been lifted to make it more widely applicable; and I believe that the same thing would be so for a pill which worked as a very early abortifacient before pregnancy could be diagnosed. One or two such com-pounds have been explored recently in Sweden but so far have not proved satisfactory, but currently it seems that the Prostaglandins used vaginally might prove to be so. I believe that there is an urgent need for systematic research in this field to study all possible compounds which are known to act at this stage, and that pharmaceutical companies, in a position to do so, should be pressed into undertaking such research.

9

The Medical Consultation

Family planning for the individual couple means not having more children than they want, though unwanted pregnancies are frequent and may even outnumber planned pregnancies. Probably most couples use birth-control methods irregularly until the first unwanted pregnancy occurs, and then become more conscientious. It also seems that most couples change methods from time to time and build up their own experience of effectiveness. The role of the doctor in giving advice should be to help the couple to choose the method which appeals to them most. Obviously many factors are to be taken into account, some of them rational and some of them extremely irrational. The degree of efficiency they require will depend on what they know of their fertility to date, whether they have had an involuntary preg-nancy, whether they were conscientious with previous methods, or whether it took them a long time to conceive when they did want a pregnancy, and whether their family is complete. Their choice will also depend on their capacity to pay, and to understand the use of the method and whether they are likely to attend for any necessary follow-ups. But there are other more emotional factors which only a doctor who is sensitive to the feelings, anxieties and doubts of his patients, and willing to give time to help them to articulate, will be aware of.

Given the opportunity, some patients discuss their sexual problems and anxieties which may or may not be related to birth-control methods, so that doctors giving this kind of help ideally should be able to deal with the associated problems their patients present; or at least they should know where to refer them. The doctor should avoid a rigid routine and should make it easier for an embarrassed patient to ask for contraceptive advice, and indeed should offer it routinely at post-natal examinations. Clearly, the doctor should be aware of the wide range of normal human sexual behaviour and be able to tolerate and accept whatever the patients bring up, should encourage them to enjoy their sex life and he must avoid increasing any feeling of guilt or anxiety over their sexual habits. However, he should not get involved unless he is able to deal with what emerges, and he should beware of probing the intimacies of people's sex lives to satisfy his own curiosity.

Choice of Method

There is no one ideal method of contraception. Such a one would have to be simple, cheap, readily available, foolproof, undetectable and require no effort; and clearly such a method is unlikely to be found in the near future, if ever. Every method has drawbacks; but as some are based on emotional factors, they do vary from one couple to another so that the doctor should be as free from emotional prejudices and preconceived ideas about what is good for his patients as is humanly possible, if he is to help the couple make their choice. If he can help them to choose what appeals most, so that they accept responsibility for their choice, they are more likely to use it conscientiously and will feel able to return for further advice if they want to change. They may not even want what they first ask for, not having realized what is involved—this is particularly likely to happen with new methods which are not so well understood. Where there are doubts it is helpful to recognize the reasons for wanting a particular method, e.g. a woman may be too embarrassed about genital examination to want the diaphragm or I.U.D. and may ask for the Pill to avoid this, or she may want an I.U.D. because no effort is involved—only to find it upsetting, as it is out of her control.

Where there are no complications and the couple can discuss and agree about what they want, it will only be necessary for one of them to come to the doctor for advice. Where there are stresses and strains or problems, where the birth-control method is used in the sex struggle, there are great advantages in interviewing both partners together.

So far we have been discussing those who actively seek advice; but just as some patients have to be persuaded into having polio injections for their children, fireguards for old people, etc., sometimes the doctor should introduce the subject of birth control and encourage action among those to whom inertia and irresponsibility come more readily than taking decisions for themselves.

Family planning advice is most necessary as a preventive medical measure, particularly among the larger families at the lower end of the social scale, for the incidence of maternal morbidity and mortality and the foetal and infant mortality all rise with increasing parity. At the time of giving such advice the effort should be taken for routine preventive measures —regular breast examination in any women over 35, gynaecological examination to detect any early disorder, and Papanicolou smear, remembering the higher incidence of abnormalities among the women of lower social grades and high parity.

Some Common Fears

In all such cases, however, there are many emotional feelings, fantasies, and anxieties concerning the use of birth control generally, or concerning particular methods which produce resistances. These anxieties should be understood when a choice is being made.

One widespread fear about using contraceptives is the fear of damaging the body in some way. This might be expressed as fear of childlessness afterwards, fear of cancer, or of interfering with nature. Some have a need to feel genitally intact and able to become pregnant—something which the 100% efficiency of the Pill threatens. There may be guilt over using contraceptives at all. Often sexual difficulties and incompatibilities, e.g. frigidity, premature ejaculation, etc., are blamed on the contraceptive method or on fear of conception; and only a method which will continue to provide this excuse will be acceptable, and any method which removes it will be intolerable.

Sometimes a husband is afraid of his wife being unfaithful, so that any method in her control may precipitate intolerable feelings of jealousy or may challenge him to greater sexual effort than he can cope with, so that he may dislike the condom but be even more against the use of anything by his wife. Because of its effectiveness, the Pill is particularly liable to produce such anxieties. Many men of course are delighted to find that the fear of conception is removed and that their sex life is improved. Some may fear that loving would degenerate into mere sexual pleasure. A husband who is unsure of himself and his ability to keep his wife may feel safest when she is pregnant, and anxious when no possibility of pregnancy exists.

Of course the birth-control method does not produce these fears; it only releases the latent anxieties or uncovers them where they have been hidden by projection on the birth-control method.

Legal Implications of Giving Advice

Attention has already been drawn to the advisability of obtaining the husband's consent before inserting an I.U.D. This does not apply to giving advice for methods, because they are self-administered by the woman and the husband has no legal right to be told anything of the interview his wife might have with the doctor, or of the method chosen, or of the advice given. Consent should also be obtained in the cases of sterilization and where there seems any prospect of legal action; it is wiser in such cases to have written consent. It is not necessary to have a husband's consent before carrying out an abortion on a married woman.

In giving advice to unmarried girls one should know their ages. Under the age of consent (sixteen years in U.K.) it is illegal to give contraceptive advice, even if the consent of the girl and her parents are obtained, although this would not apply to prescribing oral contraceptives if there were some medical reason or menstrual symptoms. This ridiculous situation does not apply to carrying out an abortion for medical reasons! If the girl is under eighteen but over sixteen, the parents should be consulted where possible, but only if the girl consents; and advice may be given to her even if she does not wish her parents to be consulted.

REFERENCES

1. MCLEAN MORRIS, J., WAGENEN G., MCCANN, T. and JACOB, D. 1967. Compounds interfering with ovum implantation and development. *Fertil. and Steril.*, **18,** 18.

X

TERMINATION OF PREGNANCY

JOHN G. HOWELLS

M.D., F.R.C.Psych., D.P.M.
*Director, The Institute of Family Psychiatry,
The Ipswich Hospital, Ipswich, England*

1

Introduction

From time immemorial means have been found to terminate unwanted pregnancies. Termination has been practised in primitive and developed societies.[35] It has been used whether it was legal or illegal. Today, as for countless centuries, organized society has to decide whether this measure is permissible, to what extent, and under what conditions. None of the issues discussed so feelingly today are new, except in that they are discussed against the background of contemporary society and in the light of developments in medical techniques. Termination of pregnancy is not a matter for the medical practitioner only; it also embraces philosophical, moral, religious, eugenic, social, political and psychological issues. A woman may well feel that the experts can be far removed from the truth if they fail to take into account her intimate, special, and profound feelings in her unique position.

The central issue in termination is that of the interests of the woman in her family and society, as against the interests of the unborn child. This dilemma has led to four general points of view on this central issue. They will be outlined and put in international perspective, before considering a number of important extra issues which impinge on the main viewpoints. Discussion follows on two special areas—the medical and psychiatric aspects. The management of termination will then be discussed and, in conclusion, an attempt made at a general appraisal.

The bias of the author is towards a liberal attitude; but, having acknowledged this, he will concentrate on putting the issues before the reader and leave him to formulate his own judgement. The coverage is international, but the recent discussions leading to the passing of the Abortion Act 1967 in the United Kingdom will allow of illustrations from practice in that country. The bibliography given here is selective. An extensive bibliography for the years 1960–67 is obtainable from the U.S.A.[17]

2

The Main Viewpoints

The reader will appreciate that each viewpoint is broadly drawn and each can have subsidiary and extra elements.

That there are No Grounds for Termination

This is one extreme viewpoint which sees the child as a human entity from the moment of conception and therefore considers his life sacred. Termination of pregnancy is the killing of an innocent human being. It asserts that to argue the viability of the child at any stage in its development is academic; every human being has a right to live; any deviation from this principle can only lead to moral compromise and undesirable consequences. Following conception, the natural course of events must be allowed to develop without unnatural intervention and the outcome must be governed by natural laws. This doctrine has an appeal in itself as well as the appeal of any absolute uncompromising attitude. It dictates decision by an obviously clear principle; it induces a feeling of security by assuming a predictability of events; it evokes sympathy by protecting the rights of a defenceless and innocent human being.

Some would adhere strictly to the above; others would depart from it when the choice is between the life of the mother and that of the child, arguing that the mother has an inherent right to live and that her destruction also destroys further potential life; in a particular set of circumstances the issue may be that of the interests of the unborn child against the rights of those yet to be conceived.

The above viewpoint is associated with that of the Roman Catholic Church since 1869 as proclaimed by Pius X. Prior to that time, Pope Sixtus V banned all abortions in 1588, but the ban was reversed by his successor, Pope Gregory XIV, in 1591. The Roman Church from 1591 until 1869[28] held that termination of pregnancy was permissible up to the time of "quickening", but forbidden thereafter. The Church does not allow termination as a method of contraception, although it accepts contraception in principle. However, it states that any method of contraception must not interfere with the natural act of intercourse as designed by God. Thus the safe period technique is accepted as a proper and natural form of contraception. "The pill", after prolonged discussion, is deemed "artificial" intervention and its use is not acceptable.

This viewpoint raises certain issues. What is a "natural" act; is *homo sapiens* not a part of nature and all his acts, *a priori*, "natural"? It raises the issue of when does the foetus have the attributes of a "human being". Its critics have pointed to its lack of realism in failing to take many of the facts of human existence into consideration, its impracticability, and thus its flouting even by Roman Catholics. A National Opinion Survey[33] in the U.K. showed that Roman Catholic women had illegal terminations in the same proportion as non-Catholic women; illegal abortion is widespread in Roman Catholic countries.

That there are Medical Grounds for Termination

For this viewpoint the term "therapeutic" abortion is often employed; it is essentially a medical viewpoint. The medical man sees himself as a healer. If healing is prevented, then there are grounds for intervention. Thus, if the life of the mother is threatened or there is danger to her mental or physical health, termination of pregnancy is deemed permissible. This is the basis of abortion law in many countries. It makes the medical man a central figure in the decision about the desirability of termination as the issues to be decided are essentially medical. Thus the doctor's position is frequently determined and defined by law.

It is possible to list physical conditions which, if they exist, may threaten the mother's life or may injure her physical health if the pregnancy is continued, e.g. cardiac failure, heart disease, hypertension, hepatitis, nephrotic syndrome, colitis, pancreatitis, post-obstetric complications, etc. Certain mental conditions may come in the same category, e.g. depression, risk of suicide, neurotic states, psychosis, mental subnormality, etc.

In determining what constitutes a "risk" or threat a doctor may be left to his own judgement. The United Kingdom Abortion Act of 1967 gives some guidance—the "risk" to life or health by continuation of the pregnancy must be greater than the risk in terminating the pregnancy. Even this formulation still calls for considerable individual judgement.

It is increasingly recognized that the foetus may be in hazard *in utero*. Thus, where there are grounds for believing that if the child is born it will suffer from severe physical or mental abnormality, then termination is desirable and permissible. Hereditary diseases must be taken into account. Indirectly the mother's health, especially her mental health, may also be at risk should her child be handicapped. If the above medical grounds are held to be valid, then usually little controversy arises in accepting clauses covering the situation of the deformed child and allowing termination because of this.

That there are Social Grounds for Termination

There are two general formulations here, one an adjunct to the medical grounds discussed above, and the other holding that social factors, in themselves, constitute grounds for termination.

The first point of view allows social factors, or the social environment at that moment to be taken into account in estimating the likely threat to the woman's life or health. It may even allow the future, or forseeable environment to be taken into account, e.g. what effect having another child might have on the mother's health in the forseeable future.

The second viewpoint regards an adverse social environment in itself as adequate grounds for termination, e.g. adverse effects on a marriage, inability to provide for more children, a turbulent emotional environment, poor material circumstances, the age of the mother, rape, etc. In a sense, most of these factors are not social but personal, i.e. they have an adverse effect on the emotional state of the mother and constitute a threat to her emotional health.

Social grounds lead to controversy. Criteria may be difficult to define; it may be feared that so many social conditions are being taken into account that abortion cannot be controlled and might become "abortion on demand". Others frankly regard legislation that includes social grounds as a means of gaining *de facto* "abortion on demand".

That Abortion should be Freely Available at the Request of the Mother

This is the viewpoint given least consideration, and yet is most widespread in the people most intimately involved, the women at risk. Indeed, given their head, there may be more abortions than births; in Hungary, for example, where termination is available on request, there are more terminations than live births. The term "abortion on demand" seems to have been introduced by its critics as a means of antagonizing the medical profession and guaranteeing little consideration or sympathy for this viewpoint. The more accurate term is "abortion on request".

Many women believe that all children should be wanted. Thus, if an unwanted pregnancy has resulted despite all the means of conception-control, then the final procedure of birth-control is termination, which should be permissible in the early months and, a smaller group maintain, in the middle months. Thus birth-control is extended into pregnancy. Women often refer to the matter as "starting a period". The woman would hold that she does not want her uterus to be trespassed upon by an unwanted pregnancy. She wishes to grow what is wanted, children should be born of love. She would particularly abhor growing a foetus forced on her, e.g. by rape. An unwanted child now may replace what may be a wanted child later on.

Supporters of this point of view hold that a woman does not usually regard the foetus in the early weeks as a child, as it is amorphous. She has no image of a child and she believes that she cannot kill something which has no reality for her. Termination, they maintain, primarily concerns women and not men, and it concerns largely married women with children; a mother does not bow to men, however learned, in her fondness for children. Acceptance of this point of view would also relieve women of the guilt forced on them by the community and on those who help her, particularly the nursing and medical professions.

Its protagonists hold that this is the only satisfactory answer to backroom or criminal abortion. When obstructions are put in the way of termination. the woman is forced to seek it by illegal means, to hide the widespread need for termination, and to subject herself to the risk of inexpert operators.

Only by having the right of decision themselves, with easy access to un-biased counselling, can women have true freedom. They maintain that liberalizing the law short of "abortion on request", even by allowing social grounds, does not eliminate backroom abortions, as for most women the impediments to seek help by legal means are too great. They point to the gross disparity between the few terminations allowed by the law and the actual widespread practice of termination by women.

Protagonists of this viewpoint regard the doctor as a counsellor and not a judge. The decision is the woman's. She feels that it is profitable to discuss the many aspects of the situation in which she is with an expert. As many of the considerations impinge on physical or emotional health, the expert is frequently a doctor, though not necessarily the one who will undertake the termination procedures.

In summary, this point of view holds that birth-control should be ex-tended into pregnancy and that a woman should have the right to ask that an unwanted pregnancy be terminated before the foetus has become for her an idealized child. We are asked to support her aspiration that all children should be wanted and loved and have an opportunity for happiness.

3

The Main Viewpoints in International Perspective

The following is an account of the position towards the end of July, 1970, a position which is continually fluctuating.

No Legal Termination

This is the situation appertaining by law in a small number of countries, e.g. Ireland, Belgium, the Philippines; in other countries the law may allow termination on medical grounds, but the climate of opinion may be such that the law is rarely employed, e.g. in France it is estimated that only 400 therapeutic abortions take place on medical grounds although the law allows termination. The position may fluctuate from time to time as mount-ing public pressure permits greater utilization of the legal position.

Termination on Medical Grounds

Here termination in general falls into two categories: (*a*) termination permissible in order to save the life of the mother, (*b*) termination permis-sible in order to preserve the health of the mother.

In 1966, 45 out of 50 States in the United States came into the first category. Until recently, it is estimated that between 1 and $1\frac{1}{2}$ million illegal abortions took place[43] as against 8,000 legal terminations. Recently the position has changed markedly as will be mentioned later, i.e. at least 13 States now have a more liberal policy and allow termination on the grounds of preserving the health of the mother, and at least three States have proceeded to the position of abortion on request. Psychiatric opinion[10] is an agreement with change towards more liberal views. Into this category also come such countries as Austria, Italy, Portugal, Spain, Turkey, India, Holland and Greece. In South America[4] in general the law allows termination to save the life of the mother, but its employment is not officially supported; it is held that thus illegal abortion in women aged 15–34 is the "first cause of death". Australia and Canada are also similarly placed, but in both countries there is a move towards the liberalization of the law and a possible approximation to the situation in the United Kingdom.

Legislation to preserve the health of the mother allows termination in France, China, Switzerland and in the German Federal Republic, where the estimated number of abortions is 1,036 legal and 1,000,000 illegal. Israel would come under this category, but because of a liberal interpretation of medical grounds and the fact that in practice account is taken of social grounds, the position in that country almost amounts to "abortion on request". (There were 26,000 abortions per year in the period 1966–68 as against 47,000 live births per year during the same period. During that period only one death due to abortion was recorded). Rumania had very permissive laws, but repealed them in 1966, and now termination is possible on medical grounds only (the grounds do include termination for mothers over 45 and mothers who have four children; the pregnancy must be under three months; early termination must take place in a specialized health unit). The following States in the United States have now liberalized their laws to conform to this category: Mississippi, Colorado, California, North Carolina, Georgia, Arkansas, Florida, Delaware, New Mexico, Oregon, Kansas and Arizona.

Termination on Social Grounds

Here also there are two categories: (*a*) where social grounds are taken into account when considering the medical grounds for termination, (*b*) where termination is possible on social grounds alone, without it legally amounting to "abortion on request".

In the United Kingdom, in the spring of 1967, the law was liberalized to allow the mother's social situation, both present and in the foreseeable future, to be taken into account when considering medical grounds for termination. Thus legal terminations have risen from 7,610 in 1967 to an estimated 75,000 in 1970. Half the terminations took place in hospital. An N.O.P.[34] survey, in February, 1970, showed that 66% of general practitioners thought that the law should remain in its liberal state, or be amended to make termination easier.

Liberalization of the law in the United Kingdom was only partial—a social clause added to medical grounds. A very liberal interpretation can lead to "abortion on request", but only if the doctor is moved to carry the law to its extreme. Some have argued that it would be more honest to admit what is necessary and provide abortion on request by law. Partial freedom still leads to backroom abortions. The estimate of at least 100,000 illegal operations per annum in the United Kingdom before the new Act, is not yet matched by the 70,000 operations estimated to be performed in 1971, i.e. a large number of women are still forced to seek illegal means, Furthermore, the illegitimate birth rate has fallen only minimally.

Before and after the new Act, large numbers of women with social/ personal grounds for termination were still denied consideration. Since the Act, married women in particular may feel neglected. Following the new Act, slightly more single than married women are having termination; it is unlikely that the purely medical grounds would be different in the two groups, but the hazardous social/personal position of the single woman is given more weight in the state of partial liberalization of the law. This arouses bitter comments such as the following from a married woman: "I have been a conscientious mother and wife, brought up a house full of children, and yet when I feel I can do best for my family by not having more children, I have less consideration than a prostitute."

In Japan 98% of terminations take place under clause 7 of their abortion law: "injurious to mother's health due to her physical and/or financial condition". There is a tendency for "designated physicians" to perform the operation almost "on request". In Sweden, Norway and Finland, in general, linked social and medical grounds are taken into consideration. The request is made to a panel; in Sweden 95% of the requests were granted. In all three countries there is a move towards further liberalization of the laws.

In Scotland, Iceland (since 1935), Argentina and Brazil it is possible under the law to undertake termination on social grounds alone, as well as medical indications. In Denmark termination is possible on social grounds on authorization of a doctor or an accredited maternity welfare organization.

Termination "On Request"

Termination on request of the woman has been possible in the U.S.S.R. since 1955. This has had no appreciable effect on the birth rate, but it is claimed that the criminal abortion rate has been abolished. After twelve weeks of pregnancy, however, termination is only possible on the grounds of the mother's health. All terminations take place in hospital.

Other countries have followed the lead set by the U.S.S.R., e.g. Hungary since 1956, (up to three months; 200,000 legal abortions in 1968), Poland since 1960, Bulgaria since 1960 (up to three months, but not for married women with no children), Czechoslovakia since 1957 (80% on social grounds alone. One in three pregnancies terminated; 100,000 terminations in 1968).

In Yugoslavia the position varies slightly in the six republics, but, in general, requests are made to "Commissions", 75–90% are granted. Medical and social grounds are taken into consideration. Permission is usually easy to obtain for the first termination and more difficult for the second. Recently there has been a tendency to be stricter in the interpretation of the law, and it is said that the criminal abortion rate has therefore gone up.

Three states in the United States now grant termination "on request". The new law comes into effect in Hawaii in March 1970 (there is a residential qualification). Maryland followed with regulations passed in March 1970 (there is no residential qualification), and the state of New York has recently passed legislation which allows termination when the woman and the doctor agree, except after the first 24 weeks of pregnancy (then it is permissible only to save the mother's life).

In some countries, e.g. Israel and Japan, the liberal interpretation of the law amounts almost to "termination on request".

Supposed Deformity of Child

In all countries where medical and social grounds permit termination of pregnancy, there is usually ready acquiescence to termination on the grounds that there is a high likelihood that the infant will be handicapped or deformed (one of the exceptions is the state of California in the U.S.A.).

Conclusion

In general, a wind of change seems to be blowing all over the world leading to greater liberalization of the law in relation to termination. This is particularly so in the United States and in the U.S.S.R. and her neighbouring countries. The same trend is evident in the United Kingdom and Scandinavian countries.

4

Related General Issues

Potential Life

One of the central issues in relation to the first viewpoint outlined above is the question of the extent to which it is permissible or desirable to destroy "potential" life. It seems to be universally held that demographic control is proper. With increasing knowledge, man now strives to limit population to a dimension that will offer the optimum conditions for his own welfare. Thus to control the number of children born, we destroy "potential life". Every act of population control, including every act of birth-control, even the "safe period" method, destroys potential life. Again, the refusal by a married couple to have children destroys potential life. One of the greatest destroyers of potential life is nature, by its process of spontaneous abortion.

Spontaneous Abortion

Spontaneous abortion is the expulsion without any outside intervention of a pre-viable conceptus in the first three months. One in three[47] of fertilized ova will never develop. One in ten conceptions[18] ends in spontaneous abortion, and the figure may be considerably higher.[48] There are grounds for believing that spontaneous abortion is more liable to occur in the case of an abnormal foetus. Many spontaneous abortions occur very early in pregnancy and will go unnoticed by the mother.

The Foetus as a Human Entity

This issue is not as clear-cut as it seems, because it involves personal, medical, legal, and religious considerations.

A woman may develop a very person-like image of the foetus from the moment of conception; it may be a psychological reality.[8] Often this psychological reality is associated with tangible evidence of pregnancy, swollen abdomen, swollen breasts, etc. For most women it is associated with "quickening"—a direct evidence of a child within the mother. For a few women this feeling never develops; right up to the act of birth itself there is denial. Awareness, reality and inescapability of the situation after birth is an important precipitant of post-puerperal depression. In a small number of women rejection of a child is permanent after its birth; when this is the case, the child merits being transferred to more accepting parents. Once the psychological reality has developed, a woman will be averse to destruction of what is now an infant. This variable factor should be elicited in any discussion of termination; once an infant is developed, the woman may wish for termination only in dire circumstances, e.g. direct and serious threats to her own life.

Nurses and doctors are members of the public, and thus share community and religious attitudes. In a special way they have direct contact with the foetus at any termination. Most doctors and nurses are probably prepared to be involved in a tedious exercise of birth-control early in pregnancy; many are sustained by a feeling of helping in the trying and difficult human circumstances of a particular case. During the later course of the pregnancy, at variable points, most would abhor the destruction of a recognizable child. There is room here for personal differences in viewpoint of individuals, which must be respected. At the point of recognizing the child, most members of the medical and nursing profession will feel it necessary to be assured that there are justifiable grounds for taking its life.

Legal definitions of viability vary. Islamic tradition maintains there is no life until 150 days (21 weeks approximately). The Shinto faith recognized life only at birth. In the State of New York it is deemed illegal to take the life of the foetus after 24 weeks; in the United Kingdom the period is 28 weeks, and the Church of England does not require baptism until then. Medical opinion denies that a foetus is capable of independent existence before 26–28 weeks. The law may be governed by the child's capacity for "independent existence" and therefore after this point its destruction is regarded as infanticide. However, the foetus usually becomes a reality to mothers and doctors long before the time accepted in such legal definitions.

All the above considerations, especially the mother's personal feelings, have to be borne in mind in a particular case. The law and medical practice, however, has to be based on generalities. "Quickening", at about 16–18 weeks, is a nodal point; this is underlined by the fact that the Church of Rome, when it accepted termination, regarded this as the "break-off" point. Aristotle[2] held the same view: "There must be a limit fixed to the procreation of offspring, and if any people have a child as a result of intercourse in contravention of these regulations, abortion must be practised on it before it has developed sensation and life; *for the line between lawful and unlawful abortion will be marked by the fact of having sensation and being alive*". (My italics.)

Many hold the opinion that it is desirable, whenever possible, to terminate before "quickening" is felt. Practical issues must be borne in mind. After about 14 weeks an abdominal operation may be necessary. In the first three months there is almost no danger, but thereafter danger and complications increase. These considerations are reflected in the practice of those countries where the law is most permissive; terminations are uncommon after three months. Thus medical, ethical and personal considerations suggest that termination should be carried out up to 12–16 weeks, after which it should be based on stringent grounds, such as danger to the health and life of the mother.

The "Back-room Abortionist"

There is a universal demand for termination, whatever "established opinion" may think. To many women the back-room abortionist is a public benefactor or benefactress. To many countries the back-room abortionist may be an asset; deprived of his or her practice, a country might be in severe straits. There is some evidence to show that some abortionists were originally themselves victims, who gathered expertise and became the sympathetic helpers of their friends. A survey in 1966[33] showed that 57% of women obtaining an illegal termination paid less than £1 ($2·5) to the abortionist. The work of the abortionist becomes less acceptable when a financial racket develops and when it takes place in circumstances that endanger the life or health of the woman. The mortality from illegal abortion is less than from legal; this is understandable as usually the legal abortion is performed on more difficult subjects. No one would deny the need to bring termination into the open where it can be conducted safely. The woman, however, will put safety second to confidentiality. Thus, only when legal abortion practice is confidential, sympathetic, and easily obtained, will back-room abortion become unnecessary. In Sweden, where the law is liberal, but not as liberal as some would require and where a formal procedure is required for abortion, Huldt[22] estimates that the criminal abortion rate has not been reduced.

Delay in Revealing Pregnancy

Study and resolution of the causes of delay may help women seek assistance in the desirable first twelve weeks. Occasionally the first "missed" period may be accompanied by some bleeding, a period assumed, and thus time is wasted. The many pressing unpleasant consequences of admitting pregnancy may make it virtually impossible for the woman to admit its existence even to herself; this denial may be very strong and, as mentioned before, it may persist until childbirth and beyond. At other times, while admitting the pregnancy to the self, the external circumstances, especially the attitude of the family, may be such as to encourage the hiding of the pregnancy. At other times the administrative circumstances are so difficult, e.g. unsympathetic authorities, as to encourage delay. Yet again, a woman's position may change with time, e.g. what was a loved child of a loved man with no need to consider termination becomes an abhorred situation if the man deserts her. Personal idiosyncracies are difficult to legislate for, but at least all the administrative procedures should be made simple, quick, confidential and sympathetic, so as to encourage early presentation.

Incidence of Termination

It has been estimated that 20–25 million abortions per annum take place in the world.[31]

It is difficult to arrive at the number of terminations performed in any country, as most are hidden; the more stringent the law, the more abortions are hidden; the number of legal terminations may be very small if they are possible only on limited grounds. In France, where there were only 400 legal abortions, it is estimated that there were 400,000 illegal terminations a year, alongside a birth rate of 800,000.[32] In the United Kingdom it is estimated that 10% of pregnancies ended in abortion before the new Act of 1967. It is even more difficult to arrive at what is optimally desirable. Liberalization of the law may, quite properly, stimulate the woman's desire for termination. Hitherto she may have accepted what was inevitable and resigned herself to having unwanted children; on eugenic grounds this is undesirable.

It is mistakenly thought that terminations are commoner in the unmarried than in the married. The reverse is true. One Survey[33] shows that 60% of illegal operations and 80% of legal operations were performed on married women.

Who Decides on Termination?

There are decisions to be properly made either by individuals, or parents, or families, or society. A woman would hold that the decision on termination should be hers. In one survey[33] only 31% thought that fathers had a right to prevent termination. A woman's body is her own and she cannot countenance trespass on it. The views of her husband or of either or both families may be antagonistic to her own and be the grounds for wishing termination. Husband or families may exert undue influence. However, usually the father or husband would be consulted by the woman. Should there be no consultation, it is unlikely that there would have been any profit in it.

A woman's true and intimate feelings cannot emerge unless she is given a confidential and tolerant hearing. It is difficult to see how any formal legal group or panel, however admirable in intention, can allow this. Observation of Scandinavian practice gives grounds for believing that panels discourage early presentation and lead to later terminations with less safety.

In the survey[33] mentioned above a substantial number of women (73%), sensibly said that they would wish to consult a doctor. It is desirable and necessary to ensure that the woman has thought about every implication of her situation, that her decision is realistic and unlikely to be regretted later. Where the law allows termination on medical, physical, and emotional grounds, then a doctor has to satisfy himself that he acts within the law and thus he makes a decision. If the law allows termination on request, then the doctor has to consider his own conscience only, and legislation should allow those who have moral or religious objections to opt out. However, such doctors may be expected to give aid in an emergency or if the mother is in danger.

In the case of a mother under 16, and usually with the girl's acquiescence, the parents should be consulted. Some hold that without her acquiescence it would be improper to consult the parents; they would undertake termination without parental consent, and certainly if in the interest of the girl's health. Over the age of 16 most people hold that the girl is capable of independent judgement, and parental consultation, unless requested by the girl, should not take place.

Early Adolescence as an Indication for Termination

Some countries allow termination in adolescents under 12, 14, or 16 years. It is held that a girl of this age would be too young to comprehend the effects of her actions and thus a pregnancy has an element of being forced. Furthermore, her tender years or circumstances make her unlikely to be a successful mother. There are clear exceptions to these general rules. Some countries regard the "tender years" as one of the conditions included under social grounds and thus independent recognition in law is unnecessary.

Rape

This is an independent ground for termination in some countries; an unwanted forced pregnancy which is abhorrent to the mother is regarded as grounds in itself. It may not always be easy, however, to establish that rape has occurred. Some countries regard rape as covered in the social grounds for termination.

Sexual Promiscuity

Some fear that a too easily available termination may encourage laxity of morals and promiscuity. However, the young are not as promiscuous as is generally believed.[42] Young people of today are also much more willing than past generations to declare openly their viewpoints and to reveal pregnancy. Thus extensive promiscuity, or illegitimate births might appear to be modern phenomena. There are very strong grounds for believing that they have always been with us in the same proportion, only more were undisclosed. Termination, however well conducted, is not an experience that women relish. The same arguments have been levelled at all the procedures of birth-control and, like all the procedures of birth-control, termination can have more advantages than disadvantages. Again, it is argued that if a woman is so irresponsible as to require a number of terminations, she is unlikely to make a satisfactory parent and thus the case for termination for such a woman is stronger.

The Unmarried Mother

The unmarried state of the mother is usually considered as one of the grounds that is covered by the social clause. The unmarried mother is more likely than the married to find herself not wanting the child. There are many exceptions to this, e.g. in some cultures pregnancy is an essential preliminary to marriage. Again, many young unmarrieds love one another and the coming product of their love makes termination unthinkable; many successful marriages start in this way. It is unwise, however, to force a marriage because of a pregnancy in the female partner; unloved partners make for unwanted children, and such a marriage is hardly the best milieu for a child. Some unmarried mothers, however, have such a capacity for mothering and strong affection for the child that they will accept it whatever their feelings for the father. Thus, even if deserted, they may, occasionally, wish to continue a pregnancy and after birth may wish to retain the child.

It is infinitely important to consider the feelings of each unmarried mother separately and uniquely. Some abhor the idea of the child, some are ambivalent, and some have the strongest maternal inclinations. Every case is unique and the mother should be given a sympathetic hearing and time to reveal her true feelings to herself. The lot of the unmarried mother is usually hard, and often made harder by the very people so quick to condemn termination of pregnancy; the morally rigid are rigid in all respects. Much can be done, and should be done, to alleviate the position of the unmarried mother and to allow her to bring up her child in the optimum circumstances for its happiness.

Adoption

This may be an essential procedure in some situations; children need to be wanted. In circumstances where a pregnancy has gone the full term and a mother has no feeling for the child, he will be infinitely happier with loving adoptive parents. In certain circumstances the love of the adoptive parents may be greater than that of the natural parents. In theory, given proper selection, no adopted child should lack affection; indeed, in general, he will be more fortunate than a child with natural parents, who is denied selection. A woman, however, cannot be expected to nurture a child through a pregnancy in order to produce children for the convenience of others. She wishes to nurture only a wanted child of her own. Herewith an apposite quotation:[41]

> She was relieved as the year passed and she didn't become pregnant, and when at last she found herself unexpectedly in this condition and was advised against having an abortion, she declared, "All right, I'll have the damned child and then I'm through." "I can't love that boy. I hated his father. I hated his father's people. I hated him before he was born, I've hated him ever since; I hate him now, and I'll always hate him."

Public Discussion

The public, and indeed the medical profession, may not always be aware of all the issues concerned with termination. Within professional bodies, special committees set up to consider such questions are often not representative of the opinions of the group they represent: elderly retired "establishment" figures are often found on these committees. Committees have two duties: (*i*) to give the people they represent an informed account of all the points of view; (*ii*) to consult these people by an unbiased questionnaire. In these circumstances it is often found that the electorate's opinion and those of its "establishment" may not coincide. In the United Kingdom, for instance, general professional opinion on termination is more progressive than that of the professional organs of opinion, e.g. a questionnaire addressed to 300 senior psychiatrists[21] in the United Kingdom revealed that 24% supported abortion on request, 56% wished for social situations to be considered, 16% wanted medical grounds only to be taken into account, and 4% had views different from the above. A National Opinion Poll in early 1970 showed that 66% of general practitioners in the United Kingdom wanted the liberalized laws left as they were, or amended to make it even easier to obtain an abortion.

5

Medical Issues

Incidence of Legal Terminations

The incidence of legal abortions per 100 live births is as follows: in the United Kingdom 6·8; in Sweden 8·35; in Japan 38·7 and in Hungary 135·6.[12]

Jurukovski[25] in a series of 18,258 Yugoslavian women showed that 72% were over twenty-five years of age and 28% under that age; 84% were married. Under a less permissive law, for instance in the United Kingdom, the number of single women may increase, e.g. 47% of legal terminations in 1968 were on single women, i.e. when there is a more stringent law, more attention is given to the precarious position of the single woman.

Risk

New techniques in medicine, including gynaecological techniques, are not without hazard; and it must be established whether the risk is a reasonable one to take and, in particular, whether the risk with abortion is less than with the continuation of pregnancy; pregnancy too has its hazards.

Illegal abortions are the main cause of maternal deaths[31] and may represent 30–50% of total maternal mortality in some countries. Death due to illegal abortion may result from embolism, rupture of the uterus (especially in the last months of pregnancy), septicemia (commonest), peritonitis, vagal inhibition of the heart (rare) and haemorrhage.

The death rate from all abortions has dropped remarkably in recent years in the United Kingdom and now averages about 35 per annum[1] in a population of 57,000,000 (0·04 per 1,000 total live births and stillbirths). This low rate is attributed to the advent of antibiotics and improved techniques.[30]

In England and Wales alone[12] during the first year of the new Abortion Act, the mortality rate for therapeutic abortion was lower than that for maternal mortality in childbirth—the maternal mortality rate for therapeutic abortions was 21 per 100,000 terminations and that for maternal mortality in childbirth was 24 per 100,000 total births.

Legal termination on high-risk patients is naturally more hazardous; the mortality rate for this group is estimated by Jeffcoate[24] to be a primary mortality rate of 1%.

However, the risk is much less for healthy patients undergoing termination in good conditions. One survey made in the year ending April 30, 1968, in the United Kingdom[23] showed 8 deaths in 27,331 operations, i.e. 0·03% approximately. The causes of the 8 deaths were: suicide after termination (2); pulmonary embolism (2); intravasation of abortifacient paste (1); anaesthetic catastrophe (1); acute myocarditis (1) and no cause assigned (1). The commonest non-fatal complications were retained products of conception, pelvic infection, haemorrhage and perforation of the uterus. Permissive legislation leads to a healthier sample of the population presenting early for termination in good conditions. For 18,758 patients undergoing abortions in hospital Jurukovski[25] gave a mortality rate of 0·01% (the two deaths were in patients with chronic heart failure).

In Czechoslovakia the mortality rate in 1963–67 was 2·5 per hundred thousand. In Hungary,[49] in 1960–63, it was 3·1 per hundred thousand; by 1964–67 the figure had decreased to 1·2. In both countries the great majority of abortions (99% in Czechoslovakia) are performed in the first three months. Lower figures are obtained in countries where a substantial number are performed after three months, e.g. in Denmark in 1950–57 (25·1 over three months) the death rate was 0·7 per thousand. Thus the stage of

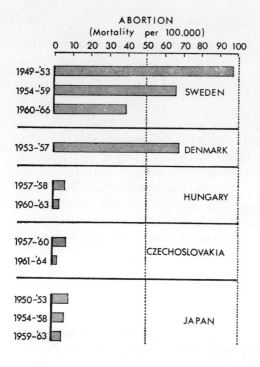

ABORTION
(Mortality per 100,000)

SWEDEN
1949-'53
1954-'59
1960-'66

DENMARK
1953-'57

HUNGARY
1957-'58
1960-'63

CZECHOSLOVAKIA
1957-'60
1961-'64

JAPAN
1950-'53
1954-'58
1959-'63

Fig. 1. Improving national mortality rates.

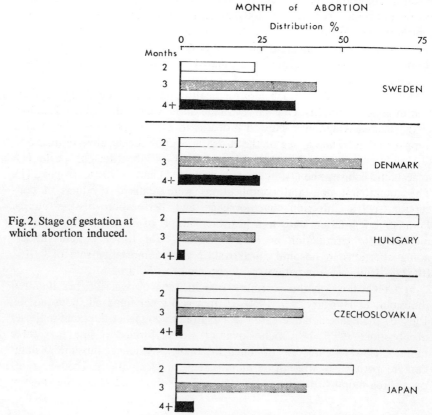

MONTH of ABORTION
Distribution %

Fig. 2. Stage of gestation at which abortion induced.

the pregnancy is a factor; in the first few months the risks are less than in the latter months. This point is made clearer by a comparison of Figs. 1 and 2.[46] Thus in Czechoslovakia now termination after the twelfth week is only possible on medical grounds, due to the finding that increased sepsis occurs with advancing pregnancy.

For healthy patients receiving legal abortions the rate of complication is 3·8%, but only 0·65% had to be readmitted to hospital for more than one day. Complications of induced abortion are secondary sterility, spontaneous abortion, miscarriage, ectopic pregnancy and slight prolongation of the third stage of labour in subsequent pregnancies.[27]

For healthy patients the risk in abortion performed in good conditions is less than the risk in pregnancy. The statistics point to the value of all terminations being conducted in good conditions under proper medical supervision in the first three months.

Illegal Methods

A variety of abortifacient drugs may be employed in the early weeks, ranging from gin to quinine and stilbestrol. Abortifacient drugs have been investigated by the Birmingham group of the Abortion Law Reform Association in the United Kingdom.[5] Failure with drugs leads to an attempt with a whole range of instruments, which in general are of two varieties: (*i*) penetrating, or (*ii*) injecting, e.g. injection of soap solution into the uterus via a Higginson's syringe.

New Techniques

Should the number of legal terminations increase, it is reasonable to expect that more thought will be given to developing new and safer procedures. In addition to procedures such as dilatation and curettage in the first trimester and, later, procedure such as open hysterotomy, amniotic fluid replacement by hypertonic saline, and intra-uterine paste, vacuum evacuation, first introduced in China in 1958, has been advocated as an improved technique. Kerslake and Casey[26] review the techniques. Dvorak *et al.*,[13] after the experience of a series of 1,500, emphasize the importance of early termination, as risk increases after the tenth week.

Of even greater value would be an effective abortifacient drug. In this connection experimentation is going on with intravenous infusions of prostaglandins.[39] In one study of 7 women (at or about the eighth week) there was a successful response in the first twenty-four hours. In 5 women (twelfth to sixteenth week) expulsion was successful in 3 of them.

Hospital Units

A permissive termination policy will make increasing demands on the medical service as patients move, desirably, from the illegal abortionist to the health service. Some argue that this creates an impossible demand on the hospital service; others regard it as manageable, and point to time saved by an effective abortion policy as fewer beds are then required to deal with the ill-effects of illegal abortion and the demand for obstetric beds is also smaller. In 1959 in the United Kingdom 70,000 women required hospital treatment for spontaneous and induced abortions. They each spent an average of seven days in hospital. After liberalization of the abortion laws in the United Kingdom in early 1970, 60% of all terminations were taking place in National Health Service hospitals, the remainder in inspected private nursing homes.[40]

It has been suggested by some that admission to highly expensive hospital beds is unnecessary. Special units[11] can be created with well trained medical staff, and they can cope with most demands; 48% of obstetricians in the United Kingdom favoured this course.[40]

Some have argued that, with training, a general practitioner can undertake the work. However, surgical intervention after the first three months is clearly a matter for surgical units in hospital or nursing home. In the United Kingdom all such units have to be registered with the central government. The medical profession must abstain from profiting from the misfortunes of patients; that this can occur within some private resources is undoubted. However, if hospitals restrict the number of patients admitted, then inevitably the burden will be transferred to private clinics. Thus a national service with the confidence of the public has much to recommend it.

Population Control

Controversy over the matter of termination of pregnancy inevitably leads to discussion of birth-control procedures. Many critics of birth-control, when faced with the less palatable process of termination, become advocates for it. Large-scale help, including both information and clinics, is required, especially in backward countries. In many countries, for instance in United Kingdom, governments have set up official birth-control clinics where advice and examination is free and aid is available at a nominal price. However, there are grounds for believing that some of the women who would benefit most are least able to take advantage of this scheme. For instance, in problem families, Howells[20] found that measures may be ineffective; one study showed that severe degrees of emotional illness found in such families lead to attitudes that make co-operation impossible, e.g. strong fears, traditional attitudes, desire to become pregnant, imposition on husband and wife of a child as an aggressive act or in order to keep the partner, apathy, inefficiency.

Diggory[11] found that in a sample in the United Kingdom of those coming for termination 30·5% used no contraception and 47·8% were unprotected at the time of conception. In a series from Birmingham, United Kingdom, the figures were respectively 45·8% and 73·5%.

More contraceptive measures usually lead to less need for abortions. If contraceptive measures are not possible, women may come to rely on abortion. Permissible abortion laws may not necessarily lead to a lower birth rate, e.g. in Russia it has not led to an appreciable fall of the birth rate. Abortion does not diminish a woman's capacity to have a child later or when her circumstances best allow of it. If contraceptive measures come into fashion, as for example in Japan, at the same time as a permissive abortion policy, the lower birth rate is assumed to be due to the abortion policy, when in all probability it is due to the contraceptive measures, the most effective controller of population.

It is estimated that there will be a world population of 6,000 million by the end of the century.[50] Abortion, even under the best care, is unpalatable, time-consuming, and inconvenient. Illegal abortion is more dangerous and more unpalatable. Thus, abortion should not be used as a means of controlling population, although it is a measure that sometimes leads to this. More effective procedures for population control are available to governments, e.g. a well organized birth-control service. Equally, denying termination should not be used as a means of increasing population. More effective means are possible, e.g. encouraging stable parents by financial incentive, housing, etc., to have more children. Such a policy produces more, and wanted, children. To restrict abortion produces more, but unwanted, children.

Sterilization

This procedure, either for male or female, can offer, in the right circumstances and ideally for a couple who already have an optimum number of children, a permanent and effective method of birth-control. In the United Kingdom in 1968, the sterilization rate for women admitted by obstetric and gynaecological wards was 4%.[46]

Medical Ethics

Some hold that medical ethics dictate that termination should be permissible only if it benefits the health of the patient in the light of all the relevant medical factors.[9] Such an interpretation would, for instance, make a plastic operation unethical. Furthermore "health" needs a wider interpretation, to include emotional as well as physical health and to include measures that promote public welfare. Again, it is not unlikely that the medical profession, like the public of which it is part, adjusts its ethical code from time to time; thus, should public opinion become more permissive, medical opinion may do likewise.

6

Psychiatric Issues

Social/Personal Grounds for Termination

In the United Kingdom before the Abortion Act, 1967, and exclusively in the area of medical grounds, one of the commonest grounds for recommending termination was psychiatric. There was considerable variation of opinion as to what constituted acceptable grounds from psychiatrist to psychiatrist and from area to area. Included, however, were the following categories.

(*a*) *Humanitarian.* The woman's torment was so compelling that phrases were used which allowed her being granted termination on grounds of danger to her mental health. This was a liberal interpretation of the abortion laws to allow forbidden personal/social grounds to be taken into consideration in practice.

(*b*) *Personality disorder, neurosis, precipitated by the pregnancy.* Because of the new situation of the pregnancy there existed a threat to the mental health, and occasionally to the life, of an otherwise healthy and stable citizen.

(*c*) *A threat to the mental health, or occasionally to the life, of a pregnant woman who already suffered from a psychiatric disorder.*

There is little doubt that most of the applicants came into category (*a*). This is supported by the fact that, since the new Act, which allows personal/social factors to be taken into account when judging the medical factors, psychiatric grounds are less often employed, i.e. social/personal factors can be taken into account *per se* when truly psychiatric factors are absent.

Clinical Grounds

These are:

(*a*) *Emotional disorder (including reactive depression).* This is the most common psychiatric illness. It can exist in the woman before her pregnancy. It can be precipitated by it. It is caused by the action of emotional stress upon a susceptible personality. Pregnancy may or may not be an added stress which damages health or even endangers life. The pregnancy can be of such consequence in a particular set of circumstances as to produce an acute neurosis in a hitherto stable person; it may even lead to suicide. On the other hand, the pregnancy can be, and sometimes is, used as a simulation of real stress. At other times a pregnancy can appear to be a stress to a woman, but on further reflection she can be reconciled to it. The true nature of the situation is a matter of clinical judgement of all the circumstances; however, the issues are so subtle that sometimes they not only lead to misjudgement, but also offer opportunities for a liberal interpretation of the law.

In summary, it can be said that emotional disorder in certain circumstances can be a threat to the health or life of a woman and so constitutes medical grounds for abortion. Sometimes psychiatric grounds are exaggerated and pressed into service as a means of circumventing a restrictive law. It is better, in the long run, to adjust the law.

(*b*) *Psychosis.* This is of two types: (1) organic: acute delirious states and dementia, or (2) functional: schizophrenia and manic-depressive psychosis. The acute organic states are physical in origin and rare; it is a matter for clinical judgement whether, when they arise, they constitute a danger to the mother. Dementia is rare in child-bearing age and would again be a matter of judgement of all the circumstances. Schizophrenia is largely unaffected by pregnancy;[45] fortunately schizophrenic women tend to be infertile. The genetics of schizophrenia are still so uncertain that the question of termination on grounds of possible hereditary transmission rarely arises. Most schizophrenic women have healthy babies. Advice can be sought from a genetic counsellor if there is much history of psychosis in the father's as well as the mother's family. Schizophrenic mothers are probably not as damaging to their children as neurotic women; they are usually neutral rather than positively harmful, but even so they are severely handicapped as parents. True endogenous depression, as distinct from the much commoner reactive depression, is probably unaffected by pregnancy; a woman heavily disposed to it, however, would find great difficulty as a mother. Each situation must be judged on its merits. The ability of a father to compensate for a mother's inadequacies would be an important factor in judging the desirability of termination in the above categories.

There is much to support the contention of psychiatrists such as Myre Sim[45] that if medical grounds for termination were based on psychiatric conditions alone, there would be a few terminations. But this would be true only if psychiatric conditions included psychosis alone. Neurosis is far commoner and includes many women with strong grounds for termination. It is imperative, however, to realize that most women seeking termination are well adjusted and thus psychiatric considerations do not apply.

(*c*) *Mental retardation in the mother.* Grounds arise on two accounts: (*i*) possible hereditary transmission to the offspring. It is a matter for genetic counselling to determine the probability of producing a handicapped child.[6] (*ii*) inability of the retarded mother to look after her child. This constitutes social grounds.

Reaction to Abortion

Here we must consider the immediate and long-term effects.

Sympathetic cheerful management can minimise the stress of the operation. There is some suggestion that following termination operations there may be more post-anaesthetic abreaction effects—depending upon the degree of pre-operative stress. Post-operative reactions call for counselling over moral, religious or social attitudes, as will be discussed later.

There is less sure agreement over the long-term effects. Some argue that the sense of guilt evoked by this destruction of the foetus may endanger subsequent mental health. A number of factors are at work—whether the feeling of guilt may be increased by doctors and nurses during the operation, by parental and familial reaction, by religious views, etc.; but the crucial factor is probably what the foetus and its father mean to the mother at that time. The average mother in the early months may have no feelings of psychological reality of the child; thus the reaction is minimal. Various studies support this contention.

Most investigations point to a minimal reaction to termination, the exceptions being studies by Ebaugh and Heuser[14] and Siegfried.[44] The latter found that 59% had some feelings of guilt or unhappy memories of the termination, yet felt it was the right course in the circumstances; 13% suffered from severe or persistent feelings of guilt, and half of these regretted the operation.

Ekblad[15] found that 25% of women experienced self-reproach or regret ("serious" in 14%), that the symptoms were generally mild, that few had consulted their doctors, and that only 5 out of 479 were unable to work. Niswander and Patterson[36] reported that two-thirds of the patients felt better immediately after termination and this percentage rose to 82.8% as time elapsed. McCoy[29] found that 73% of the patients studied were satisfied with the termination. Patt et al.[38] reported that, with rare exceptions, abortion was genuinely therapeutic. Clark et al.[7] found that of 120 patients only one was known to be emotionally worse after a termination. Whittington[51] found that the majority of 31 women who were surveyed after termination reported that they were content and mentally healthy. Baird[3] found that of 61 patients only 3 had some regrets as a result of changed circumstances. Pare and Raven[37] reported that in patients studied by them termination caused remarkably little psychiatric disturbance, provided the patient herself wanted the operation.

Reaction to Refused Abortion

This must be considered, as it relates to the mother and to the child. The continuation of the pregnancy is truly harmful to some women. Circumstances may be changed for the worse by the pregnancy; it may bring shame, desertion by the father, estrangement from the family, loneliness, loss of job, loss of career, financial difficulty, etc.

For the child it may mean persisting attempts at abortion by his mother which may or may not be successful, possible intra-uterine stress, a more difficult birth experience, rejection after birth, life with a single parent, and the stigma of illegitimacy. It can mean none of these hazards; after birth he may be accepted if his mother is fortunate enough to have good mothering capacity, or he may achieve safety and health with a substitute mother.

Available figures are not encouraging.

Hook[19] studied 249 Swedish women some years after a termination had been refused them; 23% had accepted the pregnancy, 11% had obtained an illegal abortion, 53% had a variety of "insufficient" reactions and 24% were still unadjusted at the time of the study. Clark *et al.*[7] found that of 109 women for whom termination was not recommended, 6 aborted "spontaneously", 12 obtained a legal abortion elsewhere and 20 obtained an illegal operation. Pare and Raven[37] found that 37% of women refused termination obtained it one way or another. Of the total only 49% kept the baby. One-third of the women who kept their babies regretted that termination had not been carried out. In unmarried women denied an operation, 86% got rid of their children in some way.

Forssman and Thuwe[16] conducted a follow-up study of twenty-one years on 120 children born to 197 women refused abortion. They employed a control group. They found that the unwanted children had a less secure family life in childhood, were referred more often to the psychiatric services, were arrested more often for anti-social behaviour, received more public assistance and had lower educational achievement. A high proportion (3:1) of unwanted children were reported to be living in unsatisfactory conditions, or to have been removed from them and placed in foster homes or children's homes. Of the 120 children born out of wedlock 27 were never legitimized.

These studies apply to those mothers who get as far as a psychiatrist. There are millions more who do not get this far, but, unrecorded, have to accept with their child the hazards of an unwanted pregnancy. It is here that many feel that a more liberal abortion policy, preventing unwanted children, and promoting wanted children, would have a major influence on the level of community emotional health. The presence of an unwanted child can prevent the birth of a wanted child; it may also prevent a marriage that could lead to a wanted child. Baird[3] compared, over a ten-year period in Aberdeen, the actual number of children born with the number of desired children. The number of children born was 30% more than the desired number. Of 226 women, 53 had 76 unwanted children.

Significance of Neurosis and Termination

Hook[19] made the observation that the patients most in need of termination on psychiatric grounds frequently made the poorest adjustment to it. McCoy[29] found that women terminated on social grounds made a better adjustment than those terminated on psychiatric grounds. Ekblad[15] came to similar conclusions. Jansson[23] found that not less than 50% of those who showed mental disorders after a legal termination had had previous psychiatric hospitalization. Hook[19] makes the further observation that women for whom an operation can best be justified on psychiatric grounds are more prone to adverse reaction if they do not obtain a termination.

It must be concluded that ill adjusted individuals react badly whether operations are granted or refused. Well adjusted individuals react well, whichever course is adopted. However, most women seeking termination are well-adjusted and their clinical state is not the grounds for seeking termination. Ill-adjusted individuals seeking termination require special care, whichever course is followed.

7

Management of Termination

Before Termination

By the nature of its imperfections, mankind has a habit of being involved in adverse, complex, subtle and perverse situations. Some of the factors turning around an unexpected pregnancy can be highly personal and touch on the most sensitive roots of human behaviour. A wife may find herself in a sudden, unexpected and unpremeditated situation involving husband, friends, colleagues and family. Others as well as herself can be painfully hurt. Life can turn upside down. It may seem worse than it is; it may be worse than it seems. It may be difficult to bring oneself to discuss some of these matters involving personal shame, hurt, guilt, embarrassment and humiliation, with a close friend. Discussion with a stranger may be still more difficult, unless there is a guarantee of sympathy, tolerance and confidentiality. Matters have to be broached that perhaps cannot be discussed with husband, father, mother, brother or friend. Denied the absolute condition necessary for trust, a woman may have no alternative but to seek an illegal abortion.

It follows that if the medical service is to offer the emotional as well as the physical help it must inspire absolute trust. This means a sympathetic, tolerant, unblaming, confidential milieu that allows the revelation and discussion of the innermost feelings. In most circumstances there is a great deal to recommend the family physician. There are times, however, when the very closeness of her own physician is an embarrassment, and the patient can be greatly helped if the physician is sensitive enough to refer her to a colleague. It is as serious a mistake to terminate a pregnancy that should continue as it is to continue a pregnancy that should be terminated. Only honest discussion can allow all the factors to be carefully weighed. Several interviews at short intervals may be required. When the factors are known, the practitioner's attitude should be guided by the law he is bound to observe and his interpretation of it. He must convey his opinion frankly, kindly, and with full explanation.

Speed is essential; early termination is to everyone's advantage. Procedures are easier, risks are less, attitudes are less well developed. Thus an organization that makes it quick and easy for a woman to attend, saves time.

Termination

As in a pregnancy, the psychological milieu must be considered throughout. Simple reassuring explanations are helpful. The support of relatives and friends, whenever this is possible, should be encouraged; the attitude of nurse and doctor will often dictate how easy or otherwise it is for relatives and friends to give support. Blame is destructive; understanding relieves.

Post-termination

The psychological and social situation that led to termination may still be present. Help by the physician, or referral elsewhere may be necessary. Encouragement at this point is therapeutic. The healing balm of "forgetting" should surround the termination itself. Advice on birth-control and sterilization may be apposite and welcomed.

Refused Termination

Should termination be denied, painful decisions have yet to be made—to marry or not marry, to keep the child or arrange for adoption, to tell or not tell the family, to give up a career or not, etc. The fullest understanding, and supportive obstetric and psychiatric service is called for.

8

Conclusion

The issues of termination of pregnancy are not only medical and psychiatric but also social, political and religious; and all these factors affect the law in relation to it.

Demographic control is universally regarded as desirable. Manipulating abortion policy is not an efficient procedure to this end. To prevent abortion can lead to more, but unwanted, children. Procedures available to society, such as family allowances, better housing, income tax relief, can lead to more, and wanted, children. A permissive abortion policy can lead to fewer children; but contraceptive techniques are more effective and desirable in lowering the birth rate. Termination of pregnancy is not the most effective birth-control technique. But in certain circumstances, where other techniques are not used or have failed, its employment is desirable and essential.

In general, throughout the world there is a movement towards the liberalization of the law in relation to abortion, so that birth-control can be extended into pregnancy. It is thought desirable to reduce the number of unwanted children. Other reasons are the need to eliminate illegal terminations with their attendant risks, to reduce the number of forced marriages and to relieve the anguish of women caught in an unexpected and difficult situation. There are some psychiatric grounds for termination. But the great majority of women seeking abortion are well adjusted and ask for abortion on non-clinical grounds.

The risks from termination conducted in the first three months on healthy women under proper medical supervision are less than the risk of continuation of the pregnancy. There is a proper tendency to discourage termination after twelve weeks because of the increased complication of procedures, with the consequent increased risks to the mother.

Many accept a liberal attitude to termination in the first three months, regarding the embryo as amorphous. Many hold that after sixteen weeks criteria should become strict and should normally be limited to purely medical indications as serious as a threat to the life of the mother. This is dictated by the repugnance of the nursing and medical profession and of the community in general to being involved in near-infanticide.

REFERENCES

1. Abortion Deaths. 1970. Notes and News, *Lancet*, i, 1238.
2. ARISTOTLE 320 B.C. *Politics VII, xiv*, 10. (Translated by Rackham, H. London: Heinemann).
3. BAIRD, D. 1967. Sterilization and therapeutic abortion in Aberdeen. *Brit. J. Psychiat.*, **113,** 701–709.
4. Birth Control by Catholics. 1968. *Lancet*, ii, 1196–1197.
5. BRIERLEY, A. F. M. 1966. "Abortifacients" on sale. *Family Planning*, **14,** 91–92.
6. CARTER, C. O. 1969. An ABC of medical genetics. VII—Genetic counselling. *Lancet*, i, 1303–1305.
7. CLARK, M., FORSTNER, I., POND, D. A. and TREDGOLD, R. F. 1968. Sequels of unwanted pregnancy: a follow-up of patients referred for psychiatric opinion. *Lancet*, ii, 501–503.
8. COBLINER, W. G. 1965. Some maternal attitudes towards conception. *Ment. Hyg. (N.Y.)*, **49,** 550–557.
9. Consultants' Report on Abortion. 1970. Leading Article, *Brit. med. J.*, **2,** 491–492.
10. CROWLEY, R. M. and LAIDLAW, W. R. 1967. Psychiatric opinion regarding abortion: preliminary report of a survey. *Amer. J. Psychiat.*, **124,** 559–562.
11. DIGGORY, P. L. C. 1969. Some experiences of therapeutic abortion. *Lancet*, i, 873–875.
12. DIGGORY, P., PEEL, J. and POTTS, M. 1970. Preliminary assessment of the 1967 Abortion Act in practice. *Lancet*, i, 287–291.
13. DVOŘÁK, Z., TRNKA, V. and VAŠÍČEK, R. 1967. Termination of pregnancy by vacuum aspiration. *Lancet*, ii, 997–998.
14. EBAUGH, F. and HEUSER, K. 1947. Psychiatric aspects of therapeutic abortion. *Postgrad. Med.*, **2,** 325.
15. EKBLAD, N. 1955. Induced abortion on psychiatric grounds: a follow-up study of 479 women. *Acta psychiat. scand.*, Suppl. No. 99.
16. FORSSMAN, H. and THUWE, I. 1966. 120 Children born after application for therapeutic abortion refused: their mental health, social adjustment, and education level up to age 21. *Acta psychiat. scand.*, **42,** 71–88.
17. GEIJERSTAM, G. K. (ed.). 1960–67. *An annotated bibliography of induced abortion*. Ann. Arbor. Michigan: Center for Population Planning.
18. HERTIG, A. T. 1967. In *Comparative aspects of reproductive failure* (Benirschke, K., ed.). New York.
19. HOOK, K. 1963. Refused abortion: a follow-up study of 249 women whose applications were refused by the National Board of Health in Sweden. *Acta psychiat. scand.*, Suppl. No. 168.
20. HOWELLS, J. G. 1966. The psychopathogenesis of hard-core families. *Amer. J. Psychiat.*, **122,** 1159.

21. HOWELLS, J. G. 1967. Doctors' Decisions. *Correspondence, The Times, 18th March*.

22. HULDT, L. 1968. Outcome of pregnancy when legal abortion is readily available. *Lancet*, i, 467–468.

23. JANSSON, B. 1965. Mental disorders after abortion. *Acta psychiat. scand.*, **41**, 87–110.

24. JEFFCOATE, T. N. A. 1960. Indications for therapeutic abortion. *Brit. med. J.*, i, 581–588.

25. JURUKOVSKI, J. N. 1969. Complications following legal abortions. *Proc. roy. Soc. Med.*, **62**, 830–831.

26. KERSLAKE, D. and CASEY, D. 1967. Abortion induced by means of the uterine aspirator. *Obstet. and Gynec.*, **30**, 35–45.

27. KOBAYASHI, T. 1967. Social problems of abortion in Japan. In *Fifth World Congr. of Gynaecology and Obstetrics* (Wood, C. and Walters, W. A. W., eds.). Australia: Butterworths.

28. LAMM, D. R. 1967. Quoted in *Time, 5th May*.

29. McCoy, D. R. 1968. The emotional reaction of women to therapeutic abortion and sterilization. *J. Obstet. Gynaec. Brit. Cwlth.*, **75**, 1054–1057.

30. MANT, A. K. 1969. The dangers of legal and illegal abortion. *Proc. roy. Soc. Med.*, **62**, 827–828.

31. MEHLAN, K. H. 1967. Frequency and mortality rate associated with induced abortions on a global scale (an assessment). In *Fifth World Congr. of Gynaecology and Obstetrics* (Wood, C. and Walters, W. A. W., eds.). Australia: Butterworths.

32. MICHEL, A. 1960. Quoted in a report on induced abortion. *Health Visitor, 1969*, **42**, 413.

33. National Opinion Polls, Ltd. 1966. Survey on abortion. London: Abortion Law Reform Association.

34. National Opinion Polls, Ltd. 1970. Survey on abortion. London: Abortion Law Reform Association.

35. NEWTON, N. 1966. Population limitation in primitive cultures. *Midwife and Health Visitor*, **2**, 429–431.

36. NISWANDER, K. R. and PATTERSON, R. J. 1967. Psychologic reaction to therapeutic abortion. I—Subjective patient response. *Obstet. and Gynec.*, **29**, 702–706.

37. PARE, C. M. B. and RAVEN, H. 1970. Follow-up of patients referred for termination of pregnancy. *Lancet*, i, 635–638.

38. PATT, S. L., RAPPAPORT, R. G. and BARGLOW, P. 1969. Follow-up of therapeutic abortion. *Arch. gen. Psychiat.*, **20**, 408–414.

39. Prostaglandins and the induction of labour or abortion. 1970. Leading article, *Lancet*, i, 927–928.

40. Royal College of Obstetricians and Gynaecologists. 1970. The Abortion Act, 1967. Findings of an Inquiry into the First Year's Working of the Act. *Brit. med. J.*, ii, 529–535.

41. SAYLES, M. B. 1936. *Substitute parents*. New York: The Commonwealth Fund.

42. SCHOFIELD, M. 1971. Normal sexuality in adolescence. In *Modern perspectives in adolescent psychiatry* (Howells, J. G., ed.). Edinburgh: Oliver and Boyd.

43. SCHWARTZ, R. A. 1968. Psychiatry and the Abortion Law: an overview. *Comprehens. Psychiat.*, **9**, 99–117.

44. SIEGFRIED, S. 1951. Psychiatrische Untersuchungen über die Folgen der Künstlichen Schwangerschaftsunterbrechung. *Arch Neurol. Psychiat.*, **67**, 365–388.

45. SIM, M. 1963. Abortion and the psychiatrist. *Brit. med. J.*, ii, 145–148.

46. STALLWORTHY, J. 1970. Therapeutic abortion. *Practitioner*, **204**, 393–400.

47. STEVENSON, A. C., DUDGEON, M. Y. and McCLURE, H. I. 1959. *Ann. hum. Genet.*, **23**, 395.

48. TIETZE, C. 1953. Introduction to the statistics of abortion in pregnancy. In *Pregnancy wastage* (E. T. Engle, ed.). Springfield: C. C. Thomas.

49. TIETZE, C. Quoted in *Med. Tribune, 5th June, 1969*, page 10.

50. The uses of this world. 1970. Leading article, *Lancet*, i, 1039.

51. WHITTINGTON, H. G. 1970. Evaluation of therapeutic abortion as an element of preventive psychiatry. *Amer. J. Psychiat.*, **126**, 1224–1229.

XI

SPONTANEOUS ABORTIONS AND MISCARRIAGE

EDWARD C. MANN

M.D.

Chief, Obstetrics and Gynecology,
Earl K. Long Memorial Hospital,
Baton Rouge, Louisiana
Assistant Professor of Obstetrics and Gynecology,
Louisiana State University School of Medicine
U.S.A.

1

Introduction

Spontaneous abortion may be defined as the expulsion of a previable conceptus in the prior absence of outside initiation or intervention. The expulsive process is termed *complete* if the products of conception are completely expelled; and *incomplete* if a portion (usually the placenta) remains in the uterus. Since, in the United States, the word "abortion" connotes, to the lay mind, criminal interference, the term "miscarriage" is generally used as a more "natural" synonym to describe all spontaneous abortions, whether occurring relatively early or late in pregnancy. In the British Commonwealth, on the other hand, spontaneous "abortion" usually refers to abortions occurring in the first trimester of pregnancy; and "miscarriage" to abortions occurring after the third month of pregnancy.

Although there is a single recorded case[35] of a conceptus weighing less than one pound (397 grams) which survived and developed normally, the odds for survival of a conceptus weighing even 800 grams is relatively infrequent. Accordingly, the statistical tendency is to define abortuses by weight. Thus, a conceptus weighing 400 grams (approximately 20 weeks gestational age) is, on the basis of almost certain previability, termed an abortus. Those weighing between 400 and 1,000 grams, again on the basis of improbable viability, are still termed abortuses by some institutions, and immatures by others. Since with each 100-gram increment in weight, beginning at approximately 1,000 grams, there is a significantly progressive increase in the chance for viability, prematures are usually defined in the

United States as those infants weighing between 1,000 (approximately 28 weeks gestational age) and 2,500 grams (approximately 36 weeks of gestational age).

For years the incidence of spontaneous abortion has been cited as 10% of all pregnancies. Because very early abortions may not come to the attention of reporting institutions and because recent, ostensibly more meticulously researched studies suggest that the incidence may be as high as 15%,[47, 48] the question of incidence remains moot.

2

Etiology

The great majority of spontaneous abortions occur during the first trimester of pregnancy. Since in the early months of pregnancy spontaneous abortion is almost invariably preceded by the death of the conceptus, the question of etiology hinges upon the cause of death. Many leading pathologists,[14] noting pathologic changes or anomalies in the embryo or placenta and, more commonly, hydatiform degeneration of the villi, have invoked the theory of defective germ plasm. Others,[17] have interpreted the "blighted" conceptus as an *effect* rather than a *cause*, and have sought to establish causation at an earlier remove of pregnancy when, through decidual hemorrhage and consequent aberrations of feto-maternal interrelations, the conceptus is deprived of vital transfer and organizing mechanisms, and is thus foredoomed to developmental failure and death.

While the number of possible causes for spontaneous abortion are legion, the vast majority of such causal factors occur accidentally and recur on the basis of chance alone. That accidents not infrequently occur is readily understandable when one considers the precise physiologic and temporal requisites of fertilization, ovum transport and nidation. That such accidents are largely the result of random causal factors is attested by the self-limiting nature of most spontaneous abortions. Thus, Malpas,[26] in his study of 6,000 abortions, was the first to discriminate between the habitual aborter, who aborts from truly recurrent causes, and the successive but non-habitual aborter, who aborts from chance factors which are repeated on the basis of randomicity. His findings, largely substantiated by Eastman,[9] are based upon the spontaneous cure rate in sequential abortion; that is, in the face of a previous abortion or abortions, the likelihood of the next pregnancy continuing to term without any treatment is significantly related to recurrent causal factors. Accordingly, if a woman has had one previous abortion, she has a 78% chance of spontaneous cure; with two previous consecutive abortions, she has a 62% chance; with three, 27%; and with four, only a 6% chance of carrying a pregnancy to term. In view of these findings, he concluded that the occurrence of three or more successive abortions is almost certain evidence that the sequence is due to recurrent causes and, consequently, that after a woman has had three consecutive abortions, she may be regarded as a segregated habitual aborter.

Since the vast majority of spontaneous abortions are due to non-recurrent causal factors and since the cause of a given spontaneous abortion is usually difficult to determine clinically, most investigations of spontaneous abortion have dealt with the study of the abortus by the pathologist and, more recently, by the chromosomists.[7, 38]

While the study of the abortus continues to occupy the attention of the microcopists, the study of the aborter has come increasingly, to occupy the attention of the psychologist, psychiatrist and psychiatrically-oriented obstetrician. Whereas some of us have chosen to study non-habitual spontaneous aborters[25, 34] or, to compare them, for example, with women who have undergone therapeutic abortions,[43] others,[3, 49] including the author, have chosen to study habitual aborters in whom emotional determinants, as causative agents of spontaneous abortion, can be more convincingly formulated.

The reasons for this are several. If, as a study group, only those women who have had at least three consecutive abortions are included, the investigator is almost assured of some underlying recurrent causal factor. Moreover, if the study group is carefully screened[16, 33] for discernible abortigenic pathology (such as uterine anomalies, hormonal inadequacies, tumors or demonstrable sphincteric inadequacy), there remains in an unselected study group a great majority, on the order of 85%, who abort from etiologically indeterminate causes. Such study groups, in the past, have been successfully treated by remarkably diverse regimens.

Indeed, the types of therapy to which they respond are so varied, in terms of rationale, as to be without consistency. A voluminous literature has appeared, which cites a variety of mechanismal processes which purportedly give rise to chronic abortion. Thus, briefly and incompletely, defective germ plasm, hormone and vitamin insufficiency, incapacity and malposition of the uterus, chronic infection and blood group incompatibility have all been specifically cited as antecedent mechanismal factors giving rise to recurrent spontaneous abortion.[1, 2, 6, 12, 17, 19, 22, 36, 37, 39, 40, 41, 51, 52] Evolving with these theoretical pronouncements have been specific treatment programs[4, 5, 8, 20, 23, 44, 50] which range from vitamin and hormone regimens (vitamins E, C and K; thyroid, progesterone, estrogen, relaxin and cortisone—alone or in combination) to bed rest[45] and sexual abstinence to removal of foci of infection. Each of these "specific" therapies, in the hands of certain investigators, has been productive of results which, when compared with statistically derived spontaneous cure rates, range from good to excellent.

Such success with such divergently "specific" therapies led to the premise that perhaps the curative process was mediated through some convergent factor common to all of the varied therapies and that this common factor had to do with the therapist's personality and, in turn, with the witting or unwitting psychotherapeutic use made of it in relating to abortion-prone women.

3

Investigation of Emotional Determinants

Although obstetricians and psychiatrists[3, 17, 21, 27, 46, 49] had postulated relationships between emotional factors and habitual abortion, very little validating information from a psychodynamic standpoint was reported. In an effort to establish more solidly the role of emotional determinants in habitual abortion and in a further effort to delve into the nature of such determinants, of how they might operate in the production of abortion[11, 13, 18, 21, 24] and of their modifiability, a nine-year study of over 400 habitual aborters was undertaken at the New York Hospital-Cornell Medical Center and in private practice.[28, 29, 30, 31, 32, 33] This study, the largest of its kind ever conducted, was limited to those randomly-referred women who presented histories of having had at least three consecutive spontaneous abortions. The number of consecutive abortions per patient in this group approximated 4 and reached as high as 13. Just over 75% of the group were *primary* habitual aborters, which is to say that the abortion sequence occurred in the absence of a prior term pregnancy; whereas nearly 25%, having sequentially aborted after previous parity, were *secondary* aborters.

Method

Each patient was seen preconceptionally in a series of psychiatric interviews. Interspersed between preconceptional interviews were comprehensive gynecologic, endocrinologic and radiographic examinations and, during most of the study, a battery of psychological tests (Wechsler Bellvue, Rorschach, Thematic Apperception, House-Tree-Person and Sentence Completion Tests), administered by a clinical psychologist. With few exceptions, the husband was also seen in at least one preconceptional interview.

Since one of our major premises was that "therapy", whether mediated indirectly, under the medicated guise of adiaphorous pharmacologic agents, or directly, in the manner of psychotherapy, was related to the doctor-patient relationship, we settled upon a supportively directive type of therapy. This approach, not unlike so-called adjunctive psychotherapy, was purposely chosen inasmuch as it represented a technique utilized by many obstetricians and one which was within the capabilities of many more. At the same time, the technique was extended beyond its usual evaluative limits so that it might double as a method of psycho-dynamic investigation as well as a method of therapy. While the interviews were geared to uncover basic psychodynamic information they were, from a therapeutic standpoint, utilized to acquaint the patient with the possibility of an emotional approach to her abortive difficulties and of then gaining her confidence in this approach. Although the method utilized uncovering techniques and, to a limited extent, "insight", it was for the most part an experiment in relationship therapy. That is to say, less emphasis was placed upon the "packaging" of interview material for the patient in the interpretive form of insightful disclosure than upon hearing the patient out and being available to act as confessor, supporter, provider or intercessor, as the case might be. These patients invested heavily, from an emotional standpoint, in the relationship and were generally able to turn the investment to profitable account in terms of increased self-assurance.

Following several searching interviews designed to provide the therapist with both a working knowledge, and the beginnings, of a close relationship with the patient, she was told to become pregnant when she felt ready. Once pregnant, she was seen at weekly intervals, inasmuch as early pregnancy is fraught with misgivings for such patients. During the prenatal visits, each patient underwent a routine antepartal examination which served to allay immediate fears concerning any aches or pains of pregnancy which, in retrospect, might have ominous meanings. Following examination, the patient was seen in interview for periods of time ranging between fifteen minutes and an hour, depending upon the patient's need of reassurance. Added to the weekly visit were instructions to call in the event of any alarming disturbance. Usually, after being so instructed, the patient, through contrivance or necessity, put through a test telephone call which was always taken seriously by the doctor. Once satisfied in this respect, few found it necessary to call again. Occasionally, in the predisposed patient, efforts were made to extend the limits of permissible dependency implicit in the doctor-patient relationship. Although the latitude allowed the individual in this connection was flexible, the degree of dependency beyond a reasonable point was curtailed owing to its destructiveness to the patient and to the therapeutic relationship which was designed to help the patient help herself.

This is not to gainsay the constructive value of a limited dependency relationship in the management of these patients, since many of them, for reasons to be later discussed, cannot relate confidently except in a dependent fashion. Accordingly, the patient preconceptionally and in early pregnancy was allowed to become increasingly dependent upon the therapist.

Once pregnancy had progressed to the point of near fetal viability, increasing emphasis was placed upon the unborn child, whose advent and the approaching birth served to dissolve an otherwise unhealthy transference relationship. This shift in emotional focus was mediated through the interview situations, which came to be taken less and less with the patient and more and more with the baby; through external agencies such as preparation for labor courses, and—most important—through the patient's growing pride and self-confidence in having finally progressed from unexpectant to expectant motherhood.

General Results

Of the 175 gynecologically "normal" habitual aborters treated on a psychotherapeutic regimen and followed through a pregnancy, 81% were delivered of term infants.

Our failures were instructive from several standpoints. One, for example, who had lost each of her previous pregnancies in the first trimester, did quite well throughout the first four months of her last pregnancy. At the end of that time she called, stating that she had "felt life" for the first time. When told that this was normal and in keeping with the duration of pregnancy, her reaction, instead of being characterized by elation, was one of increasing anxiety. For the next few nights she was recurrently subject to nightmarish dreams and phobic fears of being alone. Shortly thereafter, she came in tremulous and panicky with the hallucinatory complaint of hearing "little fetal hearts" all over her body. She aborted within the week.[10] Significantly, the patient's anxiety disappeared almost immediately following her miscarriage.

Others required time to unglue, as it were, a sticky dependency relationship. Some of these dropped out of the study; whereas, others continued with us, a few of whom (approximately 10%) subsequently carried a pregnancy to term.

Our successes, on the other hand, proved to be sustained by success, the abortive relapse rate having been nil. Indeed, their newly-gained "carrying power" seemed, in translated terms of ego strength, to have had an extended carrying power of its own. With the exception of one successfully treated patient, who developed post-partum depression which responded to psychotherapy, none in the group under study developed postpartal psychiatric difficulties. Instead, they addressed themselves to the long awaited role of motherhood with pride and enthusiasm. While some, by virtue of healthier personality organizations, made better mothers than others, they, on the whole, seemed to be not very far from average in their adequacy as mothers.

4

Psychopathology

The investigation leads to the following general formulations.

Familial Relationships

Mother. In general, these patients share in a dependent type of relatedness to parental figures and parental substitutes. This is most marked in their relationship to the mother who, as a rule, was the dominant, constant and dependable parent. The degree of dependency upon the mother is intense and is most remarkable for its contingency. That is to say, the mother has a needful way of habituating the patient to dependency and of then using the habituation, on pain of withdrawal, to engulf the patient in a "little-steps-for-little-feet" continuum. In this way, she continues, out-datedly, to cultivate the patient's dependency needs, which become progressively more utilitarian to the patient as she enters the prepuberal and puberal years and comes to realize, subliminally, that if her relationship with mother is to remain on an intimate basis, it must continue within a context of childlike dependency. In short, the mother is dependent upon the child's dependency and, in consequence, seeks anachronistically to preserve the relationship, to the developmental detriment of the child.

Father. The degree of detriment, particularly as it relates to psychosexual development cruxes, in large measure, upon the intercessive role taken by the father. That is to say, in the presence of a good father-daughter relationship the father can, by supportive intervention, lessen the child's dependent investment in her mother by increasing her investment in him. In the process, a buffering balance is struck, which provides the child with offsetting stimuli and incentives to more counter-dependent growth.[15] Compensatory resolution of this order is lacking in the habitual aborter whose relationship with her father is usually far less than optimal. Indeed, one of our most consistent findings was paternal absence or inadequacy.

A sizeable proportion of these patients were deprived of their fathers by death, desertion, or divorce. For the majority, however, the paternal deprivation was merely relative and took the form of inadequacy. The inadequacy usually derived from the father's loss or forfeiture of parental status. Not infrequently, his parental status was compromised by situational determinants such as chronic invalidism or by irresponsible behavior which took the form of alcoholism, gambling or philandering. More often, his inadequacy was of a comparative sort wherein, by virtue of his passivity, self-distant unconcern or ineffectualness as a provider, he invited, or at least did not contest, supersedence on the part of his wife who, by his default, assumed a matriarchal role. In some, this had less to do with the father's defectiveness than with his wife's need to dominate the marital and parental scene. Indeed, the evidence indicates that the more controlling mothers of habitual aborters bear an unconscious contempt for men and, in consequence, select husbands who will either tolerate or justify this contempt. This latter type of mother was most frequently evidenced by the secondary aborters.

Resultant Psychosexual Patterns

Be the variations as they may, there usually results a marital relationship which, at the parental remove, is weighted heavily in the direction of mother who, through necessity or design, emerges as the child's indispensable provider. In the absence of intercessive action on the part of the father, the child is typically delayed in her psychosexual maturation. Having always compliantly depended upon mother, and never having experienced a close relationship with her father, she is retarded in her heterosexual growth.

Such patients give an almost unvarying account of their adolescent years which, in effect, are but elaborated extensions of their prepuberal years. That is, at puberty, unlike their peers, they fail to develop the usual interest in boys.

Instead, their after-school hours are usually spent at home with mother. Following graduation they tend to obtain employment, remain at home, and continue the even tenor of their dependent ways. Frequently, they do not begin going out with boys until their late teens, and even then there is little of the romantic in their attachments. Often, even among the very attractive, they marry the first interested man who comes along. He is usually a reliable sort and, following marriage, becomes, in some respects, less a husband than a substitute for mother.

Although this pattern, particularly among primary aborters, is often seen in stereotyped form, it is subject to variation. The most significant variation obtains when the father assumes an intercessive role which has seductive overtones. In such instances, the father, who was unable or unwilling to relate constructively to the child in her earlier years, develops, coincident with puberty a more active interest in her. Frequently, this interest takes on a punitive form, in which the daughter, with the development of second-ary sexual characteristics, becomes, in the eyes of the father, suspect. This, at times, reaches fantastic proportions, as is exemplified by the following case history.

Case History

Mrs. S., a 26-year-old primary habitual aborter, was seen in con-nection with her presenting complaint of an inability to carry a preg-nancy to term. During her four years of marriage, she had become pregnant on four occasions, losing each pregnancy at periods of gesta-tion which ranged from two to four months. Gynecologic work-up, including a hysterocervicogram, was entirely negative. History revealed her to have been an only child, born of an alcoholic father and a possessive, overprotective mother. In recalling her childhood she re-members her mother as the dominant parental figure to whom, in the almost continuous absence of her travelling-salesman father, she was quite close. On those weekends during which the father was at home, he maintained a formal attitude toward the patient when sober, and an indifferent attitude toward her when drinking, at which time he often consigned her to backyard play while he and his wife "went to bed".

The patient's menses began at age 15 and from the outset were irregular with frequent "skipped" periods. Shortly thereafter, the father, who until then had never taken much note of the patient or her activities, would, on his visits home, question her darkly as to her heterosexual activities, and on the occasion of one of her skipped periods intimated that she might be pregnant. When the patient began dating, he was studiously impolite to her suitors and became even more accusatory of the patient. Once, after an argument with her father over her dating activities, she became "hysterical" and fainted, whereupon she was immediately taken to the family doctor for a pelvic examination to confirm the father's suspicion of pregnancy. When his suspicions were not confirmed, his comment to the patient was, "better luck than management."

Shortly after this episode, the patient began seeing her suitors, surreptitiously rather than at home and entered into her first sexual relationship. This was followed by a long period of almost compulsive sexual promiscuity, during which time she became pregnant on three occasions and underwent three criminal abortions. Following the third abortion, she "took hold" of herself, became sexually abstinent, and two years later married. Following her marriage she became vaguely preoccupied with a fateful need on her part to somehow "pay the piper" for her past misdeeds, and on the occasion of her first spontaneous miscarriage was almost relieved in her retributive belief that, to undo the three "illegal" abortions, three "legal" abortions would be necessary. Accordingly, she entered her next two pregnancies with no hope of carrying them to term and experienced their termination in spontaneous miscarriage with predestined acceptance. Having thus "balanced the books", she approached her next pregnancy with elation and high hope, only to spontaneously miscarry again in the fourth month of pregnancy. Following this latter miscarriage she became depressed and, despairing of a self-cure, presented herself at our hospital.

While the father figure in the foregoing summary plays a more obvious role in the abortigenic life of his daughter than most, he was purposely chosen to illustrate several points which bear upon the problem of habitual abortion. In the first place, the father's behavior toward his daughter, however sadistic and projective it may be, is telling in its provocative effect. It is irrational behavior, which by communicative implication is at once incitive and retributive. In this perverse respect it contains a logic all its own, which, if we may borrow from Lewis Carroll, is ironically expressed in the following lines:

> Feed pepper to your little girl
> And whip her when she sneezes.

The patient, in attempting to understand her father's behavior, comes to define its punitive denotations in terms of its spiced connotations. Accepting her father's sexual estimate of her, she then, under parental directive, one might say, compulsively acts out a sexual role which justifies this estimate. In so doing, she is obliged to keep "double-entry book" on her compulsivity. That is, she is simultaneously compelled toward sexual transgression and to punishment for her sexual transgression. In the premarital context punishment takes the form of illegitimate pregnancy and is both compounded and expiated by submission to a criminal abortion. Following marriage, and despite its sanctions, sexual activities retain their transgressive connotations, and pregnancies their punitive denotations, with the result of expiatory spontaneous abortions.

Anniversary Aborters

Before leaving the subject of expiatory spontaneous abortions, reference should be made to an almost "horoscopic" predilection on the part of many of the habitual aborters to attone, recidivistically, for past sexual misdeeds. In this connection, approximately one-fourth of the study group presented histories of pre-marital criminal abortions. This sub-group, which clinically

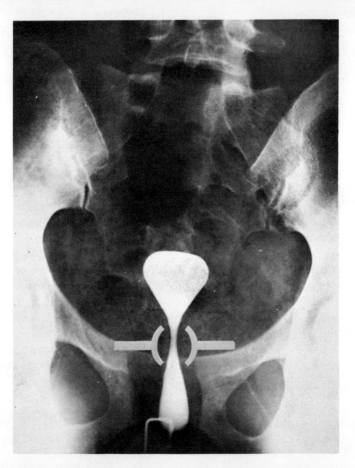

Fig. 1. This radiographic plate, when compared with Fig. 2, illustrates the determining importance of an intact isthmic sphincter in the physiology of normal pregnancy. The isthmic segment (See brackets), is a functional sphincter, clearly demonstrable in the non-pregnant state, which is essential to the prevention of gestational incontinence. The device we developed for demonstrating isthmic tone, preconceptionally, consists of a two-stage intra-uterine balloon which, when filled with a radiopaque medium, expands first within the uterine cavity then, with increasing intracavitary pressure, secondarily expands within the isthmus and cervix.

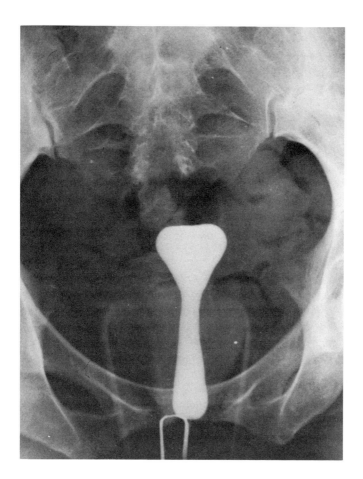

Fig. 2. This radiographic study reveals the preconceptional absence of isthmic tone. Such isthmic hypotonia, particularly in the luteal phase of the menstrual cycle, correlates very closely with the development of cervical incompetence during pregnancy. The isthmus, preconceptionally, is a functional sphincter whose tone varies according to the menstrual cycle. Thus, the isthmus normally becomes atonic during the menstrual phase of the cycle; hypotonic during the pre-ovulatory phase of the cycle; and hypertonic during the post-ovulatory phase of the cycle and during pregnancy.

Another investigative use to which the two-stage balloon has been put has been in the area of primary dysmenorrhea, where it has revealed, in the majority of instances, failure of physiologic isthmic atonia to develop with the onset of menses. Instead, the isthmus remains constricted and produces a functional barrier through which the products of menstruation are painfully forced.

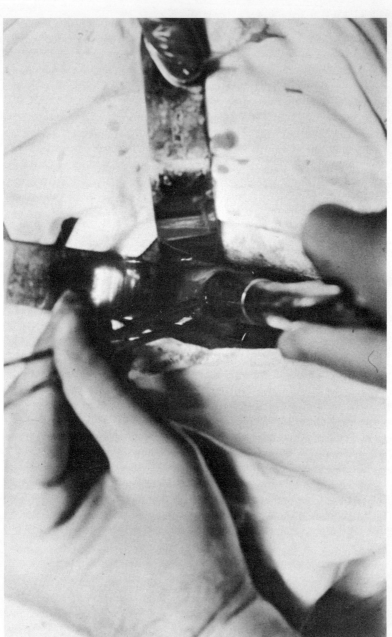

Fig. 3. Since the two-stage balloon requires fluoroscopy and rather involved manometric safeguards, a good clinical tool for determining cervical incompetence is the Hegar dilator. The isthmic segment in the post-ovulatory phase of the cycle will normally offer marked beginning resistance to a number seven dilator. If a number seven can be introduced into the isthmic segment without constrictive resistance, a diagnosis of incompetence is justified—provided concomitant endometrial biopsy or curretage reveals post-ovulatory endometrium. Anovulation, including anovulation produced by birth-control pills, results in isthmic hypotonia and renders the Hegar test unreliable.

In this illustration the isthmic-cervical segment offered virtually no resistance to a number 11 dilator. This was due to an

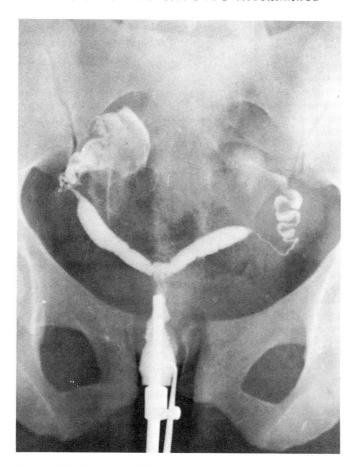

Fig. 4. This hysterographic study reveals a markedly bicornuate uterus, which is a definite but infrequent cause of chronic abortion. Hysterography is an important preconceptional diagnostic step which should always be taken in the evaluation of habitual aborters. This test, when competently performed under fluoroscopy, will disclose congenital uterine anomalies as well as such pathologic entities as submucous myomata.

was characterized by an hysterical overlay but contained few true hysterical characters, tended to convert a premarital abortion initiated from the "outside" to postmarital abortions initiated from the "inside". One patient, for example, on two successive occasions spontaneously aborted on the anniversary date of her premarital criminal abortion. Then, in the manner of a Greek tragic figure being pursued by the Furies, she attempted to circumvent destiny by becoming pregnant nine months prior to the anniversary date which would then be her expected date of confinement. When this contrived pregnancy ended in spontaneous abortion, she despaired of a self cure and presented herself at our clinic for help. Such a patient, like the

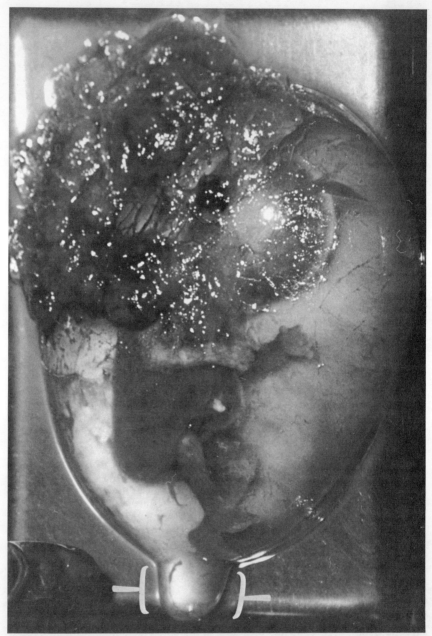

Fig. 5. This illustration demonstrates the beginning phases of cervical incompetence. Note the nippling (See brackets) of the lower pole of the intact membranes caused by herniation into the hypotonic isthmic segment. Typically, the wedging process continues downward through the endocervical canal producing cervical effacement and, ultimately, exocervical prolapse and "hourglassing" of the membranes.

In this particular instance, therapeutic abortion, by way of hysterotomy, was mandatory as a result of fulminating hypertension.

hysteric who sexualizes non-sexual situations, instead, haplessly criminalizes non-criminal situations.

This calendarical capacity to translate a psychic conflict into a somatic idiom was noted throughout the primary aborter group and was not necessarily expiatory. For instance, one rather immature aborter, fearful of her prowess as an expectant mother, recurrently aborted on Mother's Day.

Pitfalls in Psychotherapeutic Approach

Although the majority of unselected habitual aborters, most of whom are first trimester aborters, following comprehensive gynecologic evaluation are deemed free of detectable abortigenic pathology; and, although the majority of these can be successfully treated by psychotherapeutic means, *it is incumbent upon the therapist to rule out, or have ruled out for him, the presence of organic pathology.* The past history of a premarital criminal abortion, or even legitimate dilatation and curettage, may have resulted in sphincteric damage to the isthmic-cervical segment of the uterus, in which event, surgery is the definitive form of therapy. Identical damage may occur in the course of childbirth, so that secondary habitual abortion may occur in relation to trauma as well as to emotional determinants. This etiologic factor, termed "cervical incompetence", is diagnosable in the non-pregnant state (Figs. 1, 2 and 3) and, in our experience[33] occurs in only 13% of unselected (randomly referred) patients, but, in over 60% of aborters selectivity referred on the basis of a history suggestive of cervical incompetence. This condition may also occur on a congenital basis and may occur in congenital relation to a septate uterus, each of which, alone or in combination, may cause chronic abortion (Fig. 4). The syndrome of cervical incompetence (Fig. 5) typically occurs in the second or early third trimester of pregnancy and is characterized by painless, passive dilation of the cervix culminating in prolapse of the intact membranes. In the absence of surgical intervention[42] secondary uterine contractions then occur, followed by expulsion of the fetus.

Aside from this leading anatomic cause of chronic abortion were other factors, far less frequent in our study group, such as hormonal, anomalous, hypertensive, collagen, genetic and nutritional disorders.

5

Summary

Our psychosomatic experience with a large group of habitual aborters, unselectively referred on the sole basis of a history of three consecutive spontaneous abortions, more than points to a relation between emotional determinants and habitual abortion. The incidence of detectable abortigenic pathology in our unselected study group was approximately 15%. Of the

175 physically "normal" aborters treated psychotherapeutically and followed during pregnancy, 8 out of 10 successfully carried to term.

The predominating personality patterns which emerged were, among the primary aborters, an immature, dependent, self-deprecating group and a more "hysterical" acting-out group. The secondary aborters, who comprised 25% of the study group, tended to be more obsessive and vaguely dissatisfied with their marital partner. These three personality sub-groups seemed to have been related to under- and over-identification with matriarchal domination and paternal absence or inadequacy. Frigidity, with very few exceptions, was curiously inconspicuous throughout all three sub-groups.

The importance of a comprehensive preconceptional work-up to rule out organic pathology is emphasized.**

REFERENCES

1. ACEVEDO, H. F., VELA, B. A., CAMPBELL, M. T., STRICKLER, H. S., GILMORE, J., MORACA, J. I. and ARRAS, B. J. 1969. Urinary steroid profile in threatened abortion. *Amer. J. Obstet. Gynec.*, **104**, 7.

2. ASPLUND, J. 1954. Factors concerned in the causation of habitual abortion, in *La Prophylaxie en Gynécologie et Obstetrique*. Geneva: Georg et Cie.

3. BERLE, B. B. and JAVERT, C. T. 1954. Stress and habitual abortion. *Obstet. and Gynec.*, **3**, 298.

4. BEVIS, D. C. A. 1951. Treatment of habitual abortion. *Lancet*, ii, 207.

5. BISHOP, P. M. and RICHARDS, N. A. 1950. Habitual abortion, prophylactic value of progesterone implantation. *Brit. med., J.*, **2**, 130.

6. BOERO, E. A. 1935. Interruption of incompatible pregnancy before viability—a new concept and method. *Gynéc. Obstét.*, **32**, 305.

7. BOWEN, P. and LEE, C. S. N. 1969. Spontaneous abortion. *Amer. J. Obstet. Gynec.*, **104**, 7.

8. CROSS, J. V. 1946. Repeated abortions, miscarriages and stillbirths. *Lancet*, ii, 754.

9. EASTMAN, N. J. 1950. *Williams Obstetrics* (10th edn.). New York: Appleton.

10. FERENCZI, S. 1926. *Further contributions to the theory and technique of psychoanalysis*. London: Institute of Psychoanalysis, Hogarth.

11. FREIDGOOD, H. B. 1948. Neuroendocrine and psychodynamic factors in sterility. *West J. Surg.*, **56**, 391.

12. GOLDSTEIN, H., GOLDBERG, I. D., FRAZIER, T. M. and DAVIS, G. E. 1964. Cigarette-smoking and prematurity. *Rev. pub. Hlth. Rep.*, **79**, 553.

13. GREEN, J. D. and HARRIS, G. W. 1947. Neurovascular link between neuro-hypophysis and adenohypophysis. *J. Endocr.*, **5**, 136.

14. HERTIG, A. T. and LIVINGSTONE, R. G. 1944. Spontaneous, threatened and habitual abortion: its pathogenesis and treatment. *New Eng. J. Med.*, **230**, 797.

15. HILL, L. B. 1950. The importance of identification with a father figure in the psychology of a woman. *Proc. Soc. Med., Psychoanalysts, Symposium on Feminine Psychology*.

** I am greatly indebted to Mrs. Barbara Bertolin and Dr. William D. McLarn who contributed so much to the foregoing study. Their untimely deaths were truly tragic.

16. HUGHES, E. C., LLOYD, C. W. and LEDERGERBER, C. P. 1954. The role of pre-conceptional study and treatment in abortion and premature labour. In *La Prophylaxie en Gynécologie et Obstetrique*, Geneva: George et Cie.

17. JAVERT, C. T. 1954. Repeated abortion. *Obstet. and Gynec.*, **3**, 420.

18. JAVERT, C. T. 1957. Spontaneous and habitual abortion. New York: McGraw-Hill.

19. JONES, H. W., JR. and JONES, G. E. S. 1953. Double uterus as an etiological factor in repeated abortion: indications for surgical repair. *Amer. J. Obstet. Gynec.*, **65**, 325.

20. KING, A. G. 1953. Threatened and repeated abortion. *Obstet. and Gynec.*, **1**, 104.

21. KROGER, W. S. and FREED, S. C. 1951. *Psychosomatic gynecology*. Philadelphia: Saunders.

22. LASH, A. F. and LASH, S. R. 1950. Habitual abortion: the incompetent internal os of the cervix. *Amer. J. Obstet. Gynec.*, **59**, 68.

23. LUDWIG, F. 1944. The treatment of imminent abortion and habitual abortion with corpus luteum and vitamin B. *Amer. J. Obstet. Gynec.*, **47**, 581.

24. MACLEAN, P. D. 1949. Psychosomatic disease and the "visceral brain". *Psychosom. Med.*, **11**, 338.

25. MALMQUIST, A., KAIJ, L. and NILSSON, A. 1969. Psychiatric aspects of spontaneous abortion—I. A matched control study of women with living children. *J. psychosom. Res.*, **13**, 45.

26. MALPAS, P. 1938. A study of abortion sequences. *J. Obstet. Gynaec. Brit. Emp.*, **45**, 932.

27. MANDY, A. J. and MANDY, T. E. 1950. The emotional aspects of obstetric and gynecologic disorders. *Amer. J. Obstet. Gynec.*, **60**, 605.

28. MANN, E. C. 1956. Psychiatric investigation of habitual abortion. *Obstet. and Gynec.*, **7**, 589.

29. MANN, E. C. 1957. The role of emotional determinants in habitual abortion. *S. Clin., North America*, **37**, 477. Saunders.

30. MANN, E. C. 1957. Psychosomatic reactions associated with pregnancy. *Connecticut med. J.*, **21**, 962.

31. MANN, E. C. 1959. Habitual abortion. *Amer. J. Obstet. Gynec.*, **77**, 706.

32. MANN, E. C. and GRIMM, E. R. 1962. *Habitual abortion in psychosomatic obstetrics, gynecology and endocrinology*. Philadelphia: Charles Thomas.

33. MANN, E. C., McLARN, W. D. and HAYT, D. B. 1961. The physiology and clinical significance of the uterine isthmus. *Amer. J. Obstet. Gynec.*, **81**, 2.

34. MICHEL-WOLFRAMM, H. 1968. The psychological factor in spontaneous abortion. *J. psychosom. Res.*, **12**, 67.

35. MONRO, J. S. 1939. Premature infant, weighing less than one pound at birth, who survived and developed normally. *Canad. Med. J.*, **40**, 69.

36. NESER, F. N. 1959. Cervical incompetence and second trimester abortions. *S. Afr. med., J.*, **2**, 722.

37. OSMOND-CLARK, F. and MURRAY, M. 1963. Vaginal cytology in recurrent abortions. *Brit., med. J.*, **2**, 1172.

38. PERGAMENT, E., KADOTANI, T. and SATO, H. 1969. Double Trisomy in the spontaneous abortion population. *Amer. J. Obst. Gynec.*, **104**, 7.

39. RAPPAPORT, F., RUBINOVITZ, M., TOABB, R. and KROCHEK, N. 1960. Genital Listeriosis as a cause of repeated abortion. *Lancet*, i, 1273.

40. ROSZKOWSKI, I. and SROKA, L. 1962. The effect of the male factor on abnormal pregnancy. *Gynaecologia*, **154**, 321 and (1963) *Obstet. Gynec. Surv.*, **18**, 625.

41. RUFFOLO, E. H., WILSON, R. B. and WEED, L. A. 1962. Listeria monocytogenes as a cause of pregnancy wastage. *Obstet and Gynec.*, **19**, 533.

42. SHIRODKAR, V. N. 1955. Surgical treatment of habitual abortions. In *Tendances actuelles en gynecologie et obstetrique*. Geneva: Georg et Cie S.A.

43. SIMON, N. M., ROTHMAN, D., GOFF, J. T. and SENTURIA, A. G. 1959. Psychological

factors related to spontaneous and therapeutic abortion. *Amer. J. Obstet. Gynec.*, **104,** 6.

44. SMITH, O. W. 1948. Diethylstilbestrol in the prevention and treatment of complications of pregnancy. *Amer. J. Obstet. Gynec.*, **56,** 821.
45. SPEERT, H. and GUTTMACHER, A. 1954. Frequency and significance of bleeding in early pregnancy. *J. Amer., med., Ass.*, **155,** 712.
46. SQUIER, R. and DUNBAR, F. 1946. Emotional factors in the course of pregnancy. *Psychosom. Med.*, **8,** 161.
47. TIETZE, C. 1953. Introduction to the statistics of abortion. In *Pregnancy wastage* (E. T. Engle, ed.). Springfield: Charles C. Thomas.
48. TIETZE, C. and MARTIN, C. E. 1957. Foetal deaths, spontaneous and induced, in the urban white population of the United States. *Pop. Studies*, **11,** 170.
49. TUPPER, C., MAYA, F., STEWART, L. C., WEIL, R. J. and GRAY, J. D. 1957. The problem of spontaneous abortion, I.A. combined approach. *Amer. J. Obstet. Gynec.*, **73,** 313.
50. VAUX, N. W. and RAKOFF, A. E. 1945. Estrogen-progesterone therapy: a new approach in the treatment of habitual abortion. *Amer. J. Obstet. Gynec.*, **50,** 353.
51. VOS, G. H., SELANO, M. J., FALKOWSKI, F. and LEVINE, P. 1954. Relationship of a hemolysin resembling anti Tja to threatened abortion in Western Australia. *Transfusion*, **4,** 87.
52. WREN, B. G. and VOS, G. H. 1961. Blood group incompatibility as a cause of spontaneous abortion. *J. Obstet. Gynaec., Brit. Cwlth.*, **68,** 637.

XII

CRAVINGS, AVERSIONS AND PICA OF PREGNANCY

W. H. TRETHOWAN

M.B., F.R.C.P., F.R.A.C.P., D.P.M.
Professor of Psychiatry,
University of Birmingham, England

G. DICKENS

M.R.C.S., L.R.C.P., L.M.S.S.A., D.P.M.
Consultant Psychiatrist,
Rubery Hill Hospital, Birmingham, England

Then out spoke Blessed Mary so soft and so mild.
Pick me a cherry, Joseph, for I am with child.

Country Songs of Vermont
Helen Hartness Flanders

1

Introduction

Among the more peculiar manifestations of pregnancy are *cravings*,* an intense compulsive desire for any one or more of a wide variety of articles of diet, not especially craved for when not pregnant, and *aversions*, a positive and equally compelling distaste for certain kinds of food and drink, for which revulsion is not normally felt. Cravings seem usually to have excited greater curiosity than aversions, although the latter are equally common and the two are almost certainly closely related. Their intensity varies: in some cases cravings may lead to compulsive overeating (bulimia),[31] in others to excessive intake of fluid (polydipsia).[6, 13] Alternatively, anorexia in early pregnancy can occur[20] and anorexia nervosa has been described.[2] This, however, must be an exceedingly rare occurrence, as the disorder is very largely confined to unmarried virgins.

When there is a craving for some substance normally regarded as inedible the term *pica* may be preferred—sometimes known as *citra* or *malacia* in historical accounts.[10] *Geophagia* is a special form of pica, which refers to eating earth or clay, found in negro women (and men) in the United States and in Africa, and not always associated with pregnancy.[8, 9, 25, 26, 27] Similar

* Less commonly known as *longings, yens, yearnings* or *fancies* or, in Scotland as *notions*, and in France, *envie.*

dietary practices have also been recorded among primitive people in other parts of the world and in cattle.[12]

Pica of other kinds is also not confined to pregnant women, and indeed occurs much more often in emotionally disturbed children of either sex,[5, 33] in the mentally retarded, and less commonly in some deteriorated psychotic patients.

2

Historical Background

Accounts of cravings and pica go back to ancient times,[5] when attention was largely focused upon some of the more curious and bizarre perversions of appetite during pregnancy. Apart from accounts of eating earth, plaster, coal, charcoal, ashes, sand, bed-linen, and a large number of other more or less inedible substances, there exist records of women seemingly possessed of an insatiable desire to ingest not only such relatively unattractive articles of diet as live eels, lizards, frogs, spiders, flies, scorpions, lice and fleas but much more repulsive substances such as nasal mucus and faeces.[10, 13] Several writers have recorded cannibalistic cravings. Cooper[5] quotes an account, given by Hubrigkt in 1662, of a pregnant woman who, seeing a baker placing loaves in the oven, was possessed of an intense craving for three bites from his shoulder.* Following some, presumably satisfactory, financial arrangement between the woman's husband and the baker the unfortunate tradesman agreed to co-operate. It is recorded however that his stamina failed before the lady was able to take her third bite. A somewhat less extreme but equally bizarre example of a cannibalistic craving is given by Seifrit,[29] who quotes Buchan in 1803 as mentioning a "lady who longed for a hair from her husband's beard—and wanted the pleasure of plucking it out herself".

As with the Couvade phenomenon, cravings in pregnancy did not escape the notice of the Elizabethan playwrights. William Rowley in 1633, in his play, *All's lost by lust*, wrote:

> There's honourable bones a-breeding:
> my sister is peevishest piece of
> lady's flesh grown of late . . .
> Nay, she cuts her lace, and eats
> raw flesh too! What sallet do you
> think she longed for t'other day? . . .
> For a . . . what d'ye call 'em—those
> long, upright things that grow a yard
> above the ground—oh, cuckoo pintle-
> roots: but I got her belly full at last.[21]

---

* Viewed in psychoanalytic terms the symbolism of this sequence of events is remarkable!

Speculations as to the cause of cravings and pica also go back many centuries. As might be expected, early authors advanced explanations based either upon superstitious beliefs or humoral hypotheses. On the whole, the tendency was to advance some kind of physical reason. Although some such explanations are still considered feasible by certain contemporary authors, Betten, as far back as 1687, considered the cause of cravings to be entirely mental.[5]

While accounts of aversions during pregnancy, as opposed to those of cravings and pica, tend to be of more modern origin, Havelock Ellis[10] quotes Schurig in 1725 as dealing extensively with this in his book *Chylologia-* (Chapter III, *De nausea seu antipathia certorum ciborum*). In addition to more commonplace aversions which often occur today, Schurig listed absinthe, amber, roses, musk—said sometimes to have caused vomiting— rats, frogs and spiders; though it is not made explicit whether any of these were, under different circumstances, ever regarded as appropriate articles of diet.

3

Prevalence

Brought up to date, food fads and fancies in pregnancy seem to be as common as they ever were, although nowadays they usually manifest themselves in less striking ways. Most studies of prevalence suggest that between one- and two-thirds of women suffer, to some degree, either from cravings or aversions or both at some time during pregnancy, regardless of race or place. Posner et al.[27] elicited cravings in 394 (66%) of 600 lower-income, predominantly Negro, women consecutively interviewed. Ten admitted pica, nine of whom ate clay. Taggart[32] in a survey of the dietary habits of Aberdeen primigravidae found that about two-thirds developed some craving during pregnancy, mostly for foods readily available, commonly for fruit. Aversions to certain foods were found to occur as often as cravings. Marcus,[23] who investigated 80 pregnant in-patients in Manchester and obtained details referring to 225 pregnancies in all, elicited a history of cravings in 96 (42·6% of all pregnancies), aversions in 34 (15·8%) but only one instance of pica. More recently Dickens,[7] who interviewed 100 consecutive British born (including Irish) primigravidae, found 51 with cravings and 62 with aversions. Both were evident in 37 cases and neither in 24.

The frequency of cravings in pregnancy is also indicated by a study carried out in 1958 by Harries and Hughes[15] who, following a BBC broadcast, when listeners were invited to write giving details of cravings and aversions during pregnancy, analysed 509 of 514 letters reporting 820 pregnancies. These letters described 991 examples of cravings (261 for fruit) and 187 instances of cravings for substances other than food (pica). There were in addition 193 reports of substances normally liked but disliked during pregnancy.

The relatively high frequency of pica in Harries and Hughes's cases[15] was no doubt an outcome of the fact that their findings were based on the result of a volunteer survey by letter to the BBC, a method which like writing to the press, may perhaps be thought more likely to produce a large number of more curious examples derived from those eager to recount their strange experiences, than a random survey would be. Most other studies suggest, in fact, that, in women of British origin at least, the incidence of pica compared to cravings for more palatable substances is low. No example was recorded by Taggart[32] among 800 Aberdeen women attending an ante-natal clinic who discussed their diets with a dietitian, although one case came to light among another 100 who were specifically asked—a woman with an irresistible urge to eat coal and spent match-heads. Marcus[23] found only one case among 80 women who between them had had 225 pregnancies; but, although this patient sniffed coke and had a strong desire to eat it, she never actually did so. Dickens, who also made a specific inquiry into the matter, uncovered no instance in 100 patients, although 11 of the 51 with cravings did admit to pica in childhood.[7]

Finally, it should be noted that, while the matter needs further study, there is some evidence to suggest that the prevalence of cravings in pregnancy is higher in primiparae than in older women undergoing subsequent pregnancies, who, being older as a rule, tend to be more emotionally mature.

4

Onset and Duration

The time of onset and the duration of cravings and aversions during pregnancy vary. In Harries and Hughes's study[15] the stage of pregnancy when craving was experienced was recorded only in about one-quarter of the 514 letters received. Only 6 stated that craving was experienced for the full term, and 59 said that it started in the first and persisted to the fourth month of pregnancy. Marcus[23] observed in his cases that cravings, once begun, persisted throughout most of pregnancy, though with a tendency to disappear during the later months. Dickens[7] found that the onset of cravings appeared to be more or less evenly distributed throughout pregnancy, while aversions were experienced more frequently during the first trimester and progressively less so in the second and third.

Apart from an odd historical reference,[13] there is little evidence that perversions of appetite originating in pregnancy ever become permanent.*

---

* However, a lady of our acquaintance, before she ever became pregnant had an intense loathing for beer and could not even tolerate its odour. During all her three pregnancies she developed an intense desire to drink a bottle each night. After her first pregnancy was over, she did not revert to her previous distaste for beer but, although often enjoying a glass or so in between times, had no craving for it.

Cravings of a kind, however, can, it seems, occur in women who are not pregnant, though probably they are seldom striking enough to excite much attention. Such cases might conceivably turn out to be commoner if specific enquiry were more often made into the matter. For example Edwards, McSwain and Haire[8] who studied the odd dietary practices of 211 negro women in Alabama, whether pregnant or not, found that almost one-third of those who reported cravings on their questionnaires were in fact not pregnant. Indeed, in the case of those who ate cornstarch and clay, an apparently by no means uncommon practice in this particular cultural sub-group, it was found that the difference in incidence of craving for these substances among pregnant as opposed to non-pregnant women was not statistically significant. The same, however, did not apply to cravings for more orthodox articles of diet which, for certain kinds of foods at least—notably fruit, vegetables and protein foods—were craved for in a very large majority of cases only by pregnant women. This difference raises the question of whether craving for such substances as earth or clay, although somewhat increased in pregnancy, can properly be considered in the same light as the more familiar cravings also experienced much more widely by women from other cultures. There is also some evidence, which will be discussed later, to suggest that geophagia may be due to mineral deficiency in the diet of those who indulge in this practice.[1, 4, 12]

5

Food Fads and Fancies

As already indicated, the number of different items of food and drink craved for during pregnancy, or for which unaccustomed aversion is felt, is large. On grouping these together, however, certain patterns of like and dislike emerge, together with a considerable measure of agreement as to the frequency of their occurrence (Table 1). Such differences as are apparent may possibly be accounted for by differences in the manner in which the various food substances are categorized and by cultural factors related to the ethnic origin of the women under consideration.

There seems to be almost complete agreement that fruit (together with fizzy fruit drinks) is the most popular craving among all subjects.[6, 7, 8, 15, 17, 22] Cravings for sweet things other than fruit, and including ice-cream, jam, etc., and a craving for vegetables including nuts and pickles, fall almost equally into second place. Apart from the findings of Edwards and her colleagues,[8] from which it appears that a craving for meat, fish, eggs, etc. almost equals the incidence of that for fruit, protein substances are not usually nearly so highly favoured. Indeed Dickens[7] found that aversion for foods in this category was more frequent than craving (17 as against 8).

Several investigations have emphasized the occurrence of cravings for sweet, sour, savoury, or salty substances. Among fruit, apples predominate;

TABLE 1

Author	No. of instances of craving*	Ethnic origin	Fruit (fizzy drinks)	Sweets (incl. ices)	Vegetables (incl. pickles)	Meat, fish eggs	Other
Edwards et al. (1954)	129	Negro (Alabama)	37	10	16	33	4
Posner et. al. (1957)	288	Negro (Harlem)	30	23·5	13	7	26·5
Harries and Hughes (1958)	804	U.K. (Various)	35	13·5	21	10	20·5
Marcus (1965)	96	U.K. (Manchester)	32	15·5	22	10	20·5
Dickens (1971)	89	U.K./Eire (Nuneaton)	33	24	12·5	8	22·5

* Cases of pica or for substances other than food (e.g. Argo starch, Posner et. al.) are excluded. All figures, other than total numbers of instances of cravings, in percentages.

oranges rather less so. Pickles are fairly often mentioned. Vegetables are frequently preferred uncooked[18, 15] and cereal products also in a dry raw state. Indeed, Posner *et al.*, found that among his negro subjects dry foods were slightly more preferred (46%) than liquids (34%) or semi-solid substances (19%).[27] From this it may be concluded—and some subjects confirm this—that satisfaction is gained not only from taste but also from texture, there being gratification to be had from biting or chewing something which is hard or crisp.

Aversions are less well documented. Taggart[32] records a dislike for tea and coffee during early pregnancy. There may also be an aversion to fried foods and, in the later months, a preference for plain or savoury as opposed to sweet things. An aversion to tea, in particular, and rather less often to coffee, is confirmed by the findings of other investigators. Harries and Hughes,[15] giving details of 193 reports of substances normally liked but disliked during pregnancy, cited tea in 78 (40%) and coffee in 22 (12·5%). Marcus[23] made no reference to coffee but recorded aversion to tea as being fairly common (10 of 29 instances listed). Dickens[7] found that 32 of 100 subjects developed an aversion for tea or coffee, in one instance for both, and in another for coffee and drinking-chocolate. Another common aversion was for tobacco.

It may be important to note that while aversion to tea, coffee and fried foods is common, craving for these appears to be rare. Indeed, Dickens is the only investigator who recorded a craving for tea (3 instances), as opposed to an aversion (9 instances). Harries and Hughes did, however, report craving for tea leaves in 2 of their correspondents and for coffee grounds in 5.

Dickens's findings also show that cravings and aversions are for the most part antithetical. Although he discovered a number of isolated examples—not more than one or two instances in each case—of food and drink for which some women craved and others experienced aversion as a whole those items in one category were seldom to be found in the other. Only one subject craved and at a different stage of pregnancy developed an aversion for, the same article of food—tomatoes. Other kinds of differences were also apparent, for example two subjects had an aversion for boiled potatoes while another had a craving for them eaten raw.

Much the same appears to have been observed by other investigators. For example, Marcus found craving for apples in 12 cases and aversion in 1 only. Craving for meat or fish occurred in 11 instances and aversion only in 2. Harries and Hughes recorded 68 cravings for oranges but only 4 aversions. Many other less striking examples of such differences could be enumerated, together with a relatively small list of foods which appear infrequently but in the same small proportions in either category. Even when arbitrarily grouped together and tabulated, an antithesis between the various classes of food for which craving may commonly be felt or aversion experienced is still evident. This antithesis would appear to be important, as it strongly suggests that the two phenomena, cravings and aversions, are linked in that they probably stand in inverse relationship to one another.

A number of subjects had cravings or aversions, or both, for more than one food substance. Edwards and her colleagues' 55 negro women between them gave 129 examples of cravings (average 2·3 per subject) or, if pica is included, 166 (average 3·0). The three British investigators produced somewhat lower but fairly consistent figures. Harries and Hughes's 509 subjects reported 804 examples of food cravings (average 1·6 or, if another 187 examples of craving for non-food substances are included, 1·9 per subject). Marcus enumerated 137 examples in 96 women who craved (average 1·4), and Dickens 89 examples among 51 (average 1·75). Multiple aversions among Dickens's subjects were almost as common, 94 instances in 62 subjects (average 1·6). Most subjects, however, admitted either to a single craving or aversion or perhaps one of each, and a considerably smaller number to two or three. Only one subject in Dickens's series admitted to as many as 5 different cravings, though all for rather similar fruity substances, together with 1 aversion. In contrast one other subject listed 5 aversions together with 3 cravings.

The higher incidence of multiple cravings among negro women observed by Edwards *et al.* as compared with the British studies may have been in part due to the fact that a number of these women craved when not pregnant, 23 for food and 18 for non-edible substances, and that this number increased when pregnancy occurred. So great is the variation in these cases that it is difficult to decide what can be considered to be typical. The following case, however, exemplifies many of the main features under consideration.

Mrs. I, aged 18, became pregnant prematurely and shortly afterwards married her unborn child's father, whereupon she went to live with her parents-in-law. Both she and her husband worked in a hosiery factory, and she continued to do so until the seventh month of her pregnancy. She was thought to be a woman of good average intelligence. There was no history of mental illness or of any significant physical illness. Her upbringing was said to be happy, although she stated that as a child she was quite often in trouble for picking wallpaper off the walls and eating it. She was also said to be allergic to eggs. Apart from this, she apparently had no feeding difficulties and her weight had always remained within normal limits. She was somewhat sensitive and of obsessional personality, was given to mood swings, but was not otherwise overtly psychiatrically abnormal. She smoked regularly and took alcohol in moderation.

Despite the manner in which her pregnancy occurred, and her mother-in-law's initial resentment, this proceeded uneventfully, concluding with a normal full-term delivery. She did not suffer from nausea and morning sickness, though her husband did so to some extent.

In the last three months of pregnancy she developed cravings for hard sour apples, hard sour sweets, nuts and raisins. She was particularly attracted by the sensation of biting and chewing these substances. At the same time she developed an aversion for pork, however cooked. Previously this had been the kind of meat she most preferred. She was quite unable to explain this aversion beyond saying that it was "just the thought of it being pork."

Her husband, in addition to experiencing sympathetic nausea and sickness, also developed innumerable though transient cravings.

The most significant features of this patient's case appear to have been the nature of her cravings—characteristically for hard sour substances—her history of pica during childhood, and the fact that she smoked and drank. The relevance of these factors will be discussed later.

6

Pica of Pregnancy

While cravings for more or less inedible substances seem nowadays to occur less often in pregnant women in Britain and among those of comparable cultural background than historical records and some accounts from abroad seem to suggest, their number and variety may still be such as to occasion surprise. Harries and Hughes discovered that a cloak of secrecy may well surround the matter. Some women who experience a sense of shame at having such odd perversions of appetite may seek to conceal these, even from their husbands. Nevertheless 187 of their correspondents reported, in descending order of pregnancy, cravings for coal, soap, disinfectant, toothpaste, mothballs, petrol, metal-polish, tar, paraffin, wood, soil, chalk, charcoal and cinders, together with a number of other miscellaneous substances.[15] Distasteful as these may sound, a craving for them was emphasized, like that for certain foodstuffs, as being of the strongest possible intensity. Apart from geophagia, other authors mention cravings for ashes, sand and plaster;[33] whitewash, wallpaper and pencil eraser.[27, 29] No doubt a sufficiently wide and thorough search would provide many other examples. It is possible also that the current widespread immigration of women of very different cultural background into the United Kingdom may produce even more instances. Here is an example.

Mrs. M. J. a 30-year-old Jamaican, was referred during the eighth month of her fourth pregnancy on account of a compulsion to eat soap. This had been present on every occasion from the time when she first knew she was pregnant until delivery, though during the present pregnancy was somewhat less severe than during the previous three.

Her husband confirmed her craving for soap and stated that although he had made efforts to prevent this, these had been to no avail. It was also discovered that her sister also ate soap when she was pregnant and that her mother used to lick it when she too was with child.

The patient stated that she tended to eat soap whenever her stomach was upset, whereupon she felt better; although, if she ate too much, this again made her sick. She cut the soap into slices and usually ate some at least every day. Her desire to eat soap took the form of a sudden compulsion, which might come upon her at any time and sometimes woke her at night. She stated: "You can't stop it, you just have to have it—if you miss a day it's like murder!" She also said she preferred Palmolive.

Except for vomiting, which she apparently sought to control by soap-eating, the only other untoward symptom she experienced was a craving for rum early in pregnancy which however soon disappeared. The rest of her medical history was uneventful. All her previous pregnancies had been straightforward, although on each occasion she had had difficulty in expelling the placenta.

Her personal history seemed to be of some significance. Her three previous pregnancies, 6, 7 and 8 years before, were all illegitimate and by a man with whom she was living during this time. These, she said, caused her parents some distress so that at the time they expressed a wish to disown her. Things improved, however, when she got married to the man who is now her husband, this event taking place when she was two months pregnant by him.

7

Causes and Effects

From what the soap-eating lady whose case has just been recounted said about her three previous pregnancies, all of which were unplanned and unwanted, it seems feasible to suggest that her compulsion to eat soap could be regarded as a concrete expression of a symbolic need to cleanse herself of feelings of guilt, although it must not be forgotten that the fact that her mother and sister were soap-eaters when pregnant may have been a powerful determining factor. During each pregnancy, however, and particularly during the first three, she felt upset and ashamed and the thought of aborting herself was never far from her mind. Indeed, during her second pregnancy she went so far as to dose herself with quinine but only with the effect of making herself ill.

Although there may be some truth in this hypothesis, as she was seen on one occasion only, it could not be confirmed. It will serve nevertheless as an introduction to some of the theories which have been advanced to account for appetite disorders in pregnancy, although it must be admitted that at present, while theories are fairly plentiful, facts are few. Indeed the final solution of why women crave during pregnancy, suffer from pica or from aversions for foods which they normally enjoy, awaits further investigation.

Existing theories fall into four broad categories: those based on superstitious beliefs and folklore; physical explanations, which tend to ascribe pica, in particular, to a need among pregnant women to compensate for some form of dietary deficiency; psychological, including psychodynamic theories invoking insecurity, suggestion, ambivalence, attention-seeking and regression; and finally, a theory which suggests that some perversions of appetite during pregnancy are at least, in part, due to alterations in the sense of taste and smell.

Superstitious Beliefs

These chiefly surround the notion that if a certain food substance craved for is not eaten some harm will come to the child, often in the form of disfigurement.[21] Having regard to this, it is of interest to note that the French word for craving or longing—*envie*—also means a birth-mark and that the Italian word *voglia* has the same double meaning. It is reported that the mother of the Duchess d'Abrantès, wife of Marshal Junot, became highly concerned at the fact that her daughter, during her first pregnancy, experienced no longings. In one of her own pregnancies the Duchess's mother herself had apparently longed for cherries in January and, since this craving could not be satisfied, it was said that the child was born in consequence with a naevus resembling a cherry. So great did the concern of the Duchess's relatives become, that she too suddenly developed an intense longing, in this instance, for pineapple. As pineapple also was out of season, her husband obtained one only with great difficulty. When it was cut up, however, it suddenly proved so odious to the Duchess that she was unable to touch it.[10]

Although during the last century the idea that the non-gratification of longings might be attended with bad consequences to the child in the shape of disfigurement was considered to be "a popular European prejudice" (Shortland[21] found no evidence of it for example among New Zealanders in 1856), the same kind of belief is apparently to be found today among American negro women who crave for such things as red and white clay, cornstarch, flour, and baking soda. According to Edwards et al.,[8, 9] some emphatically stated that "the unborn will be marked if I don't eat it", or that the baby would be born abnormal in some other way. Other subjects not only said that eating clay kept the baby from being marked at birth, but that eating starch would "make the newborn lighter in colour, produce a healthy baby or help it to 'slide out' more easily during delivery".[25]

Aversions to certain foods may also be influenced by superstition. Edwards found that in South Carolina there is a traditional belief, once again among negro women, that milk, eggs, fish, yellow vegetables, grapefruit, tomatoes, butter, liver and beans should not be eaten during pregnancy; and in Alabama, bacon, ham and onions also. Fish is said to be especially widely taboo in a number of the Southern States, particularly if taken together with milk, even to the extent of it being thought that the ingestion of these substances might be likely to prove fatal.[8]

There is no evidence at the present time that such beliefs commonly influence or give rise to cravings and aversions among women born and reared in the British Isles, though an investigation carried out in more remote and rural areas might well bring something of the kind to light.

Physical

From the beginning, physical explanations of cravings and of pica have been popular, in the latter instance in children as well as in pregnant women. Foster[12] reported the occurrence of pica in animals, both as a natural occurrence in certain species and in certain localities, and experimentally produced by deprivation of essential articles of diet. He also described a disorder known as *leckzucht*, in which cattle begin by refusing ordinary fodder, then pass through a casual "licking" stage (from which the disorder derives its name), and ultimately develop such a depraved appetite that all sorts of alien substances are consumed. The cause of this strange condition is thought to be faulty mineral balance in otherwise normal pasture.

Foster also pointed out that in human beings pica predominates in the growth-period; hence its occurrence both in children and in pregnancy. He suggested that in humans, as in animals, the cause was essentially dietary. In 1959 the *Lancet*[1] put forward the notion that pica in children was due, at least in part, to anaemia and stated that it tended to resolve if iron was given. Although nothing was said about pregnant women, Carlander[4] later commented, in a letter from Sweden, that he had observed pica in about 100 patients, mostly women but in a few men, following gastric resection and in those who were blood donors. He too regarded pica as being associated with iron deficiency.

Similar reasons have been advanced to account for geophagia among negro women, who in the Southern States of America may often suffer from dietary deficiency.[8, 29, 33] Reports, however, are conflicting. Edwards *et al.*[9] found that while clay-eaters were often mildly-to-moderately anaemic, they showed no gross evidence of other kinds of mineral deficiency. Their main conclusion was that a desire to eat clay and cornstarch could not be explained on the basis of one motive alone. While in some women it was a traditional practice interwoven with superstition, in others its aetiology seemed to be similar to smoking, in that it gave oral satisfaction and warded off hunger. Dietary deficiency also appears to have been excluded in 394 of the 600 women with cravings studied by Posner *et al.*[27]—106 of whom ate starch, 9 clay, and 1 pencil-eraser. All received routine prenatal care, iron where necessary, and prophylactic vitamin therapy. None showed any clinical signs of malnutrition.

Viewed altogether, the case for a physical cause of pica in pregnant women, and in disturbed children also, seems slender. Even if mild anaemia is often found to be present, this could just as well be effect as cause; for, if severe, pica may possibly interfere with nutrition by reducing appetite for proper articles of diet. But more so than this, if consideration is given to the bizarre nature of some of the substances which pregnant women sometimes consume, such as those listed by Harries and Hughes[15] (e.g. disinfectant, toothpaste, petrol, metal-polish, etc.), it is quite impossible to believe that eating these, as has been suggested by some authors in the case of earth, plaster, etc., can be construed as an unconscious attempt to remedy a supposed mineral deficiency. Yudkin,[34] pursuing this argument further, neatly attacked the notion of a "food instinct" by asking whether, if eating plaster compulsively points to a need for calcium, does eating boot-polish similarly betray a physiological need for wax and turpentine!

While some might wish to entertain the hypothesis that geophagia is possibly stimulated by dietary deficiency, it is very much more difficult to apply an interpretation of this kind to a craving for edible foodstuffs most of which may form part of every day diet. Yet Jeans et al.[18] seem convinced that cravings could be explained on this basis. While observing that many pregnant women (in this instance wives of university students) had unusual cravings, they asserted that none who did so had a wholly adequate diet. Some—better fed than others—who had difficulty controlling weight, either chewed ice or nibbled raw carrot, "just to be eating something when I was hungry". These food habits were not construed as cravings. A few of the "true" dietary cravings, it was said, resulted in real improvement of the diet. Several mothers, whose "calcium and protein intake had always been low", craved ice-cream, raw potatoes and citrus fruits. Although Rust[28] and others have suggested that the eating habits of pregnant women can be improved by education, there is no evidence that, in Britain at least, the vast majority of women who receive adequate ante-natal care suffer by reason of an inadequate diet. All Dickens's cases[7] were well nourished; nonetheless, they seem to have craved no less commonly than other mothers.

Finally, it should be said, that physical theories based on diet appear to offer no explanation for the occurrence of aversions during pregnancy.

Psychodynamics

The fact that fruit is so commonly craved for seems to lend support to what might be called the "fecundation theory" of cravings, which are said to be one outcome of an ambivalent attitude of a woman towards her un-born child. According to Helene Deutsch[6] food cravings, as against nausea and vomiting, express a conflict between "destruction and preservation of the embryo". She points out that fruit, cucumbers, fish, spice, etc., are familiar to psychoanalysis as symbols of fecundation, and that a compulsive desire for them can therefore be interpreted as a symbolic repetition of the act of fecundation, "an obsessive undoing" of an unconscious wish to destroy the child.

Simplified, this theory suggests that the pregnant woman craves these foods because she unconsciously believes they may, in some magical way, protect her unborn child from her own hidden feelings of hostility.[16, 19] Regarding this, Fenichel[11] also pointed out that women with oral fixations and ambivalent attitudes towards pregnancy are those who are most liable to what he called "specific food addictions". Helene Deutsch, furthermore, postulated an "analogy between oral intake and the receptive sucking function of the vagina" with revival of the "old infantile idea of fecundation through the mouth", also put forward by Hüpfer.[16]

Like so many psychoanalytic hypotheses, the fecundation theory suffers by reason of being incapable of proof. Furthermore, it does not take into account the fact that a very large stretch of imagination is needed to regard many of the foods or other substances which pregnant women crave for as symbols of fecundity. Nor, in invoking ambivalence, and suggesting that the cravings and the vomiting of pregnancy are polar opposites—the former symbolizing protection and the latter rejection of the child—, is due account taken of the fact that such evidence as there is does not indicate that cravings are any commoner in women who vomit than in those who do not.[7, 10, 32]

However, just as Dickens was unable to find any correlation between the incidence of cravings and nausea and vomiting, neither was he able to demonstrate any significant association between the occurrence of appetite disorders and other factors which might have pointed to the possibility that some of his pregnant women could have had feelings of rejection towards their unborn children. These included such matters as whether pregnancy was planned or unplanned, whether there was undue anxiety associated with childbirth, what the attitudes of the patient's husband or family were, and whether the impact of pregnancy threatened living standards. What he did discover, however, was some very interesting evidence suggesting that in women with appetite disorders in pregnancy there is some predisposition to oral fixation; for the number who smoked, took alcohol, or had a previous history of a change in appetite in response to emotional stress, was significantly higher in those with cravings or aversions or both, than in those with no disturbance of appetite whatsoever. He also obtained 11 instances of a history of pica in childhood in the cravings group, but found no instance of this in other subjects.

Oral regression, no doubt, in part accounts for pica and for a kind of half-way phenomenon—somewhere between more ordinary cravings and pica—a desire to eat food in a form in which it is not normally eaten, e.g. raw meat, vegetables uncooked, dry cereals, etc.

Suggestion, imitation and identification are other psychological mechanisms which must be considered. Attention-seeking may also be a factor. This is exemplified by the well-known, almost classical, notion that fruit craved for is often that which is out of season and therefore the most difficult to obtain. Although in these modern deep-freeze days such cravings are probably much less frequent and much less difficult to satisfy than they used to be, their occurrence may well express a need on the part of a pregnant woman to draw her husband, and possibly her other relatives also, into a situation closely surrounding her pregnancy. In having to search with difficulty for food which is hard to obtain, the pregnant woman's husband goes some distance along the way of sharing her compulsion with her. This, together with the knowledge that in some cases expectant fathers themselves also develop cravings, indicates the relationship between appetite disorders of pregnancy and the Couvade phenomenon (see Chapter IV).

Alterations in Taste

Curiously enough, this matter has either escaped the attention it may deserve, or has been virtually neglected, by the large majority of those who have written on the subject of alterations in appetite during pregnancy. Nevertheless, it would seem to be a factor which could at least play an important part in determining the nature of the food-substance for which craving or aversion is felt.[30]

In 1935, Hansen and Langer[11] investigated the taste threshold of 28 pregnant women and compared it with that of 12 other normal women who were not pregnant, using very dilute solutions of salt, sour wine, sugar and quinine. While there were not inconsiderable variations among subjects, in nearly every case the taste threshold was raised in pregnant as compared with that of non-pregnant subjects, so that higher concentrations were almost always required for pregnant women to be able to taste the substances proffered. When the averages of the concentrations required to produce a sensation of taste were considered, it was demonstrated that the threshold to taste was raised in pregnant as opposed to non-pregnant women, in all four major modalities and in the following ascending order: sweet, bitter, sour and salt.

More recently Caresano and Minazzi,[3] using a much more precise electrical method, in which the threshold of taste was measured in terms of the amount of current required to produce a response, tested 30 subjects both when pregnant and after parturition. Once again the threshold was considerably higher and also more variable during pregnancy than after childbirth. In all cases the threshold fell remarkably rapidly, reaching its lowest level within an hour of the conclusion of labour and achieving stability within two or three hours. In discussing the significance of this, the authors came to the conclusion that the rapid fall in threshold made it unlikely that the changes in taste in pregnancy could be accounted for by hormonal influences or peripheral mechanisms, such as alterations in the lingual mucous membrane. They felt that the phenomenon could only be brought about by a sudden change in the functional behaviour of certain centres in the nervous system, e.g. in the diencephalon.

If it can be accepted as conclusive that taste is dulled during pregnancy; then this would seem almost certainly to explain the preference of pregnant women for sharp, sour, salty, spicy, or otherwise strong-tasting substances. It has been pointed out that the most common craving is for fruit, but that apples—often sour ones—and oranges, which are frequently sharp and acid-tasting, are the most popular. The same mechanism might also explain, although perhaps less convincingly, a dislike during pregnancy of certain foods, possibly more often those which are not particularly strong-tasting or are of more delicate flavour and may, if the taste sense is dulled, seem to be insipid. It may further explain the liking for hard substances which have to be chewed or bitten into, because having to do this may be a compensation for relative lack of taste.

Likes and dislikes, however, are one thing and craving and aversions, which to qualify for this designation must have a compulsive quality, are another. Although dulling of taste may well be an important factor, it is in itself probably an incomplete explanation; and several other possibilities, some of which have been discussed, may need to be invoked in order to make the explanation complete.

8

Conclusion

In conclusion it may be asked: do any of these disorders of appetite ever have harmful consequences? Isolated aversions and cravings almost certainly do not, although if overeating of a more generalized kind occurs, this may result in obesity. In contrast, if there is severe anorexia, also of a more generalized kind, nutrition may suffer.

With pica of certain kinds more direct harm may result, although this seems to be rare. Whether it does or not presumably depends on the nature of the substance and the amount ingested. It is difficult to believe that those of Harries and Hughes's[15] correspondents who recorded a craving for such things as disinfectant, petrol, or paraffin, could have actually taken very much of these substances.

Odd examples of untoward complications have, however, been recorded. The teeth of a pregnant woman who chewed two or three small pieces of coal daily for some months finally became soft and badly eroded.[22] Pleshette[26] encountered a case of pica-bezoar simulating intestinal obstruction in a woman who ate sand and ground-cement. This was relieved by oil retention enemas and colonic irrigation. There is also some conflict of opinion as to whether geophagia (which has occasionally been diagnosed radiologically[24, 26]) is harmful. Although, as mentioned, it is conceivable that clay-eaters are mineral-deficient, it is just as likely that malnutrition may be as much a result as a cause. After all, a woman who gorges herself with clay may suffer a reduction in appetite for more nutritious foods.

Similarly, eaters of clay and cornstarch have been found to be more anaemic than those who do not eat these substances. Another study of a comparable group of women did not confirm this. There seems also to be disagreement about whether toxaemia is commoner in clay- and cornstarch-eaters. Edwards et al.[9] did not find this to be so, but stated that the condition of infants born to clay- and cornstarch-eaters was poorer, with a higher stillbirth and mortality rate. O'Rourke *et al.*,[25] on the other hand, found that toxaemia was twice as prevalent in the pica as in the non-pica group. Further investigation is clearly needed to resolve these differences.

REFERENCES

1. Aetology of pica. Annotation 1959. *Lancet*, ii, 281.
2. BROEDERS, G. H. 1967. Anorexia nervosa in pregnancy. *Med. T. Verlosk.*, **67**, 272.
3. CARESANO, G. and MINAZZI, M. 1965. Taste sensitivity in pregnancy and puerperium. Electrogensimetric study. *Ann. Ostet. Ginec.*, **87**, 298.
4. CARLANDER, O. 1959. Aetiology of pica. *Lancet*, ii, 569.
5. COOPER, M. 1957. *Pica*. Springfield, Illinois: Charles C. Thomas.
6. DEUTSCH, H. 1947. *Psychology of women*, Vol. 2 *Motherhood*. London: Research Books, Ltd.
7. DICKENS, G. and TRETHOWAN, W. H. 1971. Cravings and aversions during pregnancy. *J. psychosom. Res.*, **15**, 259–268.
8. EDWARDS, C. H., McSWAIN, H. and HAIRE, S. 1954. Odd dietary practices of women. *J. Amer. diet. Ass.*, **30**, 976.
9. EDWARDS, C. H., McDONALD, S., MITCHELL, J. R., JONES, L., MASON, L. and TRIGG, L. 1964. Effect of clay and cornstarch intake on women and their infants. *J. Amer. diet. Ass.*, **46**, 109–115.
10. ELLIS, H. 1900. *The psychology of sex. Vol. 3, Part 1*. New York: Random House.
11. FENICHEL, O. 1945. *The psychoanalytic theory of neurosis*. London: Routledge & Kegan Paul.
12. FOSTER, J. W. 1927. Pica. *Kenya E. Afr. med. J.*, **4**, 68.
13. GOULD, G. M. and. PYLE, W. L. 1898. *Anomalies and curiosities of medicine*. London: Rebman Publishing Co.
14. HANSEN, R. and LANGER, W. 1935. Changes of taste in pregnancy. *Klin. Wschr.*, **14**, 1173.
15. HARRIES, J. M. and HUGHES, T. T. 1958. Enumeration of the "cravings" of some pregnant women. *Brit. med. J.*, **2**, 39.
16. HÜPFER, S. 1930. Über Schwangershafts-geluste. *Int. Z. Psychoanal.*, **16**, 105.
17. HYTTEN, F. E. and LEITCH, I 1964. *The physiology of human pregnancy*, Chap. 5. Alimentary Function. Oxford: Blackwell.
18. JEANS, P. C., SMITH, M. B. and STEARNS, G. 1952. Dietary habits of pregnant women of low income in a rural state. *J. Amer. diet. Ass.*, **28**, 27.
19. KROGER, W. S. and FREED, S. C. 1951. *Psychosomatic gynecology, including problems of obstetrical care*. Philadelphia and London: W. B. Saunders.
20. LANTUÉJOUL, P. 1957. Anorexia in the first months of pregnancy. *Progr. Med.*, **85**, 403.
21. LEAN, V. S. 1904. *Collectanea*, Vol. 2. Bristol: Simpkin, Marshall & Co.
22. LEVINE, L. and GOODWIN, R. M. 1949. Oddity of pregnancy. *New Eng. J. Med.*, **24**, 1010.
23. MARCUS, R. L. 1965. Cravings for food in pregnancy. *Manchester med. Gazette*, **44**, 16.
24. MENGEL, C. E. 1964. Geophagia diagnosed by roentgenograms. *J. Amer. med., Ass.*, **187**, 955.
25. O'ROURKE, D. E., QUINN, J. G., NICHOLSON, J. O. and GIBSON, H. H. 1967. Geophagia during pregnancy. *Obstet. and Gynec.*, **29**, 581.
26. PLESHETTE, N. 1953. Pica-Bezoar simulating intestinal obstruction during pregnancy. *Harlem Hosp. Bull.*, **6**, 137.
27. POSNER, L. B., McCOTTREY, C. M. and POSNER, A. C. 1957. Pregnancy craving and Pica. *Obstet. and Gynec.*, **9**, 270.

28. RUST, M. 1960. A survey of food habits of pregnant women. *Amer. J. Nursing*, **60,** 1636.
29. SEIFRIT, E. 1961. Changes in belief and food practices in pregnancy. *J. Amer. diet. Ass.*, **39,** 455.
30. SUVOROVA, N. M. 1959. The state of the gustatory sensitivity in normal and pathological pregnancy. *Akush. i. Ginek.*, **6,** 33.
31. SZECSI, K. 1961. Gracidin therapy of bulimia of pregnancy. *Orv. Hetil.*, **102,** 647.
32. TAGGART, N. 1961. Food habits in pregnancy. *Proc. Nutr. Soc.*, **20,** 35.
33. WELLER, S. D. V. 1963. Pica. *Curr. Med. Drugs*, **3,** 1.
34. YUDKIN, J. 1966. Man's choice of food. *Lancet*, i, 645.

XIII

THE PSYCHOPATHOLOGY OF VOMITING OF PREGNANCY

LEON CHERTOK

M.D.

Director, Psychosomatic Department,
Institut de Psychiatrie La Rochefoucauld,
Paris, France

1

Introduction

Our present-day understanding of the vomiting of pregnancy is a result of the perspectives opened up in recent years by the evolution of psychosomatic medicine. Apart from the inherent limitations of endocrine, humoral, toxic, and other such theories as to the aetiology of this condition, the latter do not, for example, take into account the facts that *not all* pregnant women vomit, that pregnant animals do not vomit, and that among some peoples vomiting of pregnancy is unknown.[4]

Review of the Literature
The long and curious history of the treatment of vomiting of pregnancy bears eloquent witness to the considerable importance of psychological factors in this condition. All kinds of empirical, and indeed exotic, modes of treatment have at various times been tried and applied, and it is significant to note that, among these, there occurred cases of "spontaneous" placebo effects.[2]

Towards the mid-nineteenth century, some of the earlier writers on severe vomiting of pregnancy had occasion to notice the personality, "nervous temperament",[14] and "pathological nervous state"[10] of the pregnant women concerned. Some authors took into account psychological factors, and spoke of "moral" (i.e. mental) conditions.[17] Finally, under the influence of psychoanalysis, attention was directed to attempting to understand the psychological significance of the symptom. Mild vomiting was also included in these studies, on the assumption that the only difference between this and severe vomiting was one of degree.

From the psychoanalytically oriented point of view, vomiting represents the expression of affective (emotional) states.[12, 16] It is taken to have the general meaning of symbolic rejection,[11, 13] an oral attempt at abortion.[19, 22, 24] Adopting the view that the woman who vomits has, in a sense, chosen to vomit and not to miscarry, Helen Deutsch[9] has pointed out the rather ambivalent attitude in such cases in the mother-child relationship.

In addition to these deep-lying psychological motives, the pregnant woman is faced with a number of conflicts and problems which, while being on a more "superficial" psychological plane, are nevertheless obviously of considerable practical importance, and thereby also affect the mother's attitude to the child: e.g. those concerned with financial difficulties, the fear of responsibilities, marital problems, the fear of being disfigured by pregnancy or of consequent illhealth, the need to give up professional activities and to reduce one's leisure time, etc.[18]

Experimental studies of vomiting during pregnancy had hitherto failed to confirm the existence of any relationship between vomiting and the rejection of the child or of motherhood.[1, 8, 15, 21] It is, however, the view of Chertok, Mondzain and Bonnaud,[3, 4, 5, 6] on the basis of more recent research, that these studies do not justify the conclusion that no such relationship exists. In fact, in these earlier studies, the problem does not seem to have been formulated sufficiently clearly, and in particular, would appear to have been defective in the following respects.

1. The criteria for the selection of samples are vague. The same sample may include primiparous and multiparous women of very different ages, of different races, and from different socio-economic and cultural backgrounds, as well as women suffering from mild or severe vomiting—in fact, a heterogeneous population.

2. The basis for the assessment of rejection is not indicated sufficiently clearly: as a result, we do not know whether this attitude was openly admitted by the women concerned, or whether it was deduced by the investigator —and if so, how much interpretation by the investigator was involved.

3. In general, it is by no means clear at what stage of pregnancy the investigation was undertaken, nor whether account was taken of the influence of any possible retrospective rearrangement of data, where the investigation was carried out subsequent to the period of vomiting.

2

Present Study

The present writer and his colleagues[3, 4, 5, 6] have attempted a new approach to the problem of vomiting of pregnancy, formulating, as far as possible, precise working hypotheses, and clearly defining the conditions of investigation.

Already in various earlier papers, we reassessed the factors most frequently mentioned in the literature in relation to the vomiting of pregnancy: viz. the mother's attitude toward the child; frigidity; the mother's personality (mother image); the husband's attitude and personality; and practical socio-economic difficulties. To these we added the following items: the mother's experience of the first foetal movements (quickening); the incidence of psychosomatic symptoms other than vomiting; and (where relevant) the result of preparation for childbirth.

The general hypothesis is retained, that there is a relationship between vomiting of pregnancy and the mother's attitude to the child. Clinical experience, however, by no means supports the view that—as might have been thought—the attitude most likely to provoke the symptom is one of rejection. Thus we have been struck, in the course of our clinical observations, by the fact that in France *unmarried mothers rarely vomit*. This is confirmed by Sendral;[23] and yet it seems a reasonable assumption that unmarried mothers should, in general, tend to reject motherhood.

Similarly Nordmeyer,[20] in Germany, reported that, of 85 women who sought an abortion, *not one* vomited. It is, therefore, interesting to find that in Switzerland unmarried women *do* vomit: this can possibly be explained by the fact that in that country abortion is more readily accepted, officially and socially, for reasons of health.

Already in 1962, the author and his colleagues[4] noted with considerable interest that the "ambivalent attitude is found only in those pregnant women who vomit, and with an extraordinary degree of reciprocity, all women who vomit have an ambivalent attitude." They added the following comment.

"This might be interpreted as follows.

The woman who does not vomit either blooms fully through her pregnancy, which enables her to live deeply her desire to have a baby, or refuses the pregnancy with such intensity as to deny its existence, abstaining from the social right to vomit.

Vomiting thus seems to be a means of expressing the inner struggle of contradictory tendencies, and not a pure and simple expression of the refusal of maternity."

We were, therefore, led to the conclusion that it is not marked rejection which tends to induce vomiting, and consequently we attempted to define more precisely the mother's attitude towards the child, by taking into account not only clear-cut attitudes of wanting and rejecting, but also an "ambivalent" attitude.

Method

The present research involved 100 primiparous women, followed from the third month of pregnancy until childbirth. Ages ranged from 18 to 38 years, with a mean age of $24\frac{1}{2}$ years. It should be stated that in this research no attempt was made to study a random sample; the criteria of selection were simply the following: (1) primiparae, (2) married and of French origin, (3) having attended the maternity department concerned before the third month of pregnancy.

The data were obtained from "semistructured" (semi-formalized) psychological interviews, in the course of which the various problems of pregnancy and childbirth were dealt with. More specifically, an analysis was made of data concerning vomiting and the mother's attitude towards the child. Attention was necessarily limited to conscious attitudes expressed verbally, for it was clear that the data were not such as would allow any adequate assessment of more deep-seated attitudes. In particular, the mother's attitude toward the child was assessed early in pregnancy, i.e. during the actual period of vomiting. It is for this reason that the data obtained from the first interview, in the third month of pregnancy, were taken as the principal basis for determining the original attitude of the women, independent of the influence of those surrounding them and of later evolutionary changes.

In the present research, in the first place, *vomiting* was defined as rejection of gastric content; no account was taken of simple nausea. Of the 100 women studied, 68 vomited during pregnancy.

The usual, mild vomiting was observed clinically in 54 (79%) of the 68 women who vomited. In the remaining 14 cases (21%) the vomiting was more severe, but not serious enough to require hospitalization. In no case was there severe, persistent vomiting in the "classical" sense—i.e. hyperemesis such as might endanger the mother's life.

The following *criteria for research* were isolated and defined:

Attitude toward the child. Conscious, verbally expressed attitudes on the mother's part were defined in three distinct categories:

1. Child wanted. This category included all instances where the women verbally expressed their desire for motherhood. In such cases pregnancy was eagerly awaited, sometimes watched for, and its confirmation was greeted with joy.

2. Child rejected. Women in this category immediately and unequivocally expressed their rejection of motherhood. Pregnancy was regarded as a catastrophe, accepted only because of external social pressures (husband, family, etc.), and in fact felt to be imposed by force.

These first two attitudes, of wanting and rejecting the child respectively, have in common the fact that they are *clear-cut* and unambiguously expressed verbally.

3. Ambivalent attitude. This category included women in whom opposing tendencies co-existed. These women were partly pleased, and partly annoyed, by their situation. At any given time, either attitude might predominate, but the other was always present, particularly in conversation.

In a preliminary pilot study, an attempt was made to discover a relationship between vomiting in pregnancy and the (verbally expressed) attitude of the mother toward the prospective child, from an analysis of the records of 50 women. This preliminary survey revealed a positive relationship between vomiting and ambivalence on the mother's part. This finding was confirmed by a subsequent study of 50 additional case records.

Frigidity. We classified as frigid those women who asserted that they did not experience any pleasure in the sexual act, and for whom sexual relations constituted a purely "marital duty".

Mother image. We considered only the *negative* aspects of the mother image, and recorded as such:

—an anxious, pessimistic or domineering, unloving character on the mother's part;
—a previous pathological obstetrical history, experienced as a younger woman;
—the influence of prejudicial information concerning pregnancy and motherhood;
—psychological trauma consequent upon the mother's permanent or protracted absence.

Husband's attitude. The husband may assume a *positive* role, in a harmonious couple for whom the child is often a fulfilment. He may, on the other hand, assume a *negative* role, through his hostility or ambivalence towards his wife's pregnancy, or otherwise, by his *non-participation* in his wife's life and problems, and their evolution.

Socio-economic difficulties. It was essentially *housing problems* (inadequate or insanitary housing, etc.) which presented themselves in the course of our investigations.

Experience of first foetal movements (quickening). We distinguished:

—a positive experience: an emotionally pleasurable occasion;
—a negative experience: a disagreeable, or even painful, occasion;
—a neutral experience, without any particular emotional impact.

Psychosomatic symptoms (other than vomiting). We regarded as such *all functional symptoms*, whether painful or not (e.g. vertigo, severe headaches, lumbar pains, etc.).

Results of preparation for childbirth.[7] In those women who had undergone preparation for childbirth, an evaluation of the latter was made, after parturition, in terms of a successful or unsuccessful result (complete or partial).

It now seemed advisable to combine the results obtained from the two samples. At this point two questions arose—the first concerning the *homogeneity* of classification of the two successive groups studied, and the second concerning its *objectivity*.

1. It was feared that, as the criteria of judgment became more closely defined with use, so also might they have become distorted. Furthermore, because of our growing interest in the vomiting of pregnancy, the tendency of our interviews was to improve the quality of our enquiry on this subject. The later case-records are clearly more complete, and more detailed and precise, than the earlier ones, with respect to the symptom of vomiting of

pregnancy. It is necessary, therefore, to ask ourselves whether the results obtained in the two respective groups are in fact homogeneous.

2. Again, the same group of investigators had carried out the two successive analyses (i.e. those, respectively, of the pilot study, and of the subsequent survey of 50 additional cases), and had participated in the formulation of the hypotheses. There was, therefore, a distinct possibility that the interpretation of the results, in the second analysis, might be biased in the direction of the earlier hypotheses and findings.

The solution to the first problem was achieved by use of an odd-even statistical control. This not only guaranteed homogeneity of classification and justified the combining of the two samples, but also answered the possible objection as to a heterogeneous selection of the two samples.

The second problem was solved by submitting the records of the 100 cases to three independent, external judges—psychologists from outside the research team, who had not participated in the actual investigation. These were provided with the criteria for classification, formulated in such a way as to reduce to a minimum the role of subjective interpretation. The judges worked independently, and their separate judgments were brought together only for a final synthesis. Since provision was made for only two possible alternative answers ("Yes" and "No") to each item, it was agreed that, where judgments differed, that of the majority would be accepted. Needless to say, the judges carried out their task in complete ignorance of the hypotheses formulated by the research workers, as well as the previous results obtained. As an additional . precaution, vomiting was removed from the items for judgment. In this way, the possibility was eliminated that the judges might be reformulating working hypotheses on the basis of their own observations, thereby introducing the defect of secondary subjectivity.

Results

The data tabulated below represent, in the case of each specific criterion, the assessment of the research team (Tables I–VII), and the majority assessment of the external judges (Tables Ia, IIa, IIIa, b, IVa–VIIa, VIII). These data were subjected to the χ^2 test.

1. *Attitude toward the child.* We have mentioned elsewhere[3, 6] the reasons which induced us, for convenience in statistical analysis, to combine the respective attitudes of wanting and rejecting the prospective child, in a single category of "*clearly defined attitudes*".

From Table I, which is based on the research team's assessment, it will be seen that there is no relationship between vomiting on one hand, and a clearly defined attitude of acceptance or rejection by the mother on the other hand; but that there *does* exist, in support of the hypothesis advanced, a correlation between vomiting and an *ambivalent* attitude. A χ^2 test confirmed the positive correlation between *vomiting and ambivalence*, at a ·02 level of significance.

TABLE I

Attitude toward the child, and vomiting
(Research team's assessment)

	Clearly defined attitude	Ambivalent attitude	Total
Vomiting women	31	37	68
Non-vomiting women	24	8	32
Total	55	45	100

Table I*a*, which represents the majority assessment of the external judges, does not, however, provide confirmation of a correlation at the same level of significance. In this instance, the relationship between vomiting and ambivalence, while not statistically significant, nevertheless shows the same trend. Among those who vomited, 36 women (53%) were assessed as ambivalent, as compared with 12 (38%) of those who did *not* vomit.

TABLE I*a*

Attitude toward the child, and vomiting
(External judges' assessment)

	Clearly defined attitude	Ambivalent attitude	Total
Vomiting women	32	36	68
Non-vomiting women	20	12	32
Total	52	48	100

It should be noted that these results are derived from a majority assessment of the divergent individual evaluations made by each of the external judges. The findings of one of these gave a positive correlation, at the ·05 level of significance. While the other two judges' findings were not statistically significant, they did in fact give consistent confirmation of the same general trend. At all events, the majority assessment, therefore, could not but partly obscure the correlation observed by the first judge.

During the meeting between research personnel and external judges, for the purpose of synthesizing the data obtained, a careful study of individual assessments showed that one of the judges tended to regard as rejection maternal attitudes that the others considered as ambivalent. In this instance, the judge concerned adhered very closely to the very first attitude manifested by the woman—one which she herself conceived, in retrospect, as her reaction to her first awareness of pregnancy.

On the other hand, a second judge assessed a large number of women as ambivalent. He considered as rejection only those attitudes persisting at the time of interview, regarding as ambivalent those cases in which initial rejection is converted to acceptance under external (personal and environmental) pressures.

These two judges adhered very closely to the criteria as defined, while, however, each applying them to a different stage of pregnancy.

The third judge provided more interpretative assessments, integrating the different types of attitude observed at the various stages. It may be noted that it is his assessments which provided proof of our hypothesis at the most satisfactory level of statistical significance, and are most consistent with those of the research team.

2. *Frigidity*. Neither of the following Tables II and IIa reveals any correlation between vomiting and frigidity.

TABLE II

Frigidity and vomiting
(Research team's assessment)

	Frigid	Non-frigid	Total
Vomiting women	32	36	68
Non-vomiting women	11	21	32
Total	43	57	100

TABLE IIa

Frigidity and vomiting
(External judges' assessment)
(13 cases excluded for lack of information on this criterion)

	Frigid	Non-frigid	Total
Vomiting women	15	40	55
Non-vomiting women	9	23	32
Total	24	63	87

3. *Mother image*. The assessment by the research team, of "poor mother image", as undertaken in our first analysis, was an *overall* assessment. The data thus obtained are shown in Table III.

TABLE III

Poor mother image (overall assessment) *and vomiting*
(Research team's assessment)
(10 cases, of which 8 of vomiting, excluded)

	Poor mother image	Other cases	Total
Vomiting women	37	23	60
Non-vomiting women	18	12	30
Total	55	35	90

The criteria of assessment submitted to the external judges were, however, subdivided into the following components: psychological, obstetrical, and traumatic. Where the presence of *one single component* gave rise to the assessment of "poor mother image", the data summarized in Table IIIa were obtained.

TABLE IIIa

Poor mother image (one component) *and vomiting*
(External judges' assessment)
(2 cases of vomiting excluded)

	Poor mother image	Other cases	Total
Vomiting women	28	37	65
Non-vomiting women	15	18	33
Total	43	55	98

Where not one, but *two components*, were taken into consideration, the data shown in Table IIIb were obtained.

TABLE IIIb

Poor mother image (two components) *and vomiting*
(External judges' assessment)
(4 cases of vomiting excluded)

	Poor mother image	Other cases	Total
Vomiting women	10	53	63
Non-vomiting women	4	29	33
Total	14	82	96

Neither the research workers, nor the external judges, were able to find any correlation between vomiting and a poor mother image.

This apparent concordance of the statistical results does not, however, bring out the relative difference in emphasis between the assessments of the external judges and those of the research team. Generally speaking, the external judges proved less severe than the research workers, in their attitude toward the mothers of our pregnant subjects. It is our opinion that there entered into the picture, here, important variations in the evaluation of the mother image. These variations are no doubt dependent upon the difficulties of defining mother-daughter relationships, and the delimitation of their role.

4. *Attitude and role of husband.* The trend towards a negative correlation between vomiting and the "husband's positive contribution", which would seem to emerge from the research team's analysis (Table IV), finds confirmation in the external judges' assessment (Table IVa).

TABLE IV

Attitude of husband and vomiting
(Research team's assessment)

	Positive contribution	Other cases	Total
Vomiting women	34	34	68
Non-vomiting women	22	10	32
Total	56	44	100

TABLE IVa

Attitude of husband and vomiting
(External judges' assessment)
(8 cases, of which 7 of vomiting, excluded)

	Positive contribution	Other cases	Total
.Vomiting women	43	18	61
Non-vomiting women	26	5	31
Total	69	23	92

5. *Housing problems.* As shown in Tables V and Va, there appears to be no correlation between vomiting and housing problems.

TABLE V

Housing problems and vomiting
(Research team's assessment)

	Housing problems	Other cases	Total
Vomiting women	24	44	68
Non-vomiting women	12	20	32
Total	36	64	100

TABLE Va

Housing problems and vomiting
(External judges' assessment)
(2 cases excluded)

	Housing problems	Other cases	Total
Vomiting women	23	44	67
Non-vomiting women	8	23	31
Total	31	67	98

6. *Psychosomatic symptoms* (other than vomiting). The external judges (Table VIa) found a tendency toward a correlation between vomiting and other psychosomatic symptoms. Preceding findings on the part of the research team (Table VI) tended, in fact, to show that, on the contrary, women who did not vomit presented more psychosomatic symptoms of other kinds than those who vomited—thus suggesting the hypothesis that these symptoms serve a substitutive role.

The contradictory results obtained from the two analyses merely show that the criteria for scoring have been differently applied in the two respective cases. It is, therefore, not possible at the present time to draw any conclusions whatsoever from our analyses, as to a possible relationship between vomiting and other psychosomatic symptoms.

TABLE VI

Psychosomatic symptoms (other) and vomiting
(Research team's assessment)

	Present	Absent	Total
Vomiting women	57	11	68
Non-vomiting women	31	1	32
Total	88	12	100

TABLE VIa

Psychosomatic symptoms (other) and vomiting
(External judges' assessment)
(1 case of vomiting excluded)

	Present	Absent	Total
Vomiting women	61	6	67
Non-vomiting women	25	7	32
Total	86	13	99

7. *Results of preparation for childbirth.* The data obtained (Tables VII and VIIa) show that there is no correlation between vomiting of pregnancy and the successful or unsuccessful result of preparation for childbirth.

TABLE VII

Preparation for childbirth, and vomiting
(Research team's assessment)
(76 = number of prepared women)

	Success	Failure	Total
Vomiting women	26	25	51
Non-vomiting women	15	10	25
Total	41	35	76

TABLE VIIa

Preparation for childbirth, and vomiting
(External judges' assessment)
(61 = number of prepared women available for interview)

	Success	Failure	Total
Vomiting women	19	18	37
Non-vomiting women	15	9	24
Total	34	27	61

8. *Experience of first foetal movements (quickening).* Table VIII represents the findings of the external judges alone. The research team had originally directed its analysis towards investigating the possibility of a correlation between the mother's first awareness of the foetal movements (quickening), and the cessation of vomiting. In fact, it was not possible to

substantiate any such correlation. However, in the course of our analyses another hypothesis emerged, viz. the possible relationship between vomiting and the nature of the emotional experience of quickening. It is this hypothesis which we submitted to the external judges, for their considered assessment.

From Table VIII it will be seen that, if one considers on the one hand positive and neutral experiences, and on the other hand negative experience, there is a very definite trend towards a *positive correlation* between vomiting and a *negative experience of quickening*.

TABLE VIII

Experience of first foetal movements, and vomiting
(External judges' assessment)
(12 cases excluded—6 in each group)

	Positive experience	Negative experience	Neutral experience	Total
Vomiting women	30	13	18	61
Non-vomiting women	19	2	6	27
Total	49	15	24	88

3

Conclusions

The main findings of the author's research team, which received substantial confirmation from the assessments of three external (independent) judges, were concerned with the establishment of correlations between various psychological factors and the vomiting of pregnancy. They may be summarized as follows:

1. a positive correlation between vomiting and the mother's *ambivalent* attitude towards the prospective child.
2. a positive correlation between vomiting and the mother's *negative* experience of the first foetal movements (quickening).
3. a negative correlation between vomiting and the husband's "positive contribution" to the marital partnership.

In particular, the results of this research suggest, therefore, a connection between vomiting and the ambivalent attitude of the pregnant woman toward her child. Contrary to earlier assumptions, however, the results show, in support of the author's hypothesis, that it is not rejection in itself that tends to provoke the symptoms, but a more complex attitude in which the tendency toward rejection conflicts with opposite tendencies (toward desire and acceptance).

Vomiting may therefore represent the expression of a conflict between wanting and rejecting the child. While this conflict may become manifest in other psychosomatic symptoms, vomiting would appear to be the most widespread form of expression in this particular instance.

It can readily be imagined that ambivalent women, as we have described them, i.e. those who have no clearly defined attitude toward the child, are more liable on the one hand to disturbance by unconscious conflicts, and on the other to socio-cultural influences. It can equally well be imagined that the conflict itself is more severe in ambivalent women.

4

Summary

Our present-day understanding of vomiting of pregnancy is a result of the new perspectives opened up by psychosomatic medicine.

The relationship between vomiting of pregnancy and the attitude toward the child (as also other factors) was studied in 100 primiparous women, of whom 68 suffered from vomiting. Verbally expressed attitudes were studied by "semi-structured" (semi-formalized) interviews.

The results show a positive relationship between vomiting of pregnancy and an ambivalent attitude on the mother's part toward her prospective child.

REFERENCES

1. BERNSTEIN, I. C. 1952. An investigation into the etiology of nausea and vomiting of pregnancy. *Minnesota Med.*, **5**, 34.
2. CHERTOK, L. 1965. A historical note on placebo effects in vomiting of pregnancy. *J. Amer. med. Ass.*, **194**, 473.
3. CHERTOK, L., MONDZAIN, M. L. and BONNAUD, M. 1962. Désir d'enfant et vomissement. *Proc. 3rd World Congress Psychiatry* (Montreal, June 1961), **2**, 1022 (General sessions).
4. CHERTOK, L., MONDZAIN, M. L. and BONNAUD, M. 1962. Psychological, social and cultural aspects of sickness during pregnancy. *Activ. nerv. sup.*, **4**, 394.
5. CHERTOK, L., MONDZAIN, M. L., and BONNAUD, M. 1962. Recherche sur les facteurs psychologiques du vomissement gravidique: contribution méthodologique. *Bull. Inst. nat. Hyg.*, **17**, 975.
6. CHERTOK, L., MONDZAIN, M. L. and BONNAUD, M. 1963. Vomiting and the wish to have a child. *Psychosom. Med.*, **25**, 13.
7. CHERTOK, L., BONNAUD, M., BORELLI, M., DONNET, J. L. and REVAULT d'ALLONNES, C. 1969. *Motherhood and personality: psychosomatic aspects of childbirth*, London: Tavistock Publications.
8. COPPEN, A. J. 1959. Vomiting of early pregnancy: psychological factors and body build. *Lancet*, i, 172.
9. DEUTSCH, H. 1947. *The psychology of women: a psychoanalytic interpretation*, **2** (Motherhood), 112, 113, 119. London: Heinemann.
10. DOLÉRIS, J. A. 1896. (Intervention dans la discussion de la communication de L. E. Damany: les vomissements incoercibles au début de la grossesse—Séance du 16 Avril, 1896, de la Soc. d'Obstét. et de Gynéc. de Paris). *Ann. Gynéc. Obstét.*, **45**, 402.

11. FERENCZI, S. 1952. In *First contributions to psycho-analysis* (transl. by Ernest Jones). London: Hogarth Press.
12. FREUD, A. 1946. The psychoanalytic study of infantile feeding disturbances. *Psychoanal. Study Child*, **2**, 119.
13. FREUD, S., and BREUER, J. 1895. *Studies on hysteria*. In Freud, S., *Complete psychological works: Standard Edition*, **2**, London: Hogarth Press. 1955.
14. GUÉNIOT, A. 1863. *Les vomissements incoercibles pendant la grossesse* (Thèse d'Agrégation). Paris: Martinet.
15. KLEIN, H. R., POTTER, H. W. and DYK, R. B. 1950, *Anxiety in pregnancy and childbirth*. New York: Hoeber.
16. MASSERMAN, J. 1946. Psychogenic vomiting. *J. nerv. ment. Dis.*, **103**, 224.
17. MATHIEU, A. and ROUX, J. C. 1904. *Maladies de l'appareil digestif*. Paris: Doin.
18. MENNINGER, W. C. 1943. The emotional factors in pregnancy. *Bull. Menninger Clin.*, **7**, 15.
19. MÜLLER, E. H. 1908. Beiträge zur Kenntnis der Hyperemesis gravidarum. *Psychiat. neurol. Wschr.*, **10**, 102, 125, 134, 149, 156, 164, 190.
20. NORDMEYER, K. 1946. Zur Ätiologie der Hyperemesis gravidarum. *Dtsch. med. Wschr.*, **71**, 213.
21. ROBERTSON, G. 1946. Nausea and vomiting of pregnancy. *Lancet*, i, 336.
22. SCHWAB, M. 1921. Die Ursache des unstillbaren Erbrechens in der Schwangerschaft. *Zbl. Gynäk.*, **45**, 956.
23. SENDRAL, L. 1915. *Sur les vomissements gravidiques: celles qui vomissent, celles qui ne vomissent pas* (Thèse No. 14). Montpellier.
24. WEISS, E. and ENGLISH, O. S. 1957. *Psychosomatic medicine*, 3rd edn., p. 382. Philadelphia: Saunders.

XIV

PSYCHOPATHOLOGY OF TOXAEMIA OF PREGNANCY

C. A. Douglas Ringrose

M.D., F.R.C.S.(C)

Edmonton, Alberta

Canada

1

Introduction

Description and Distribution

Toxaemia of pregnancy is a disorder, unique to the human species, that occurs in the last half of pregnancy in one pregnancy out of fifteen. There are two gradations of the condition. Pre-eclampsia is characterized by a blood pressure exceeding 140/90 mm of mercury with abnormal edema and/or albuminuria. Eclampsia is present when convulsions are super-imposed. At times the disorder can occur with pre-existing hypertensive disorders. The disease is more common in the underprivileged, the un-educated and the indigent. There is also a higher incidence in the very young and the very old primigravida. Prenatal care reduces the incidence of pre-eclampsia and virtually abolishes eclampsia.

The patho-physiology has been exhaustively studied and consists of abnormal sodium and water retention and vaso-spasm with the resultant well known clinical picture. Characteristic reversible renal lesions have been described,[23] and are likely secondary to the vaso-spasm. Toxaemic lesions elsewhere are not specific or invariable and are probably secondary to hypoxia and electrolyte imbalance.

Etiology

Organic theories on the etiology of toxaemia have been very numerous and the comment of Zinke,[27] expounded fifty-eight years ago, retains con-temporary pertinence. He stated: "We know something of the causes but precious little of the character of the poison or its origin, notwithstanding the extensive and continued investigations by good men the world over." The role of toxin producer has been assigned to many organs or organ combinations. At times hyperfunction of the organ has been implicated and at other times, hypofunction has been blamed. The etiologic "organs" have included breasts, pituitary, adrenal, placenta, uterus and kidneys.

Sellheim[16] felt that mammary toxins were responsible.

Hyperplacentosis due to over-activity of the Langhans layer and over-production of chorionic gonadotrophin has been postulated by some[10] and refuted by others.[25] On the other hand, placental ischemia has been said to produce malfunction of enzymes engaged in deactivating pressor and water-retaining substances. These substances escape into the circulation and produce hypertension and make vessels more permeable.[14] Kaku[11] and Magara[13] favor a placental substance as a cause of toxaemia. Renal ischemia has been proposed by Sophian[22] as the etiologic agent, whereas others considered this a result rather than the cause of the disorder. The adrenal cortex and the adrenal medulla have been implicated due to overproduction of products by some, and underproduction by others.[2, 8, 14]

The anterior and posterior pituitary have likewise been involved by the theorists.

A patient's blood type was once considered important in predisposing her to toxaemia, but later reports have refuted this view. A primary cerebral dysrhythmia has also been proposed as a cause of eclampsia.[19, 26]

No organic theory has persisted in the face of critical appraisal.

2

Psychopathogenesis

A number of authors have recognized the important role of the emotions and the personality in the development of toxaemia of pregnancy. Dieckmann[6] has written: "The fact that intelligent prenatal care, even under poor nutritional conditions, has resulted in a decreased incidence of eclampsia and severe pre-eclampsia together with a marked decrease in maternal mortality from the toxaemias of pregnancy, usually eclampsia, demonstrates that pre-eclampsia-eclampsia is preventable. The perfect control would be constant twenty-four hour observation and complete control of the ingestion of food and fluid in the pregnant woman from the first month, together with the elimination of all factors which increase tension." Brown[3] has observed that more than two prenatal visits virtually prevents eclampsia, suggesting that even the most superficial doctor-patient relationship has prophylactic value. Soichet[21] has stated that toxaemia is a somatic solution to conflict. He feels that the patient considers herself guilty in the eyes of the unborn baby. This stimulates destructive forces latent within the woman and toxaemia results. He notes that toxaemia is unusual in schizophrenics because a different solution to their conflicts is employed. Salerno,[20] however, claims that toxaemia occurs frequently in schizoid patients and represents a patho-physiological response to prolonged stress. Holland and Bourne[9] state that emotional tranquillity and complete physical rest is the ideal for which to aim in the control of pre-eclampsia. Coppen[5] feels that pre-eclamptics are more masculine than the control group.

In assessing the role of the mind in the genesis of toxaemia of pregnancy one can utilize retrospective or prospective techniques.

Retrospective Assessment

The Minnesota Multiphasic Personality Inventory test was given to 41 patients who manifested toxaemia of pregnancy; 28 were given the test in the antepartum period and 13 received the test immediately post-partum. Thirty-two had pre-eclampsia, 7 had hypertension with superimposed pre-eclampsia and 2 had eclampsia. The age distribution of these patients is outlined in Table I. There were 12 primigravida, 8 were gravida two, 2 were

TABLE I

AGE DISTRIBUTION OF TOXAEMIC PATIENTS

Age Range (In Years)	No. of Cases
10 — 15	4
16 — 20	10
21 — 25	7
26 — 30	5
31 — 35	8
36 — 40	4
41 — 45	3

gravida three, 2 were gravida four and 17 were gravida five to seventeen. Twenty-two were single, widowed, separated or divorced, and 19 were married. There was a past history of toxaemia in 10 of the 29 multiparous women. In 11 of the 41 toxaemic patients, a family history of hypertension was elicited. An assessment of weight gain in these 41 women indicated that 12 gained between 21 and 30 pounds. Sixteen gained less than 20 pounds and 13 patients gained more than 30 pounds.

The Minnesota Multiphasic Personality Inventory consists of 566 statements, which are answered true or false depending on the patient's opinion of herself. The answers are then evaluated, and by comparing the responses to the normal parameters laid down by experience 10 personality factors can be evaluated. The tests are also evaluated for reliability of response and validity (the L, F and K scores). A question score consisting of all the "cannot say" responses is also obtained. The personality factors evaluated are: hypochondriasis (Hs), depressive (D), hysteria (Hy), psychopathic deviate (Pd), interests (Mf), paranoia (Pa), psychasthenia (Pt), schizophrenia

TABLE II

PERSONALITY ASSESSMENT OF 41 TOXAEMIC PATIENTS

	PRE - ECLAMPSIA	HYPERTENSION + PRE - ECLAMPSIA	ECLAMPSIA	% of total
Abnormal.... .... (trait or traits above 70th percentile)	14	4	1	46
Borderline Abnormal......... (trait or traits between 61st and 70th percentile)	15	3	1	46
Normal.......... .... (all traits below 61st percentile)	3	0	0	8

(Sc), hypomania (Ma), and sociability (Si). Liberal variation is permitted, as the answers are considered normal if they fall between the 40th and 60th percentile and abnormal if they fall outside the 30th or the 70th percentile. The M.M.P.I. results on the 41 patients are summarized in Table II.

Results of Retrospective Study. Nineteen personalities had frankly abnormal traits, 19 had borderline abnormal traits, and only 3 personalities were definitely normal. The incidence of each abnormal and borderline abnormal trait is shown in Table III. No particular abnormal personality pattern appears to predominate.

TABLE III

INCIDENCE OF A NORMAL AND BORDERLINE ABNORMAL
PERSONALITY TRAITS (M. M. P. I.) IN A GROUP OF 41
TOXAEMIC PATIENTS

TRAIT	Number of occurrences in abnormal range	Number of occurrences in borderline abnormal range
Hypochondriasis	4	7
Depression	2	12
Hysteria	4	6
Psychopathic deviate	7	11
Interests	6	12
Paranoia	0	14
Psychasthenia	1	7
Schizophrenia	6	7
Mania	6	9
Sociability	0	11

Prospective Assessment

It is well known that the unmarried mother, particularly in the younger age groups, has a higher than average tendency to develop toxaemia. Accordingly, it was decided to utilize the Minnesota Multiphasic Personality Inventory to test a group of young unmarried mothers from a Salvation Army Hospital. The group was predominantly from the middle economic class. They usually lived at the hospital during the last half of pregnancy and had regular prenatal examinations. The test was given to 41 consecutive, unselected patients and was administered in all cases before the onset of symptoms of toxaemia. Subsequently, 8 developed pre-eclampsia and 14 manifested incipient pre-eclampsia. Incipient pre-eclampsia was diagnosed if the subjects developed abnormal edema and had a weight gain of two pounds or more in one week. Nineteen showed no evidence of toxaemia. The ages of these 41 unmarried mothers are as follows: 2 were between eleven and fifteen years, 31 were between sixteen and twenty, and 8 were between twenty-one and twenty-five.

Prospective Study Results. Nine of the 14 patients with incipient pre-eclampsia (64%) had abnormal personalities as evidenced by reliable, valid records with a score or scores above the 70th percentile. Of the 8 patients with pre-eclampsia, 6 (75%) had abnormal personalities. In contrast, only 6 in this group of 19 unmarried mothers who did not develop pre-eclampsia (32%) had abnormal personalities. The incidence of each abnormal factor is outlined in Table IV.

TABLE IV

INCIDENCE OF ABNORMAL PERSONALITY TRAITS

Category	H_8	D	Hy	Pd	Mf	Pa	Pt	Sc	Ma	Si	Normal
No pre-eclampsia (19 cases)	0	0	0	5	1	2	1	2	3	1	13
Incipient pre-eclampsia (14 cases)	1	2	0	6	3	3	2	6	2	1	5
Pre-eclampsia (8 cases)	0	0	0	5	1	1	0	1	2	0	2

There were no scores below the thirtieth percentile. Multiple abnormal factors were present in some records. In the pre-eclampsia group, 5 personalities were abnormal in the psychopathic deviate area, 2 in the manic category, and 1 each in interest, paranoia and schizophrenia. Among the incipient pre-eclamptics, 6 were abnormal in the schizophrenic category; 6 in the psychopathic deviate area; 3 in interest and paranoia; two each in psychasthenia, mania and depressive; and 1 each in hypochondriasis and sociability. Of the 6 abnormal personalities in the group of 19 who did not develop pre-eclampsia, the incidence of abnormal factors was psychopathic deviate 5; mania 3; paranoia and schizophrenia 3 each; interest, psychasthenia and sociability 1 each. Statistical analysis of the correlation between emotional instability and toxaemia reveals that there is only one possibility in twenty that these results could occur by chance alone.

Additional Evidence

In the course of using auto-hypnosis as a tool for shortening labor, it has been observed that toxaemia is virtually abolished.[18]

The use of hypnosis during parturition is an ancient practice which has recently manifested resurgent interest. It is likely that the natural childbirth methods of Read[17] as well as the psycho-prophylactic relaxation techniques of Lamaze[12] and similar programs in Russia,[15] United States,[1] Eastern Europe[7] and China[4] utilize hypnotic phenomena. The hypnotic relaxation is taught initially toward the end of the second trimester and reiterated on three or four pre-natal visits during the remainder of the pregnancy. Prior to this, the physiologic changes that occur during pregnancy and delivery are explained. Labor is portrayed as a natural, normal phenomenon entailing vigorous activity by the automatically working uterus with resultant muscle soreness and fatigue. This strenuous muscular exertion by the uterus is portrayed as analogous to the soreness in the leg muscles of a long-distance runner towards the end of a race. The doctor's role is said to be similar to the coach of an athlete, assisted in his function by the nursing personnel and the husband when possible.

As a result of the auto-hypnosis conditioning, the labors in primigravida age eleven to twenty were 64% as long as a corresponding control group. In primigravida twenty-one to thirty years of age, the labors were 74% as long as the control group. In women para one to para four, aged twenty-one to thirty years, the average labor in the hypnosis conditioned group was 65% as long as the control group. The incidence of toxaemia of pregnancy in utilizing this regime was less than 2% and exclusively of a very mild variety.

3

Management

The etiology of toxaemia of pregnancy has not been satisfactorily explained by any organic theory. Evidence has been presented in favor of personality decompensation during pregnancy as a cause of toxaemia. This psycho-somatic theory is shown in Table V, which lists the negative influences that can affect the pregnant patient. Personality tests such as the M.M.P.I. may help elicit the high-risk patient and permit the use of more intensive prophylactic measures. The type of personality deviation that predisposes toxaemia was not constant. Good prenatal care has long been recognized as a potent prophylaxis against the development of toxaemia. In 1812 Leglay enunciated the following principle which is still germane.[24] He wrote: "Have indulgence for the pregnant woman's complaints, listen to her desires with complaisance, console her and, in place of the severity of the doctor, adopt rather the affectionate tone of her friend or her father." When toxaemia is encountered, the beneficial effects of rest, sedation and delivery are well

TABLE V

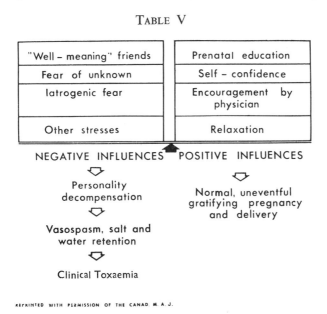

"Well – meaning" friends	Prenatal education
Fear of unknown	Self – confidence
Iatrogenic fear	Encouragement by physician
Other stresses	Relaxation

NEGATIVE INFLUENCES   POSITIVE INFLUENCES

Personality decompensation

Normal, uneventful gratifying pregnancy and delivery

Vasospasm, salt and water retention

Clinical Toxaemia

established. Supplementary treatment has concentrated on "removing the toxin". In the past, purgatives, diaphoretics, venesections, and the withdrawal of spinal fluid have all been utilized and subsequently abandoned. Currently diuretics are in vogue to induce more rapid efficient production of urine with rich sodium content.

4

Summary

Toxaemia of pregnancy lacks an organic etiology despite intensive efforts by distinguished scientists utilizing sophisticated methods of investigation. It does, however, fulfil requirements for a psychosomatic disorder. In women who develop toxaemia there is frequently a pre-existing concealed personality abnormality. Such a personality copes with stress less efficiently, and decompensation can result in toxaemia. Any treatment of toxaemia to be successful must bolster the patient's confidence and abolish her fears. The use of hypnotic techniques appears to offer excellent prophylactic possibilities in this regard.

REFERENCES

1. BLACK, M. E. 1961. Psychorelaxation management for labor and delivery. *Clin. Obstet. Gynec.*, **4**, 108.
2. BROWNE, F. J. 1958. Aetiology of pre-eclamptic toxaemia and eclampsia. *Lancet*, i, 115.
3. BROWN, W. E. 1958. Toxemia of pregnancy. Haas Memorial Lecture, Univ. of Michigan.
4. CHEN, W. C. 1957. Relaxation during parturition. *Chin. med. J.*, **75**, 337.
5. COPPEN, A. J. 1958. Psychosomatic aspects of pre-eclamptic toxaemia. *J. psychosom. Res.*, **2**, 241.
6. DIECKMANN, W. J. 1952. *The Toxemias of pregnancy* 2nd edn. St. Louis: Mosby.
7. FIJALKOWSKI, W. 1965. New ways of psychophysical preparation for childbirth. *Amer. J. Obstet. Gynec.*, **92**, 1018.
8. GORDON, E. S., CHART, J. J., HAGEDORN, D. and SHIPLEY, E. G. 1954. Mechanism of sodium retention in pre-eclamptic toxemia. *Obstet and Gynec.*, **4**, 39.
9. HOLLAND, E. and BOURNE, A. W. 1955. *British obstetrical and gynaecologic practice.* Vol. I. Philadelphia: Davis.
10. JEFFCOATE, T. N. and SCOTT, J. S. 1959. Some observations on the placental factor in pregnancy toxemia. *Amer. J. Obstet. Gynec.*, **77**, 475.
11. KAKU, M. 1953, Placental polysaccharide and the aetiology of the toxaemia of pregnancy. *J. Obstet. Gynaec. Brit. Emp.*, **60**, 148.
12. LAMAZE, F. 1958. *Painless Childbirth.* London: Burke.
13. MAGARA, M. 1950. A study on the cause of toxemia of pregnancy *J. int. Coll. Surg.*, **14**, 215.
14. MASTBOOM, J. L. 1952. The importance of adreno-cortical steroids for the development of toxaemia of late pregnancy. *Gynaecologia*, **134**, 217.
15. Maternal & Child Care. 1960. Report of medical exchange mission to the U.S.S.R. *U.S. Public Health Service Publication.* No. 954.
16. PAGE, E. W. 1953. *The hypertensive disorders of pregnancy.* Springfield, Illinois: Charles C. Thomas.
17. READ, G. D. 1933. *Natural childbirth.* London: Heinemann.
18. RINGROSE, C. A. D. 1966. Auto-hypnosis as an adjunct in obstetrics. *Med. Trial Technique Quarterly*, **13**, 21.
19. ROSENBAUM, M. and MALTY, G. L. 1943. The importance of adreno-cortical steroids for the development of toxaemia of late pregnancy. *Arch. Neurol. Psychiat.*, **49**, 204.
20. SALERNO, L. J. 1958. Psychophysiologic aspects of the toxemias of pregnancy. *Amer. J. Obstet. Gynec.*, **77**, 1268.
21. SOICHET, S. 1959. Emotional factors in toxemia of pregnancy. *Amer. J. Obstet. Gynec.*, **77**, 1065.
22. SOPHIAN, J. 1955. Myometrial resistance to stretch the cause of pre-eclampsia. *J. Obstet Gynaec. Brit. Emp.*, **62**, 37.
23. SPARGO, B., MCCARTNEY, C. P. and WINEMILLER, R. 1959. Glomerular capillary endothelioisis in toxemia of pregnancy. *Amer. Med. Assn. Arch. Path.*, **68**, 593.
24. TAUSSIG, F. J. 1937. The story of prenatal care. *Amer. J. Obstet. Gynec.*, **34**, 731.
25. THEOBOLD, G. W. 1953. Sympathetic nerves and eclampsia. *Brit. med. J.*, **1**, 422.
26. WHITACRE, F. E., LOEB, W. M. JR. and CHIN, H. 1947. A contribution to the study of eclampsia. A. consideration of 22 cases. *J. Amer. med. Assn.*, **133**, 445.
27. ZINKE, E. G. 1906. The treatment of puerperal eclampsia, *Am. J. Obstet.*, **53**, 226.

XV

PSYCHOLOGICAL MANAGEMENT OF THE PRE-NATAL PERIOD

STEPHEN HORSLEY

M.R.C.S., L.R.C.P.

Consultant in Social Psychiatry
Sheffield
England

1

Introduction

A new principle in pre-natal care is the inclusion of systematic psycho-logical screening during the first routine examination of every expectant mother. Although the all-important emotional components of interpersonal relations during pregnancy and labour were demonstrated many years ago by Read[30] his innovations were repudiated by colleagues who ignored the crucial significance of psychological factors. Creak,[14] Sutherland[36] and Tait[38] were among the first in England to recognize that the ante-natal clinic provided a unique opportunity to observe the attitudes of the mother-to-be towards childbirth and motherhood. This concept was developed by Prince,[28] who stressed that total care of the expectant mother must include "full attention to her mental hygiene from the moment of her coming under ante-natal care until the time when her relationship with the baby is ade-quately established."

It is no longer in dispute that the "maturational crisis" of a normal first pregnancy induces profound changes in a mother's personality. Yet, only a decade ago, writing on *The management of pregnancy*, Alan Brews[5] clearly implied that the fundamental aim of this great branch of obstetrics . . . (ante-natal care) . . . was the preservation of the *physiological* aspect of pregnancy and labour.

One or two relevant questions will indicate the potentiality of some far-reaching changes in the pattern of contemporary medical care during pregnancy and parturition. The first question is, what should be the future goal of a comprehensive maternity service; and the second question is, what are the unfulfilled needs?

In his inaugural address, delivered at Oxford, to the Royal College of Midwives, Professor John Stallworthy[34] defined the goal of modern obstetrics as "the provision of such care for the women of the country that their pregnancies would be wanted, and planned; and would be supervised in such a way as to foster the unity of their homes, reduce to a minimum the incidence of scars on body or mind, and ensure as far as humanly possible that the infant would be healthy and unimpaired during the process of pregnancy and birth." Recognizing that the expectant mother needs far more than efficient ante-natal care, Stallworthy pleads for changes in the traditional outlook on such important issues as sex education, family planning, and the relationship of the husband, wife, midwife and doctor during pregnancy and labour. Sheer clinical efficiency saves life, but often fails to preserve peace of mind when a stereotyped pattern of medical care gives too little thought to the vitally important changes evoked by the developmental crisis of pregnancy.

The most urgent of the defects needing to be put right is the almost total lack of systematic attention to the psychology of normal pregnancy and, as a corollary, the relative absence of comprehensive teamwork which will be seen to be essential for the management of the stresses of normal pregnancy and for the prevention of mothering breakdown. The need for a comprehensive approach to pregnancy research was indicated by Illsley[19] in his study of the social background to first pregnancy; and, in a further paper on the social aetiology of foetal damage, he showed that a search for single causes was likely to be fruitless. But pregnancy research is still fragmentary and sometimes misdirected in its failure to correlate obstetric, psychological and social factors. Thus, although a number of obstetricians and midwives are beginning to show some interest in the psychology of pregnancy, their concern is opportunist rather than systematic. It is rare for obstetricians to seek psychiatric consultation in a purely preventive sense; and the usual reason for referral is the hope that the psychiatrist will remove a difficult patient from the maternity unit. Physicians and obstetricians share a natural reluctance to call in the psychiatrist too soon: but, when treatment is indicated, delay is futile and it completely excludes the possibility of preventive psychiatry. The new role of the consultant in psycho-obstetrics has yet to be defined.

2

General Issues

In the department of obstetrics, where the pressure of work seems to limit what can be done, the need for further evaluation of priorities is imperative. This in turn requires the cooperation of people with the ability to sift evidence from many fields. Modern medical practice is turning increasingly towards the basic principles of public health, particularly primary prevention, supported by early diagnosis and prompt treatment: but in obstetrics, the focus of prevention is often restricted to the obvious issues of maternal and infant mortality, and to the hazards of prematurity and infant morbidity. Less clamant issues tend to be relegated to the neglected regions variously designated "emotional hygiene" or perhaps "pregnancy fears" and sometimes "psychological requirements".

Feelings Disregarded

The intelligent modern mother is often critical of the doctor who merely writes his notes but never tells her anything about her pregnancy. She is also highly critical of so-called "relaxation classes", when they concentrate exclusively on the mechanical aspects of childbirth without giving any information on "how the mother may expect to feel". There are still some hospitals where attitudes of relative insensitivity in the staff may engender such comments as: "It seems that the mothers' feelings are totally disregarded."

Lonely and Frightened

Commenting on the increasing recognition of the psychological aspects of childbirth, McDonald[22] pinpoints the "quality of kindness" as a decisive factor in the contribution of the individual midwife to the outcome of labour. Professor Norman Morris[23] has indicated many serious gaps in our knowledge and understanding of the emotional needs of the average woman during pregnancy, labour and the puerperium. One difficulty is that the psychology of pregnancy is still bedevilled by sentiment and untested assumptions which must be replaced by objective study of the hard issues. The lack of any such study is evident from the Report of the Maternity Services Committee[31] which spares three lines to state: "The psychological requirements of the mother should not be forgotten, and time and opportunity should be given to allow her to discuss her problems with her doctor and midwife." Similarly, the Standing Maternity and Midwifery Advisory Committee[32] reports tersely: "The psychological outlook of the mother and her emotional state are sometimes ignored." Again, in a personal communication, Professor Scott Russell observes that "owing to the numbers coming to the clinics it is difficult, if not impossible, to provide anything approaching an ideal service from the point of view of the patients' emotions."

The immediate problem is *how* to provide sufficient extra personnel competent to ensure effective psychological screening of every primigravida during her first routine prenatal examination.

Feasibility of Routine Psychological Screening

Soviet Russia appears to be the only country to make ante-natal care obligatory and to include psychological assessment in the general history and examination. In Great Britain there is still resistance to the introduction of psychological screening as a routine procedure. The first barrier arises from false assumptions concerning any such enquiry into a person's emotional and psychological background. A different problem arises from shortage of professional staff, and it is obvious that there will never be enough doctors and psychiatrists to undertake routine psychological care of every expectant mother. Any large-scale plan to incorporate psychological management as part of the ordinary work of a maternity department would require numerous unqualified staff to assist the specialist establishment.

Several original reports of major advances in this field by Cohen et al.[18] strongly support the contention that psychological screening in the antenatal clinic can be carried out effectively by students and non-psychiatric personnel in obstetrics, paediatrics and nursing. Another equally important possibility appears in Cohen's demonstration, that students in training can learn quickly the principles of therapeutic intervention in the case of those expectant mothers found to be at high risk. Cohen also makes it clear that psychiatric treatment is not indicated in most of the stresses of pregnancy in which the therapist's role is an essentially practical one of providing, according to circumstances, any one of the following:

(a) educational help to compensate for lack of experience;
(b) authoritative support to cope sympathetically with any irrational fears arising from old wives' tales or other horror stories;
(c) the possibility, in cases of sheer socio-economic hardship, of calling in the appropriate officer of the health and social security services.

The question of feasibility is answered by Cohen's observation that his trainees, using a fourteen-point "Pregnancy Profile Questionnaire" are able to complete the screening procedure in a matter of 12–14 minutes during the routine history-taking for each new patient at her first clinic visit.

Whither Psycho-obstetrics?

Blanket phrases such as "psychological aspects of pregnancy" and "psychological preparation for labour" cover so many different conceptual aims that it is imperative to separate these aims into distinct groups, comprising:

(a) psychophysical methods of relieving pain in childbirth;
(b) identification and management of psychiatric disorders during pregnancy;
(c) psychological assessment and management of normal pregnancy.

This chapter is concerned primarily with the psychological management of normal pregnancy; but, as some overlap is inevitable, brief reference is made to each of these separate branches of psycho-obstetrics.

Psychophysical Preparation for Childbirth

The most comprehensive review of the contemporary trend is Lee Buxton's[7] *A study of psychophysical methods for the relief of childbirth pain.* Buxton considers more than twenty different techniques of psychophysical preparation used in America, England, Europe and Russia for the relief of pain during childbirth; and he shows that these techniques fall roughly into four main categories according to which aspect of training is thought to be the most important. Buxton differentiates these techniques as follows: (i) natural childbirth; (ii) autogene training; (iii) hypnosis; and (iv) psychoprophylaxis. Each of these still has its adherents, but the diversity of techniques which have multiplied since Read[30] published his first book has very largely been replaced by the method of psychoprophylactic preparation of childbirth.

Psychoprophylaxis originated in Soviet Russia about twenty-five years ago through the work of Nikolayev,[24] Velvovsky,[40] and others who applied Pavlovian concepts of conditioned reflexes to *prevent* pain, and to remove fear and tension from childbirth. Lamaze[20] was one of the first visitors to Russia to make a serious study of the psychoprophylactic method and, when he introduced the method to France in 1952, it was an immediate success. Since that time, schools of psychoprophylaxis have appeared in many parts of Europe, but it has only recently been accepted in England, where it is being taught by the National Childbirth Trust.

The psychoprophylactic method is a form of intensive training given during the final weeks of pregnancy. The training consists of from six to eight lectures, combined with exercises to acquire skill in three procedures said to be helpful in preventing or reducing pain. These are:

(a) deep rhythmical breathing during uterine contractions;
(b) abdominal effleurage in rhythm with respiration;
(c) pressure on the anterior superior iliac spine, and on the rhomboid muscles.

The Russians claim that the method gives a painless labour, but they admit that it is not always completely successful, and in such cases it is customary to give a conventional analgesic. Nevertheless, it is believed in Russia that failures attributed to the method are due to inadequate training of the doctors, midwives and patients.

The psychological implications of *l'accouchement sans douleur* have been criticized by Chertok[9] who observed that the anxieties of pregnancy have deep roots in the woman's early psychosexual relationships with parents, siblings and friends. A further criticism of the method (as practised in England) is its failure to pay any attention to the psychosocial needs of the expectant mother. Unfortunately, with its exclusive emphasis on the relief of pain and fear, the method fails to cope with "primordial affective experiences" which continue to have long-lasting effects on the mental health and equilibrium of the whole family.

Identification and Management of Psychiatric Disorders in Pregnancy

Prior to 1937, when expectant mothers were referred on account of acute mental illness to the author's out-patient clinic, it was the established practice to admit these women as voluntary patients to the county mental hospital for observation. Many were suffering from suicidal tendencies and acute depression which, in most cases, cleared up spontaneously very soon after delivery; but in the thirties there was much resistance from people who objected on sentimental grounds to the idea of a baby being born in a mental hospital. In 1937, with the availability of chemical convulsants such as cardiazol (leptazol), triazol, and picrotoxin, the author began to treat most of these patients in the wards of a general hospital or in the outpatient department.[16] Similarly, when electro-convulsive therapy modified by muscle relaxants became available in the early 1940s, the author continued to treat cases of early and acute psychiatric illness without transferring these patients to a mental hospital.

A decade ago, a sabbatical year spent in a group practice which handled some 300 confinements annually made it possible to give close attention to every expectant mother believed by her usual medical attendant to suffer from emotional or psychiatric disability. Those so referred comprised a group of 42 young married women, each diagnosed by one of the practice partners as "neurotic" or as "psychiatrically unreliable". Each of the selected group was offered appointments which combined the routine of pre-natal care with time and opportunity to discuss at leisure and in detail such vital data as: personal and family history, education, occupation, relation-ship with husband, family and friends, attitudes to sex and conception, to pregnancy, birth and breast-feeding. This work gave results far beyond the simple provision of medical support for the vulnerable patients in a typical group practice. In terms of "mere mending" offered to allegedly unstable women during their pregnancies, the project was effective in the practical sense that every mother in the selected group enjoyed a relatively easy delivery at home. In terms of "crisis theory" the project appeared to indi-cate the possibility of preventive intervention within the exigencies of a busy general practice.

Types of Psychiatric Problems

The borderline between normal depression and its pathological equivalent is difficult to define, but there is no doubt that the great majority of depres-sive reactions will be treated by the family doctor. The causes of depression have been classified by Watts[41] under the following five headings:

1. *Physiological depression.* This occurs during the first trimester with irritability, tears, and a tendency to "fly off the handle" but it occurs also shortly after delivery as "four day blues".

2. *Socially determined depression.* This is common in the unmarried, but it is common also when pregnancy occurs too soon after delivery (when some mothers feel deep shame at what the neighbours will think).

3. *Depression due to physical causes.* Physical causes must be considered in the differential diagnosis which includes a heterogeneous group of physical agents, ranging from acute virus hepatitis and other viral infections to the

deficiency diseases such as pellagra, and gross brain damage from head injury and brain tumour.

4. *Psychogenic depression.* Depression due to bereavement during pregnancy is always a major crisis with far-reaching hazards, especially the risk of mothering breakdown and consequent developmental problems in the infant.

5. *Endogenous depression.* In its classical form endogenous depression is unmistakable, nevertheless, the writer agrees with Watts[41] that endogenous depression is probably the most common and often the least recognized depressive disorder occurring in the community.

There is probably no psychiatric disorder peculiar to pregnancy in which, although mild depressive reactions are common, the acute and suicidal forms are rare. In fact, suicide is much less likely during pregnancy than during the puerperium: moreover, because the response to treatment is good, there is seldom any justification for therapeutic abortion on account of threatened suicide. However, it is worth considering the findings of Burke,[6] who studied 58 women of child-bearing age admitted to hospital on suspicion of self-poisoning. Burke found that only 7 of these women were pregnant at the time of admission: "They were all in the first four months of pregnancy; most of them were young and unmarried."

In the case of schizophrenia it is commonly observed that the illness tends to recede during pregnancy, only to reappear during the puerperium. Baker[1] remarks that many women with schizophrenia seem to conceive with ease and, being aware of their better health during pregnancy, many of them welcome childbearing. The onset of an acute schizophrenic episode is nearly always an indication for prompt admission to a psychiatric unit where electro-convulsive therapy, together with full doses of a tranquillizer, is often the quickest way to cut short the acute phase of the illness. On the other hand, although the presence of schizophrenia during pregnancy should always be regarded as an indication for psychiatric attention, the majority of this uncommon group of patients can be managed by supportive therapy in the out-patient department.

In addition to the functional psychoses (manic-depressive psychosis, and schizophrenia) and the rare organic psychoses, it is necessary to consider the needs of the very much larger group of mildly neurotic reactions appearing during pregnancy in women who are normally non-neurotic. The marked increase of minor neurotic disorders during pregnancy may be correlated with Bibring's[4] research, which indicates that normal pregnancy is a crisis situation in which important personality changes may be expected.

The psychology of normal pregnancy involves a study in human relations in which, as Philipp[26] observes, many minor problems are "only a bridge for making contact". The plain truth is that until psychological assessment is recognized as an essential part of routine pre-natal care, there will always be preventable tragedies—referred too late to the department of psychiatry.

The majority of psychiatric problems occurring during pregnancy will involve whole families in consequences such as marital tension, mothering breakdown, and developmental failure in the child; and the majority of these family troubles can be traced to neglected stresses associated with pregnancy.

Stressful Pregnancy

Hitherto, the incidence of pregnancy stress has been largely a matter of speculation based on retrospective studies made only when mothers attended welfare clinics to seek advice about behavioural problems in young children. These studies revealed problems of two quite different types, each belonging to a separate age-group: thus, young mothers tend to bring physically and intellectually normal children in the mistaken belief that they are "backward" or that their behaviour is "abnormal", when in fact the only discoverable abnormality is the mother's inability to form a warm relationship. In contrast, older mothers who have experienced severe preconceptual stress are thought to have a higher incidence of mongol infants than other mothers of similar age, and Stott[35] contends that emotional stress during the second and third months of pregnancy increases the risk. Again, Drillien and Wilkinson[15] suggest that preconceptual endocrine disorder may also be an aetiological factor in mongolism.

Prospective studies of pregnancy stress which began as pilot projects in Nebraska (Cohen)[10] and later in England (Horsley[18]) have led to long-term follow-up observations, which may provide data for the evaluation of prenatal screening. These parallel studies provide the present conceptual model for the psychological management of the pre-natal period.

3

Psychological Assessment and Management

Psychological management of pregnancy is likely to be inadequate unless it begins at the first pre-natal visit, which offers a unique opportunity to record details of the expectant mother's developmental history and family background. On this first visit she is likely to be more forthcoming than after a subsequent examination at which she may feel that the doctor is too busy to be bothered with details. In taking her personal history from childhood to adolescence, it is useful to enquire about close relationships, boy friends, sex, and whether she likes being married. If this question is asked at the right moment, it releases one or more well-defined groups of ideas about marriage and parenthood. An opportunity must be made to discuss old wives' tales and other superstitions. For example, a common fear is that the expectant mother must on no account stretch . . . (because she has been told that this will twist the cord round the baby's neck). Supernatural hazards are better voiced, and, if the young woman speaks of the fiction that dreams of rats portend a death in the family, she may be helped by a free discussion of birth and death. Other common superstitions concern the effect of looking at beauty or ugliness, the significance of cravings, and the quaint notion of "eating for two". Some couples have a frightening belief that birthmarks are produced by intercourse.

What does she Need?

Criticizing childbirth ritual, Lomas[21] penetrates the benevolent façade of contemporary society to reveal the neglect of the personal and psychological in favour of the physical and mechanical. Lomas suggests that society's failure to give peace of mind to the parturient mother stems not only from a relative ignorance of the mother's psychological needs and aims but also from "an unacknowledged antipathy" towards them. If any system of screening is to be meaningful, it is necessary to understand a little of what the mother's symptoms imply that she needs. But the writer would emphasize that effective screening does not require special training in psychoanalytical concepts and techniques. Indeed, as Cohen et al.[13] have shown, there are serious drawbacks to ante-natal screening procedures based on psychopathological concepts, whereas it is probably more meaningful and practical to formulate a simpler "developmental, adaptive model".

Personal Judgments, or Structured Questionary?

A major difficulty confronting research in psychiatric epidemiology lies in the individual variation of any routine assessment, whether of the sick or the "not yet sick". Consequently, it may be found that the use of a structured formulary can be more reliable for the purpose of recording basic data than the personal judgments of different clinicians. Ten years ago the amount of dependable information on the psychology of pregnancy was very small; but a remarkable acceleration in this field has occurred during the past five years. This progress is due largely to the research of Cohen et al.,[13] whose studies of pregnancy stress have been carried out by staff who did not have special training in mental health. This necessitated the discarding of any screening item found to be awkward or obscure to non-psychiatric personnel; and this lesson can be applied elsewhere by psychiatrists working as team-members with obstetricians and paediatricians. The writer's own Pregnancy assessment record was designed originally without reference to Cohen's Pregnancy profile questionnaire, but now that the advantages of simplification have been established, the writer acknowledges Cohen's influence in the modified record card to be described.

Pregnancy Assessment Record

The record card in current use has been modified during the course of a long-term prospective study of the mental development of a cohort of young children. In an initial pilot study, rather on the lines of Caplan's Jerusalem project,[8] the writer's immediate aim was to detect "carriers" of unhealthy attitudes and so, in the course of the screening process, to develop a therapeutic relationship with expectant mothers, in the hope that this would reduce the hazard of future mothering failure. A significant observation in this study was the frequency with which stress factors are completely overlooked when routine history-taking and examinations are conducted in the usual way (focused almost exclusively on physiological wellbeing). Hence, as a basic assumption, it was held that, whenever the expectant mother was given both time and help to speak freely of any events which for her might be stressful, if it was found that her stresses were severe or multiple, she was *ipso facto* at high risk.

Contribution of Public Health Nurses

Neither the detection of "carriers" nor the identification of "high risk" mothers can be achieved by doctors alone. Accordingly, in an attempt to provide effective screening on a larger scale, groups of health visitors and midwives were invited to cooperate in the use of a questionary for identifying and collating pregnancy stresses. Although the resultant collaboration proved the value of close cooperation between the department of obstetrics and the preventive psychiatry unit (in which the health visitor plays a key role), there were still some unresolved difficulties. The first problem was how to extend the project to cover the whole of a defined population, and the next was how to translate the observations of the field workers into analysable data. At this juncture, a suggestion by Scott[33] led to the use of a diagrammatic scheme for the guidance of public health nurses in classifying the sources of stresses, the affected parent, and the signs and symptoms to be observed. Scott indicated the potential value of classification into:

(*a*) Four types of groups of stresses, comprising
    1. the unfortunate pregnancy (accidental hazards);
    2. irresponsible pregnancy (personal insufficiencies);
    3. factors preventing proper communication;
    4. gynaecological (reproductive) factors.
(*b*) Pathology of stresses, in four groups correlated with those indicated in (*a*).
(*c*) Signs to be observed in three different areas, viz.
    1. in the home;
    2. in the father;
    3. in the mother.

In the following scheme shown in Fig. 1, I have made only minor modifications to Scott's original outline.

In the light of experience it is recognized that the initial plan was impracticable in that it was too dependent on the limited number of carefully selected personnel whose training included some experience in mental health counselling or psychotherapy in a clinic for child and family psychiatry. A serious criticism of the pilot project is its extravagant use of professional

Four main areas of stress	Pathology of stress	Signs and symptoms in three areas
I. The unfortunate pregnancy (accidental hazards)	Husband dead or drafted away. Physical accidents to either partner. Economic reverses, job redundancy. Eviction through no personal fault.	I. *The Home:* unprepared { housing clothes equipment; other children neglected, adopted, or in care
II. Irresponsible pregnancy (personal insufficiencies in either partner)	Husband absconded, uninterested, unfaithful, ill, unemployed. Wife unready, too young or too old (unwanted accident) total change of environment; immigrant. Either partner with a personality disorder. Adoptive parents who adopt for the wrong reasons.	II. *The Husband:* evasive, not cooperating, hanging about all day; reversal of roles with wife; not involved with neighbours.
III. Factors preventing proper communication	*Too little* communication due to mental illness, especially states of depression and schizophrenia, mental subnormality, perfectionism. *Too much* communication, with excessive parental dependency on child (lonely mother in top flat) and in some cases of amphetamine addiction.	III. *The Wife:* tense, unhappy, apathetic, no anticipatory pleasure, uncommunicative, ashamed; not answering the door; evasive about, or hostile to, husband; not involved with neighbours.
IV. Reproductive factors	History of abortion, infertility, or complications in pregnancy, labour and puerperium; elderly (last chance), previous death of child (rhesus factor).	

Fig. 1. *Classification of pregnancy stresses.*

Basic Data   *Case ref.:*

Dates of:	*Potential Stresses*
(a) birth	(1) old for childbearing
(b) marriage	(2) unmarried*
(c) expected date of delivery	(3) shotgun wedding
(d) whether planned/unplanned?	(4) attempted abortion or
(e) if planned, how long trying to conceive?	miscarriage*
	(5) relative infertility
Family history:	(6) any serious illness or
(f) parents' ages, health (mental/physical)	abnormality
(g) siblings' ages, health, marriage, etc.	....
....	(7) maternal or sibling
....	obstetric complications
(h) family history of obstetric trouble	....
....	(8) broken home in child-
....	hood
(i) death, divorce, remarriage of parents	(9) bereavement during this
	pregnancy*
Psychosocial supports:	(10) economic insecurity
(j) husband's age, health, occupation and	(11) no emotional support*
whether unemployed	(12) no support*
(k) husband's attitude to wife before, and	....
during pregnancy	(13) no communication*
....	(lonely or isolated in
(l) husband's absence due to death, desertion,	in top flat)
drafting overseas, etc.	
....	
(m) how often does she see her mother, or	
other close relative?	
(o) racial intolerance?	
(p) psychiatric illness in either partner?	
Subjective factors and changes perceived by	(14) hazard of those fears
the woman:	which are commonly
(q) bizarre appetites, craving, irritable,	concealed unless she is
altered affections, more emotional	given help to reveal
....	them
(r) pregnancy sickness (time and degree)	
....	
(s) sleep and dreams	
(t) what sex does she hope for, and what name	
or names has she chosen?	
....	
(u) what are her feelings about breast-feeding	
and other bodily functions?	
(v) any other problems?	
....	

Fig. 2. *Pregnancy assessment record.*

time and, in view of Cohen's evidence,[11] it may be questioned whether the doctor-patient interview (in which only two or three patients are seen in one hour) can now be justified.

It is of the utmost urgency to develop and extend this research specifically in the adaptational process of pregnancy, in the field of family psychiatry generally, and in the overall discipline of preventive psychiatry. The modified assessment record card (Fig. 2) provides a practical instrument which can be used by any of the medical and nursing staff already concerned in prenatal care. Most of the details on this card are clear without explanation; but some briefing may emphasize the need for cultivating staff attitudes of perceptive attention to a woman's spoken, or unspoken, communication. Bentall and Fairs[3] express similar views: "Personal relationships with the mother are of more importance than anything else in encouraging a happy and satisfactory outcome."

Scoring and Analysis of Data

When the basic data are being recorded on the pregnancy assessment card, it will be evident whether any potential stress factor is present. Scoring is simple: one point for each stress factor, except those marked in Fig. 2 with an asterisk—these receive two points. In the analysis of records there is a differentiation into three levels of risk:

(a) low risk   zero to one point;
(b) high risk   two points;
(c) very high risk   three points or more.

This rough separation into three groups provides a useful guide as to which expectant mothers should have priority in the allocation of limited resources. The emotional insecurity arising from multiple stresses must receive the same consideration and skilled attention generally accorded to the physical hazards of the complications of pregnancy. In other words, the identification of a mother as being at "very high risk" should lead to immediate and continued psychotherapeutic care by a member of the consultant staff (and by one who is already recognized by the patient to be a member of the obstetric department). Referral elsewhere, to a psychiatric unit, is contra-indicated unless there is no proper provision within the pre-natal unit. Not every very high risk patient requires psychotherapy, but every one should be re-assessed periodically by a competent psychotherapist, who must have continuity of responsibility throughout pregnancy and the puerperium. Similarly, all high risk cases should be considered by the consultant staff in order to decide jointly how to meet the needs arising from different types of stress. Then, according to circumstances, the appropriate member of the multidisciplinary team may provide educational help, sympathetic support, material aid, and in cases of severe emotional distress arrangements may be made for individual or group psychotherapy. Even the "low risk" mother should not be denied the benefit of proper psychological management during pregnancy and parturition.

4

Strategy of Psychological Management

In an earlier paper[17] the writer showed that pregnancy is a time of changing feelings, heightened sensitivity, and increased susceptibility to any crisis. Characteristic changes appear in early, middle and late pregnancy; but because of cultural reticence in many women and in their doctors, the variety of changes in sexual appetite and feelings during pregnancy are seldom given more than the most cursory attention. This conspiracy of silence can be overcome by allowing the shy victim time to talk with a counsellor who understands the nature of her difficulties; and only then is the expectant mother likely to accept the upsurge of irrational feelings about childbirth and to learn that the crisis of a normal pregnancy can become a vital growing point in self-understanding.

The potentiality of this "living learning situation" may be found to be dependent on the basic supports of husband, relatives, and all the professional attendants, each of whom plays a fundamental role. But, before considering the people in supporting roles, it is necessary to examine more closely the emotional and psychological needs of expectant mothers.

Emotional Changes of Pregnancy

There is more disagreement about the emotional needs of expectant mothers than about any other aspect of obstetrics. Perhaps the general practitioner who has known the family for many years is the most likely person to become aware of emotional changes, and of their significance. The family doctor sees very few major psychoses, but he will undoubtedly see a great many of the milder emotional disturbances of pregnancy which, because they are so common, are sometimes disregarded. But to ignore these "signals" can have grave repercussions for the future health and happiness of mother and child. Therefore, any doctor or midwife who provides pre-natal care *must* ensure that every expectant mother is given ample opportunity to speak freely of whatever anxiety or fear she may have. The way in which these emotional communications are handled will have profound and lasting effects on every member of a family, and this is why emotional problems in expectant parents must be identified, so that appropriate adjustments may be made while there is yet time.

Emotional Changes as Signals

The events of pregnancy and childbirth always arouse intense emotion, and in considering the question of home or hospital delivery it is always advisable to assess the woman's emotional state before making a decision.

Emotional security for most women is greater at home, but *recent* changes of environment may isolate and disturb a young wife despite the acquisition of every modern aid to housekeeping. In contrast, when anxieties are concealed by denial (or by the taboo on expression of any feeling), the resultant emotional barrier may indicate a difficult delivery, or a stormy puerperium. Denial of any emotional change may also be a sign of grave portent, especially if this is associated with refusal to attend classes for preparation for childbirth or to cooperate in pre-natal care. And in terms of vulnerability, women who fail to keep their appointments at the ante-natal clinics must be regarded as "very high risk" cases to be "chased diligently" by midwife or health visitor.

Emotional Changes as Signs of Imminent Breakdown

Threats of suicide are fairly common, especially in the unmarried, during the first trimester: but most of these are found to be attention-seeking signals. A far more serious warning exists in the rare instance of severe insomnia when this occurs together with quiet depression and total loss of interest. In such cases it is of course essential to ask definite questions about the presence of depression and its duration, intensity and rhythm; questions should also elicit whether there are suicidal thoughts, a feeling that life is no longer worth living, or a longing to get away from everything. Although suicidal attempts are rare during pregnancy, severe depression may occur and it must always receive psychiatric treatment (preferably by modified E.C.T.). One other pointer suggested by Tod[39] is that pathological anxiety during pregnancy heralds post-partum depression.

Other Psychological Needs

The expectant mother needs more than economic and material support. She needs more than medical and nursing attention. In particular, she needs the emotional support which only her husband can give. And the family doctor may help indirectly by giving some attention to the husband who is then enabled to provide more effective support for his wife. This is why it is important that the doctor should arrange a joint interview with the patient and her husband. It is important to tell husband and wife together that many perfectly normal women become moody and irritable during pregnancy; they nearly all become more sensitive, and many need help in understanding the sudden changes of feeling which seem to threaten marital harmony. Ignorance of these alterations of feeling can have serious consequences towards the end of pregnancy when it is normal for a woman to become more passive in every way, but also more in need of affection. Most husbands try to anticipate their wives' need for extra comfort and consideration; but one who has become estranged at an early stage of the pregnancy may fail in this critical time of his wife's greatest need.

Supporting Roles

Psychological management of pregnancy concerns—in addition to the expectant mother—her husband, other relatives, doctor, and midwife. It is anachronistic to exclude any one of these from the general strategy of management, but it may be useful to reconsider each in a separate role.

1. *The husband.* In his Reith Lecture, Medawar remarked that we in Great Britain "did not begin to record the ages at which mothers bear children until 1938 . . . ; and we still do not record the age of the father." The writer's established practice is to record the dates of birth of both parents; time will show whether paternal ages are significant. Knowledge of the age of both partners may indicate potential hazards if there is a marked discrepancy. Qualities to be considered in a husband are:

(a) personality and maturity. Does he give emotional support, or does he need it?

(b) attitude to wife's pregnancy, and to her sensitivity, her irritability and her moods. Does he lose interest if his wife loses her looks, or her ardour? Is he self-centred, or is he more concerned with helping his wife?

(c) the amount of support he gives: economic, emotional, and physical.

(d) couvade! Is the husband so incapacitated by "his" pregnancy sickness and other symptoms that he fails in his male role?

2. *The relatives.* In a first pregnancy the patient's mother wields great influence both at a conscious and at an unconscious level. Long-forgotten hates and resentments may reappear and, in the case of an only child, there may be the added fear of complications which have been said to be the reason for no siblings. In the case of an immature personality, fears tend to be related to the maternal pattern and, at the first emotional upset, the immature bride is likely to run home crying to her mother: but the only hope of any worthwhile relationship in the future will stem from the bride's ability to face independence—leaning temporarily, if she must, on her husband. Conversely, if the bride is a more mature woman with a secure family background, she may enjoy a vivid independence yet still welcome the moral and material support which her own mother may be able to give. In-laws play a similar supportive role when the marriage and pregnancy are accepted happily; but the crisis of serious psychiatric illness may release a damaging search for a scapegoat, and, in this situation, the doctor must intervene to emphasize the futility of blaming either partner and to stress the need to re-open communication in face-to-face confrontation in which all the participants are willing to see other points of view.

3. *The doctor.* The brash beginner, conscious of his packed waiting-room, may be tempted to make a spot diagnosis and to reinforce this with brief advice and a prescription which only confirms the patient's worst fear of some serious physical abnormality. Alternatively, if the doctor mis-

takenly tells a patient that her morning sickness is psychological, she may at once draw her own conclusion that he regards her as a psychiatric case. Clearly the family doctor must be approachable, and he must recognize the overriding importance of giving his patient the feeling that he has time to listen sympathetically to fears which she may never again express in words.

Much is learned from one's first experience of a potentially dangerous clinical problem. Nearly forty years ago, during the vogue for twilight sleep, during a resident post in the maternity wards of a northern general hospital, the author unwisely gave intravenous nembutal to a forty-year-old primigravida whose labour promised to be prolonged and difficult. Delivery followed quickly and easily, but the apparent success of the narcosis was marred by the immediate sequel. On regaining consciousness and being shown her perfectly normal baby, this patient began to rage and shout that she had been deprived of the most important joy in her life. She refused to have anything to do with her baby, and for several days she was gravely ill with post-partum haemorrhage and acute delirium.

The modern practitioner will manage the psychological problems of pregnancy far better if he recognizes his own conscious attitudes and his unconscious reactions to the emotional upsets of his patients. According to his attitude to psychological medicine, he may be tempted to hope that early signs and symptoms of emotional disequilibrium are *merely* a passing phase; or, if he is more knowledgeable, he may recognize the minor disorders of pregnancy as the patient's tentative "bridge of communication". Unfortunately, in contemporary medical practice there is often so much discontinuity that the patient loses the vital opportunity to confide in "her own doctor", and this need for continuity of professional care is one of the strongest reasons for encouraging and extending the concept of general practitioner obstetricians working with other colleagues in group practices. Ideally, every group practice should have regular clinical meetings with obstetricians, paediatricians, and psychiatrists; or the practice should include these specialists in the partnership.

4. *The midwife.* The midwife who only sees her role in a one-to-one relationship with her patient may wish to challenge the opinion of Sir John Peel[25] who states convincingly: "The all-purpose midwife is really as out of date as the all-purpose doctor in 1968." The modern midwife is one of a multidisciplinary team, and her role must be re-examined in a context which embraces relationships beyond the immediate responsibility for delivery.

Because of her physical closeness to the patient, a simple human relationship in which the midwife has a special responsibility for the "maintenance of the patient's individuality" (Tacchi[37]), her impact is immeasurable, whether she happens to be identified by the patient as (i) a hostile mother-figure, (ii) a comforting mother-figure, or (iii) a rejecting spinster. A relevant question may sharpen this issue! What is known of the effect of clashes of personality between expectant mother, midwife, husband, and doctor? There are special needs in the midwife-patient relationship when this concerns an immature personality, especially if there are constant demands for a mother-figure on whom to rely. In such circumstances, whether in relaxation classes or in the labour ward, so long as authority is maintained, the immature girl can be made to conform. And this often achieves what is conveniently described as a "normal" labour in which the patient does very little to help herself. But what of the future? The clinging mother is herself still at heart a clinging child with none of the healthy independence which she must acquire before she can give any comfort or security to her own baby. And what are the midwife's feelings about the patient? These may be a guide to the normality, or abnormality, of the patient who, if happy, may radiate joy, if unhappy, may communicate profound gloom, and if schizophrenic, may make any conversation seem odd or irrelevant.

The influence of the midwife on the actual process of delivery is very considerable and, as Beazley[2] has observed, the incidence of painful labour is undoubtedly greater whenever less interest is shown in the problem. Her responsibility extends far beyond the perinatal period in which she is most involved; and therefore, if we are to recognize the importance of continuity of care, it is essential to include the midwife in the general strategy of pre-natal and post-natal management. In particular, there are endless opportunities for public health nurses and midwives, if they recognize values beyond mere relaxation and exercises in the classes for preparation for childbirth. These ante-natal classes vary enormously in content and quality: anatomy and physiology may be taught with zest, while the emotional stresses of pregnancy are often disregarded, or mishandled in such a manner as to cause trouble in the future mother-child relationship. For example, if there is an authoritarian gap between midwife and mother, this can be a real obstacle to acceptance of new values and beliefs. The mothercraft class provides a seed-bed for prejudice and concealed stress, but it is rich in potential for the health visitor or midwife who can bring together the forces of creative tension by applying Lewinian theory: "Complete acceptance of previously rejected facts can be achieved best through the discovery of these facts by the group members themselves. Then, and frequently only then, do the facts become really *their* facts (as against other people's facts)." An alternative to the *antitherapy* of autocratic instructional classes would be to include group psychotherapy as part of the process of preparing high-risk mothers for childbirth.

5

Group Psychotherapy

The phrase "group psychotherapy" is often misapplied to non-therapeutic, and even to antitherapeutic, situations in which selected groups of young mothers meet for purely instructional purposes when they may be harangued by midwives, health visitors, or physiotherapists in the course of preparation for childbirth. The therapeutic possibilities of mothercraft groups are of considerable interest, and there is no doubt that the participants are peculiarly sensitive to a "living learning situation" for which they happen to be both physiologically and psychologically in a unique state of readiness to respond. This is why it may be of supreme importance to ensure that the management of these primarily educational groups is in the hands of people who are properly prepared to give adequate attention to the "hidden" communications which are blocked by autocratic attitudes in any group leader.

Health visitors and midwives who take charge of the new psychoprophylactic classes and other forms of preparation for childbirth must receive regular support from a group psychotherapist or a consultant in community psychiatry. Incidentally, there is no more rewarding field for group psychotherapy than with young expectant parents especially during the first pregnancy.

Curiously, this age of mini-skirts and sexual licence has done little to modify prudish attitudes to breast-feeding. And when a group of young women begins to discuss breast-feeding and other bodily functions, the members often express astonishment at their own sense of freedom to cross the threshold of taboo. Again, when they talk about frigidity and other neurotic problems, the fading of inhibition allows them to speak frankly about their choice of partner, their sex education, and the pleasures and disappointments of sex when their desires wax and wane at different times during pregnancy.

Group discussion of sex education still reveals the abysmal ignorance of many young couples whose parents never offered any information, while other parents flatly refuse to answer their daughter's questions, and some utter the awful warning: "If you get a baby, don't ever come home again." Not surprisingly, many young women in such a group speak bitterly of their parents' lack of sympathy or understanding. On the other hand, the most determined views are expressed on the intention to give the new baby a better and happier life.

The commonest subject to be ventilated spontaneously is the fear that the baby might be backward or damaged and, when such anxieties are mentioned, it may be of special importance to explore feelings of guilt which always persist after an earlier abortion, and also after an attempted abortion. Then, when the group reveals its fantasy life, hopes and half-concealed fears may be expressed in quaintly vivid analogies—as when one primigravida, who had been trying anxiously for seven years to conceive, related a dream about a ferret which was "snuggling too close" to her bosom. Her evident anxiety about the dream led another member to reveal that she too had dreams of "little furry animals" which she recognized as ferrets: and in one such dream she was not expecting a baby, but ferrets: she commented spontaneously, "That does not make sense, because I don't like ferrets." The whole group went on to discuss the significance of dreaming about small animals and water.

An interesting but puzzling observation made by the group was that towards the end of the second trimester nearly every member ceased dreaming. This consistent change in the dream life of the expectant mother appears to be part of an alteration in the sleep pattern during successive stages of pregnancy. The mechanism of sleep disturbances in pregnancy is uncertain, but the frequency of sleep disorders must be considered in the overall strategy of management.

Group psychotherapy may be analytical or supportive, and the choice of method will depend partly on the needs of its members but also on the availability of a group psychotherapist. The simpler form of supportive psychotherapy is suitable for a selected group of expectant mothers meeting once a week to discuss jointly with the doctor and health visitor any of the changes of feeling, appetite, anxiety and mood, which often lead to marital tension and misunderstandings. The mutual support generated by such a group releases an unprecedented flow of completely uninhibited conversation in which shyness and fear are replaced by a sense of relief that "secret" anxieties are common to others. Incidentally, this type of group work is an invaluable opportunity for the young health visitor or midwife to experience and to understand more about the psychology of pregnancy than she could learn from any number of academic lectures.

6

Conclusion

Systematic psychological screening in normal pregnancy is still a novelty which may be contrasted with the failure of the health services to provide any generally established pattern of psychological management. In England a few such projects have been reported, but unfortunately the literature does not always distinguish carefully between fact and theory, some of which is highly equivocal.

The standard textbooks of obstetrics pay scant attention to the psychological needs of the average woman; and the standard textbooks of psychiatry contribute virtually nothing to the very real problem of the psychological management of normal expectant parents. However, in the wilderness of obstetric and psychiatric literature, there is a small but very helpful book concerned primarily with psychiatric disorders in obstetrics. In this book Baker[1] does in fact provide a wealth of practical guidance for doctors and midwives whose work is mainly in the field of normal obstetrics.

The present study confirms that it is possible to incorporate a system of psychological screening and management as an integral part of pre-natal care. The study shows that an approach which freely opens up communication between expectant mothers and their professional attendants also has the long-term value of encouraging further consultation after delivery. And the study indicates that women who receive extra support through psychological management appear not only to enjoy easier labour, but also to have fewer behavioural problems with their infants. But the unnecessary use of anaesthesia and analgesia, even to the point of complete amnesia, tends to make nurses and doctors indifferent to the psychological needs of the woman in labour.

The research value of this prospective study can only be assessed after long-term follow-up of comparable cohorts of women and children. But one factor which appears to merit immediate attention is the quality of maternal responsiveness which emerges during the process of screening and counselling. Maternal responsiveness is thought to be an important vehicle for future face-to-face communication. The mother who learns to share her difficulties by frank discussion, learns also to confront her day-to-day problems in ways which maintain "open contact" whether this be with her doctor, her midwife, her husband, or her child. But mothers whose "minor complaints" are disregarded or relegated to the oblivion of anaesthesia may be at risk in their future role at any point in the continuum from maternal responsiveness to mothering breakdown.

Prugh and Harlow[20] suggest that marital conflict and similar stresses during pregnancy may lead either to "distorted relatedness" in which the mother fails to perceive the infant as a separate person, or to "insufficient relatedness" in which the mother may be emotionally cold with nothing left to give. Another aspect of pregnancy stress has been considered by Prechtl,[27] who shows that psychological stresses during pregnancy could be aetiological factors in brain lesions; but Prechtl has been one of the first to admit that a weak point in his argument is the lack of knowledge of the mothers' personalities before they had their babies.

The role played by a mother's previous experience seems to be an important determinant of her responses to the developmental crises of pregnancy and parturition. In a preliminary analysis of the interview data taken from the present study it appears that traumatic episodes in childhood and adolescence may damage the future responsiveness of an expectant mother to her infant. Even more damaging are personal experiences of sexual terror, gynaecological disorders, and obstetric complications; and a still more serious hazard is the absence (for any reason) of male attention and support. On the other hand, it is evident that early experience of an affectionate mother-child relationship may accelerate the development of maternal responsiveness.

The inherent disadvantage of retrospective assessment led Cohen[12] to design a major prospective study to assess pregnancy stress and its potential influence on maternal attitudes which might be expected to influence normal growth and development in the infant. In his earlier pilot studies Cohen[11] shows that even minor stresses during pregnancy appear to disrupt the normal process of maternal adaptation to the foetus and thus to affect the future mother-child relationship.

In the United Kingdom this work depends largely on voluntary effort which is only effective when those concerned can be spared from other duties: hence in five years a mere 480 primigravidae have received the close attention now regarded as essential for adequate pre-natal care. But this random sample of only 480 is a very small fraction of the primigravidae attending a central clinic serving a general population of half-a-million. Even so, as a result of our experience we believe that the screening procedure described (together with the provision of appropriate counselling, social support, education, and sometimes psychotherapy) represents an important advance in the management of pregnancy.

In contrast, with proper support to ensure adequate staffing (first at the University of Nebraska, and later at the University of Pittsburgh) Cohen has made a detailed study of approximately 1350 pregnant women; moreover, in their discussion of the implications for current obstetric practice and for long-term research, Cohen et al.[13] show that approximately 58% of women seen in a University Pre-natal Clinic should be considered as "high risk" cases.

Using different criteria the author identified a lower incidence of women at high risk: low risk = 53%; high risk = 33%; very high risk = 14%. Nevertheless, this restricted study provides substantial confirmation of Cohen's findings that a large proportion of primigravidae is at high risk.

These parallel studies in the U.S.A. and in England point clearly to the urgent need to provide psychological screening and appropriate management during the routine care of every expectant mother.*

Finally it is pertinent to recall the words of Grantly Dick-Read in his classic *Childbirth without fear*: "Her mind is of even greater importance than her physical state; for motherhood is of the mind, and the body is usually subjected to the mental processes, unless any gross abnormality exists. There is a vast territory around and about maternity which is still unexplored."

REFERENCES

1. BAKER, A. A. 1967. *Psychiatric disorders in obstetrics.* Oxford & Edinburgh: Blackwell Scientific Publications.
2. BEAZLEY, J. M. 1968. Labour pain—how much are midwives to blame? *Nursing Mirror*, **1**, 19.
3. BENTALL, A. P. and FAIRS, D. J. 1967. Planning a new maternity hospital. *Nursing Times*, Vol. 63, 1198.
4. BIBRING, G. L. 1959. Some considerations of the psychological processes in pregnancy. *Psychoanal. Stud. Child.*, **14**, 113.
5. BREWS, A. 1957. *Eden & Hollands manual of obstetrics.* London: Churchill.
6. BURKE, M. F. 1968. Suicide in pregnancy. *Brit. med. J.*, **1**, 49.
7. BUXTON, C. L. 1962. *A study of psychophysical methods for relief of childbirth pain.* Philadelphia and London: Saunders.
8. CAPLAN, G. 1964. *Principles of preventive psychiatry.* London: Tavistock Publications.

* I acknowledge my indebtedness to Professor Richard Cohen for the opportunity to read advance copies of three original papers on the gradual evolution of his screening technique for the identification of pregnancy stresses.

9. CHERTOK, L. 1959. *Psychosomatic methods in painless childbirth.* Paris: Pergamon Press.
10. COHEN, R. L. 1966. Pregnancy stress and maternal perceptions of infant endowment. *J. ment. Subnorm.*, **12,** 18.
11. COHEN, R. L. 1966. Some maladaptive syndromes of pregnancy and the puerperium. *Obstet. and Gynec.*, **27,** 562.
12. COHEN, R. L. Experiences of pregnancy: some relationships to the syndrome of mental retardation. In *Psychiatric approaches to mental retardation.* (F. Menolascino, ed.). New York: Basic Books. (In press.)
13. COHEN, R. L. *et. al.* 1968. The incidence of significant stress as perceived by pregnant women. (Personal communication.)
14. CREAK, M. 1956. In *Child Health and Development* (R. W. B. Ellis, ed.). London: Churchill.
15. DRILLIEN, C. M. and WILKINSON, E. 1964. Emotional stress and mongol births. *Develop. Med. Child Neurol.*, **2,** 140.
16. HORSLEY, J. S. 1940. Convulsion therapy of early mental illness in out-patient clinics. *Med. Press and Circ.*, **203,** No. 5255.
17. HORSLEY, J. S. 1964. Emotional hygiene in pregnancy and the puerperium. *Publ. Hlth.*, **78,** 273.
18. HORSLEY, J. S. 1969. *Key concepts in community psychiatry.* London: Tavistock Publications. (In press.)
19. ILLSLEY, R. 1961. The social aetiology of foetal damage. *J. Ment. Subnorm,* **7,** 86.
20. LAMAZE, F. 1956. *Encyclopedie médico-chirugicale.* Paris.
21. LOMAS, P. 1964. Childbirth ritual. *New Society* (31 December).
22. MCDONALD, J. 1969. The quality of kindness. *Nursing Mirror,* **128,** 40.
23. MORRIS, N. 1960. Human relations in obstetric practice. *Lancet,* i, 913.
24. NIKOLAYEV, A. P. 1961. The present position and the prospects with regard to painless childbirth in the U.S.S.R. *Vestiv. Akad. med. Nauk,* **2,** 64.
25. PEEL, Sir JOHN. 1968. The future of the maternity services. *Nursing Mirror,* **127,** 27.
26. PHILIPP, E. E. 1964. Minor disorders of pregnancy. *Brit. med. J.,* **1,** 749.
27. PRECHTL, H. F. R. 1963. In *Determinants of infant behaviour,* Vol. 2. (B. M. Foss, ed.). London: Methuen.
28. PRINCE, G. S. 1962. The prevention of mental ill health. *R. Soc. Hlth. J.,* **2,** 117.
29. PRUGH, D. G. and HARLOW, R. G. 1962. Masked deprivation in infants and young children. In *Deprivation of Maternal Care.* Geneva: W.H.O.
30. READ, G. D. 1933. *Natural Childbirth.* London: Heinemann.
31. Report of the Maternity Services Committee. 1959. London: H.M.S.O.
32. Report of the Standing Maternity and Midwifery Advisory Committee. 1961. London: H.M.S.O.
33. SCOTT, P. D. 1968. Preventive psychiatry. (Personal communication).
34. STALLWORTHY, J. 1969. Changes in midwifery—progression or regression? *Nursing Mirror,* **128,** 34 .
35. STOTT, D. H. 1963. How a disturbed pregnancy can harm the child. *New Scientist,* **320,** 13.
36. SUTHERLAND, R. 1956. In *Child health and development* (R. W. B. Ellis, ed.). London: Churchill.
37. TACCHI, D. 1965. Progress in antenatal care. *Nursing Mirror,* **121,** 155.
38. TAIT, H. P. 1956. In *Child health and development.* (R. W. B. Ellis, ed.). London: Churchill.
39. TOD, E. D. M. 1964. Puerperal depression. *Lancet,* ii, 1264.
40. VELVOVSKY, I. Z. 1949. [Quoted by Chertok, Ref. 9.]
41. WATTS, C. A. H. 1966. *Depressive disorders in the community.* Bristol: John Wright & Sons.

CLINICAL

Peri-Natal

XVI

PSYCHOPROPHYLAXIS IN OBSTETRICS
A SOVIET METHOD*

I. Z. VELVOVSKY
Ukrainian Institute for the Advancement of Doctors
Kharkov, U.S.S.R.

1

Historical Development

In 1920 K. I. Platonov, the renowned Soviet psychiatrist and founder of the Kharkov Psychiatric School, together with a group of pupils, which included the psychiatrists I. Z. Velvovsky and P. P. Istomin, started to investigate the application of hypno-suggestion in painless childbirth. Eminent obstetricians and gynaecologists like A. P. Nikolayev and V. I. Zdravomyslov also became interested in this field and were soon to be followed by many other clinical workers.

What was new in the Soviet approach was the attitude to hypnosis and suggestion. The Soviet workers firmly supported I. P. Pavlov's postulates and steadfastly rejected all misgivings emanating from the School of Charcot, which suggested that some damage may be caused by suggestion under hypnosis. These misgivings were reflected even in the proceedings of the Innsbruck Congress of Obstetricians and Gynaecologists in 1922.

But already in 1926, the author of this chapter was disappointed in hypno-suggestion as a general method of painless childbirth, and he started to develop an approach which linked obstetrics and gynaecology on the one hand, and psycho-neurology on the other. By 1930 the author had reached his own formulations in "Psycho-gynaecology" and "Psycho-obstetrics" and laid down the principles of the psychoprophylactic system of painless childbirth.

However, it was only after the last World War that the author was able to organize a Department of Women's Psycho-Neurology in a Central Clinic of a psychoneurological and neuro-surgical Hospital of the Ministry of Transport of the U.S.S.R. in Kharkov, which was under his leadership. The Department of Women's Psycho-neurology which he organized included psychoprophylactic consultations and a maternity home which paid particular attention to the psychological needs of the patients. Here in 1947–49,

---

* Translated by the late N. Kinalewsky, Foxhall Hospital, Ipswich, Suffolk.

with the co-operation of two obstetrician-gynaecologists, V. Ploticher and E. A. Shugom, the theoretical aspects of a "Psychoprophylactic System of Painless Childbirth" were finally developed and its practical applications introduced into practice.

In 1949, in addition to the acknowledgement of Professor Platonov and of many other psychiatrists, obstetricians and gynaecologists of Kharkov, this system received also the support of obstetrician-gynaecologist A. P. Nikolayev, a most distinguished specialist in this field. He has now become the highest authority in this field, a founder member of the movement, and an enthusiastic propagandist. Further, this system has received the approbation of the Scientific Council of the Ministry of Health of the U.S.S.R., of the Presidium of the Academy of Medical Sciences and of many other Institutes. It was legalized in 1951 by the Ministry of Public Health of the U.S.S.R. as the leading system of painless childbirth in the U.S.S.R. It has been adopted by many eminent obstetrician-gynaecologists of the U.S.S.R. among whom we may list A. P. Nikolayev, G. S. Salganik, P. A. Beloshapko, M. A. Petrov-Maslakov, I. F. Jordania, F. A. Syrovatko, V. N. Shishkova, M. I. Donigevich, N. P. Lebedev, I. P. Yakovlev. A number of neurophysiologists and psychiatrists, as for example A. O. Dolin, S. N. Astakhov, R. A. Zachepitsky, have produced a series of valuable works, investigations and monographs, delving deeply into the problems involved in this type of psychoprophylaxis.

In 1952, the acceptance of the Soviet system abroad was assisted by Fernard Lamaze of France, and we would like to acknowledge the role he played. Thereafter the Soviet method of psychoprophylaxis of labour pains quickly received fame and recognition, spreading into many countries of Europe, Africa, Asia and South America.

2

Basic Concepts of the Soviet Psychoprophylactic System

The theoretical foundations and methodological principles of the system of prophylaxis described above were defined by the author when he came to scrutinize in a new light the nervous mechanisms of pregnancy and childbirth. For this purpose the author has compared the evolution of the process of reproduction with the evolution of the higher nervous system from fish to man. This comparison was done following the principles of the evolutionary process of reproduction as described by F. Engels in his *Dialectics of Nature* and, adhering, for the neuro-dynamics of reproduction, to the teachings of I. P. Pavlov's school on higher nervous activity and cortico-visceral structures. Without considering the above-mentioned works and without formulating a special "Psycho-neurology of Women" the author could not have reached his formulation of the psychoprophylactic system. Furthermore, without considering these basic factors, which led the author to his conclusions and formulations, it is impossible to understand the essence of the Soviet psychoprophylactic system, its modern progress and the trend of women's psycho-neurology.

These points will not be elaborated here, but the reader is referred to our books, one of which is written in collaboration with other authors and published in English[4] and Spanish[5]; we would also like to refer the reader to a collection of articles[2, 3] which discuss our findings more fully. Here we will briefly comment on the main formulations.

The comparison mentioned above has shown that "true" pregnancy and delivery (i.e. the implantation of the ovum, the formation of the placenta, labour and lactation) are functions of animals that have reached a level of development at which they have developed a brain where the cortex of the latest convolutional structure (the neocortex) interacts with the adjacent subcortex of the neostriatal type (the neostriatum). Completeness and relations with the outside world are secured by the cortex. Beginning from the implantation of the fertilized ovum, pregnancy and labour follow the laws of the automatic neuro-dynamic system (as conceived by Pavlov, there is positive induction of the subcortical system and negative induction, i.e. development of inhibitory states of the cortex). The cortex, however, can still influence pregnancy, and indeed its presence is linked with the phenomenon of "true" pregnancy. Pregnancy and labour should be analysed from the positions of Pavlovian nervism by being conceived as a completely combined chain of unconditioned reflexes, i.e. instinctive, and conditioned reflex activity. Considering pregnancy and labour from a neuro-dynamical point of view, the author applied neuro-dynamical interpretation to the process of pregnancy and of the labour (the contractions, the pauses, the bearing down, the speeding up, the presentation of the foetus, rotation of head and so forth).

During normal labour the basic processes operating in the central nervous system of women are *balanced within certain limits*. It is perfectly evident, however, that these complex neurodynamics are sensitive to the slightest changes during labour, and are therefore unstable. The phenomena of inhibition and excitation in the cortex and the subcortical structures may either intensify or weaken, irradiate or concentrate. Normally, both these processes are reversible and quantitatively limited. The dynamic changes occurring in them may be caused by numerous factors, in particular by the nature and force of the stimulations coming from the birth canal, from the internal organs, and, lastly, from the external environment through the first and second signal systems.

The liability and mobility of the basic nervous processes may be responsible for the multiform peculiarities of pregnancy and labour. In addition to the properly balanced operation of the complex unconditioned chain reflexes, dynamic changes, and even coarser deviations, may occur in any link of the reflex arcs. These deviations may be transient or protracted and stable. The obstetric deviations and complications in labour are well known to obstetricians, but the *deviations in the neuro-dynamics of labour* have until now failed to attract due attention.

When wide circles of practising obstetricians become cognizant of the fact that pain may also form in the cerebral cortex, it will be clear to them that the presence of local material factors during labour need not necessarily produce pain and, on the other hand, that pain may arise centrally and cortically without the presence of special local pain factors.

Looking at these processes as resulting from the reflex system, the author could find no grounds for considering as unavoidable the appearance of pain during the physiological course of labour, in spite of the natural strain.

But if there is pain, the author separated pain due to disorders of labour dynamics in its motor function which would be common, i.e. the labour pain that occurs as mass phenomenon in physiological labour, from those the author named "peripherogenic" or "receptogenic", i.e. those pains which appear during labour because of the failure of the amniotic sac to break, asynclitism (Naegele's obliquity, Litzmann's obliquity), rigidity of the cervix of the uterus, narrow and deformed pelvis, and other circumstances connected mainly with the obstruction of the motor function. These latter pains denoting pathological labour, however, play a certain part in the development of so-called historical pain of "labour psychofixation".

The reasons for labour pain as a mass phenomenon during physiological labour are divided by the author into two groups:

(i) excessive aggravation of neuro-dynamical interaction in the system of the cortex-subcortex;

(ii) the historical psychofixation of the act of labour as a painful act, and as an act of suffering which induced negative emotions to pregnancy and made it a mass phenomenon.

In relation to (i) it can be said that the following circumstances contribute to the appearance of pain reactions to the stimuli of normal labour:

(a) variations in the cortico-subcortical and intracortical induction processes;

(b) changes in the threshold of excitation and in the tone of the cerebral cortex;

(c) formation of states of "excitatory weakness" in the cerebral cortex;

(d) emergence of phasic states in the cerebral cortex and, particularly, development of paradoxical reactions;

(e) changes in the conditioned reflex bonds of the cerebral cortex and in the normal relationship of the signal systems;

(f) revival of trace reactions from preceding painful labour.

During a complicated and aggravated course of labour, under great strain or even overstrain of the nervous system, pain develops more easily in persons with a weak and easily excitable nervous system and unbalanced signal systems. In such parturient women pain may arise sooner and in response to weaker stimuli, and may at the same time be more sharply pronounced and more unbearable than in persons with a strong and well-balanced type of nervous system. The basic nervous processes running an inert course, the pain phenomena will probably become more firmly fixed, something which will condition their appearance in subsequent parturition.

From (*i*) and (*ii*) above, it is clear that normal physiological pregnancy need not be a painful act; and on that basis is built the psychoprophylactic system of the prevention of suffering during physiological labour, and this is accepted as the basis of the Soviet System.

Only since we formulated in the light of I. Pavlov's teachings the basic postulates concerning the origin and development of childbirth and the pain that accompanies it, have we been able to approach the solution of the problems of preventing rather than relieving labour pain.

By psychoprophylaxis of labour pain we imply a system of measures aimed at preventing the appearance and development of labour pain and effected through influences exerted on the higher divisions of the central nervous system.

The principal part of this method is prevention and elimination of the causes underlying the disturbances in the physiological balance of the higher divisions of the nervous system, leading to the emergence of pain.

The basic aim and fundamental objective of the system of psychoprophylaxis of labour pain is not only individual labour pain relief but, as we have repeatedly indicated, an endeavour to do away with labour pain and the misgivings of women in childbirth as a mass phenomenon.

The ultimate aim of the new system is a striving to reach a point when the most important biological and social function—reproduction of the human race—may not be accompanied by suffering and distressing experiences and labour pain may be forgotten in normal childbirth as a grave survival of the past.

3

Outline of the Principles and Structure of the Soviet Psychoprophylactic System

In order to prevent the phenomena of pain during normal labour it is necessary to have a *SYSTEM* composed of a minimum of two linked parts:

(*i*) Psychoprophylactic preparation of pregnant women for labour.

(*ii*) Psychohygiene of lying-in women in the maternity home.

Both (*i*) and (*ii*) are intended to guide pregnant and "lying-in" women according to the basic principles of modern obstetrics.

A pregnant and lying-in woman must also of course be guarded against aggravation and complications, especially pathological complications of pregnancy and labour. Similarly, psychotherapy may be required for morbid mental phenomena that disturbs the normal course of pregnancy, e.g. hyperemesis gravidarum and toxemias of pregnancy.

(i) Psychoprophylactic Preparation

A careful and profound study of the expectant mother's anamnesis by the physician is particularly important for the system of psychoprophylaxis. History-taking in the system of psychoprophylaxis is noted for the fact that it is not confined to ascertaining the living conditions, development, past illnesses and special data of an obstetrical nature. It is necessary to obtain data on the pregnant woman's home conditions, her family relations, and of her own, her husband's and close relatives' attitude to the pregnancy, the forthcoming labour and the future child. Great importance is attached to the analysis of the woman's experiences during her pregnancy, her ideas of childbirth and her frame of mind in connection with the impending labour and motherhood. Accurate ascertainment of the influences exerted on the expectant mother by the people surrounding her (husband, relatives, friends, etc.) is very important. It is also important to take into consideration her usual mode of behaviour: capriciousness, liability, aggressiveness, irritability, and inability to endure pain or, on the contrary, self-control, composure, etc.

Properly organized, the ante-partum psychoprophylactic preparation of pregnant women should begin during the very first visit to the maternity health centre. Only in this case will the lessons be of a nature generalizing, consummating and consolidating all of the preceding work and only in this case may they be reduced to four in number, i.e. correspond to the usual number of visits to the maternity health centre which the pregnant woman must make during the last month.

Under the circumstances, however, when the pregnant woman is prepared only during the last stage of pregnancy, a minimum of six sessions is obligatory.

The first session is individual, the subsequent sessions being conducted in groups of several women each. The groups are organized in accordance with the cultural level of their members.

The objectives of the pedagogical part of the preparation may be formulated as follows:

1. To eliminate the negative emotions of the pregnant woman and the excessive orienting reactions of the parturient woman by explaining and disproving the erroneous ideas of, and attitudes to labour and by instilling appropriate, scientifically-substantiated views and conceptions of labour. The woman should become familiar with the atmosphere of the maternity home, and the special medical equipment of the labour room.

2. To acquaint the woman with all the basic phenomena of labour so as to impress on her the fact that these phenomena are normal; deprived of the element of surprise they will not frighten her.

3. To teach the pregnant woman proper conduct during labour so that she may follow instructions properly. To teach her special pain-prevention techniques. This ensures the accomplishment of normal activity during

labour (position, breathing, bearing down, etc.) and results in a saving of energy.

A question not infrequently asked is: "Why are these lessons regarded as instruction rather than 'suggestion' or 'autosuggestion'? What is the difference?"

To be sure, suggestion plays a big part in a large number of phenomena. But can the ideas of *education, instruction, enlightenment and propaganda* be replaced by those of *suggestion and autosuggestion*?

In referring to correct preparation for painless labour, we speak not only about school education, but also about teaching, tutorage and training, in order to get women accustomed to intelligent, physiological and technically correct behaviour of women as such.

In relation to details of such teaching which is carried out not as a primitive suggestion during weaker background of activity of the cortex (hypnosis in different stages), but as "Education of an intelligent act, built on all possible association, when the cortex is strong and having high tonus" (I. P. Pavlov).

Here we will say that we are discussing a pedagogical system, which is not based on suggestion in the hypnotical stage as developed by Read in his relaxo-suggestive system, which is opposite to the principle of the Soviet psychoprophylactic system, in spite of the fact that some of his technical methods may sometimes seem to have some similarities with our system.

(ii) Psycho-hygiene

In the second period, i.e. in the maternity home, the main principle is active observation of the obstetric course of labour by the clinical staff. Doctors and midwives quickly recognize signs of anxiety, complications and pathology; if these signs appear, they must be quickly removed and the situation corrected. In addition, it is also necessary to keep observation on the woman and to remind and encourage her to use fully and correctly the knowledge which she acquired during her preparation period; she will be advised to behave according to the instructions and training she received. The doctor must be an active leader, a mentor and a conductor of labour behaviour, as well as being alert as an obstetrician.

In accordance with the basic lines of the system of psychoprophylaxis of labour pain, it is necessary to do the following in the maternity home:

1. Safeguard the parturient woman's peace of mind and prevent the emergence of any disturbing and depressing reactions in the process of labour.

2. Stimulate the parturient woman's behaviour in such a manner that she may be able, under the supervision and control of the physician and midwife, actively, consciously and skilfully to make use of the information and techniques learned by her during the preparation at the maternity health centre.

3. Manage labour, preventing and eliminating possible deviations and complications in its development.

We urgently insist that the personnel observe all these principles with the maximum of attention precisely in normal labour, as against the old ideas, according to which the obstetrical personnel was actively mobilized only when labour took a pathological course. The vigorous activity of the personnel precisely in normal labour characterizes the prophylactic trend in its management. This trend and the ensuing demands made by the personnel permit the real management of labour and the psychoprophylaxis of labour pain to be inseparably connected with it.

During the excitation of the subcortex in labour, the negative induction of the cerebral cortex is to a certain extent a natural phenomenon. It is our aim, however, not to let these natural processes become excessively strong. Thus we are striving to prevent the normal labour stimuli, which usually remain below the threshold of excitation of the cerebral cortex, from acquiring the strength and nature of threshold and superthreshold stimuli. It is this that constitutes the most important aim of the entire system of pain-prevention.

To achieve the aforesaid aim, it is necessary to teach the parturient woman to master and perform some active and not very strenuous motor techniques in order to stimulate irradiation of a light excitation of the cerebral cortex, i.e. its alert tone. This is necessary to reduce the negative induction of the cerebral cortex and decrease the excitation (positive induction) of the subcortex. We believe it necessary to maintain a requisite level of the threshold of excitation of the cerebral cortex by a moderate mobilization of the parturient woman's motor and allied sensory functions. This is why we use "pain-prevention techniques", to which special attention must be devoted during the preparation.

In principle it makes no difference what motor techniques are used. Other motor techniques, which act as "sensomotor" techniques, could be used as successfully as those of our complex, provided they are connected with labour. By way of example we shall examine one of our techniques aimed at mobilizing the attention. We teach the women to pay attention to the first signs of labour, orient themselves to it and "check" on it.

For this purpose it is recommended that the pregnant woman time her pangs and the intervals between them by the clock. This concentrates her attention and prevents the development of the processes of disorderly orientation and of the guarding reflexes.

The parturient woman's systematic observation of her labour from its first signs to the strains aids in "corticalizing" her behaviour. Without this, as often happens, labour assumes many features attesting the excessive excitation of the subcortex and weakened control over it by the cerebral cortex.

During the pangs, active inhalations and exhalations play a similar physiological role, but by mobilizing motor acts. In our nomenclature they are known as the "first pain-prevention technique".

The cortex is activated to an even greater extent by the "second pain-prevention technique" which consists of a complex of acts. This technique mobilizes the respiratory motorium, the motorium of the forearms, wrists and arms and their co-ordination. It is but natural that such an element of higher nervous activity as attention operates here, too.

In our opinion this complex aids in raising the tone of a considerable portion of the cerebral cortex and in preventing excessive development of inhibition. We believe that this excitation may irradiate to adjacent zones of the cerebral cortex.

We therefore think that in the question of preventing labour pain, according to the psychoprophylactic system, it is not a matter of removing or controlling the pain that has already emerged, but one of preventing its appearance.

The main, dominating and leading principle in our system, is to increase the activity of the positive inductive processes in the cerebral cortex in order to achieve a rise in its tone and provoke a moderate excitation in it rather than inhibition.

All the foregoing considerations show objectively that psychoprophylactically prepared women whose cerebral cortex is in an active state react differently from unprepared women, whose cerebral cortex is more or less inhibited. The method of psychoprophylaxis of labour pain normalizes the reactivity of the nervous system and the course of somatic processes by activating the regulatory cortical mechanisms. The labour of psychoprophylactically prepared women runs a painless course or, to be exact, without the usual reactions to pain.

Will not stimulation of the cerebral cortex to activity retard the development of the labour process and change its course for the worse? This is a legitimate question. But the facts obtained in observing the course of labour in many thousands of parturient women warrant another conclusion, namely, that the activation of the cerebral cortex to the extent required by the system of psychoprophylaxis does not disturb the course of labour.

This may be explained by the fact that the cerebral cortex has the properties not only of inhibiting and disinhibiting certain mechanisms but also of regulating and stimulating them. The higher the development of the animal, the more clearly do these active functions of the cerebral cortex come to the fore as regards such phenomena which, at a certain stage of its phylogenetic development, occur automatically and do not depend on their active regulation by the cerebral cortex. Owing to its particular development in man, many functions are increasingly subject to the influence of the cerebral cortex.

It is necessary to remember that the system of psychoprophylaxis works successfully with the physiological processes of labour, both motor-activity and neuro-dynamics. This is why, when there is restlessness, signs of breaking down, disturbed motor-activity, the sharpening of vegetative reactions (which should not arise if the mother is well-versed in the principles of psychoprophylaxis), the obstetrician has a tendency to "reinforce" painless labour by employing at once pharmacological agents, such as analgesic drugs.

The appearance of anxiety in a woman who has been well and correctly prepared must immediately alert the obstetrician to investigate the situation by external methods, and, where necessary, by internal examination. In cases where there is an appearance of such complications as jamming of the lip of the uterus, presence of unopened sac and any other disturbing factors, then it is necessary to take all possible steps, including operative and pharmacological intervention, *but only if there is real need for it.*

With the creation of an active state of the cerebral cortex by our methods no paradoxical pain reactions to the normal stimulations from the physiologically operating processes will be able to emerge. However, adequate pain reactions to harmful stimuli attesting deviations from normal and a development of a pathological course of labour will emerge in the cerebral cortex. Deviations from the normal course of labour will infallibly evoke in the parturient woman, prepared according to our system, signals of uneasiness and pain, whereas with other methods of pain-relief such signals may not appear.

The emergence of a pain signal stimulates the obstetricians to watch the parturient woman especially carefully, and urgently demands a timely and precise diagnosis of the complication, as well as interference necessary to remove the pathology.

From our point of view, it is absolutely inadmissible to use analgesic drugs in order to "reinforce" painless labour, as it is proposed particularly by Professor Foy here in the U.S.S.R. It is inadmissible because it may veil arising anxiety, not to mention that it is quite impossible to guarantee that any unjustified drug administration will not be traumatic.

With respect to the main mass of parturient women whose labour proceeds physiologically, we therefore deny the necessity of combining the method of psychoprophylaxis with analgesics. However, if deviations from normal labour have developed or some form of pathology has manifested itself during the course of labour and requires special obstetrical interference, we are impelled by the force of circumstances to inhibit, i.e. to "treat" the pain. In such cases the use of pharmacological agents, including general anaesthesia, and all varieties of hypnotic suggestion (hypnonarcosis, narcohypnosis, etc.) is indicated. But these no longer constitute psychoprophylactic pain-prevention in normal labour; they are therapeutic measures and interferences required by the failures to prevent pain caused by complications and the pathological course of labour.

It should not be assumed, however, that the system of psychoprophylaxis produces no effect in complications or pathology of labour. As the clinical analysis cited below shows, the system is effective in such cases also.

Lastly, there are rare cases in which we believe the use of pharmacological agents in addition to the psychoprophylactic preparation to be helpful even in obstetrically normal labour. This is sometimes necessary when the neuropsychiatric status of the parturient woman deviates from the normal.

Apart from the tendency to reinforce the prophylactic system by pain-killing drugs, we must mention another tendency which we consider erroneous. This is the tendency to regard the usefulness of gymnastic elements as the most important factor in painless childbirth; there is a tendency even to re-name the psychoprophylactic system as "physioprophylactic method".

With the aim of sharing our knowledge and making our efforts better known to clinical workers, we offer here a brief description of the psychoprophylactic system from the beginning of preparation in the last four, six and seven weeks of pregnancy.

In our method we have introduced breathing exercises and other exercises of a gymnastic nature. During preparation these exercises serve as a medium for psychologically influencing the patient and encouraging and potentiating physical effort; used during labour, they are important as stimulators of an alert state in the cerebral cortex; furthermore, they prevent the weakening of this state. *By themselves, without psychological preparation and potentiation, the gymnastic measures do not have any painless effect during the process of labour.* We do not deny their general hygienic effect, but this is more noticeable, of course, if those methods are not introduced as late as during the last week of pregnancy, but much earlier during the term of pregnancy and for the full duration of it.

Our observations of 2,000 childbirths in a maternity hospital and the information at our disposal of more than 100,000 psychoprophylactically prepared cases of childbirths, managed by our pupils and followers in other institutions, attest the possibility of producing a positive effect in 95% of parturient women without the additional use of any pharmacological agents whatsoever.

4

Further Development and Perspectives

During the last years of our psychoneurological and gynaecological practice, we have come to realize the importance of insisting on introducing the psychoprophylactic system, not during the last weeks of pregnancy but at the beginning, as soon as a woman comes for the first consultation to make sure that she is pregnant.

During the last years we, together with our collaborator the obstetrician and gynaecologist G. H. Baltpurvin, have devised and described a system working from the very beginning of the pregnancy, during the full duration of it until labour, and even embracing the post-natal and lactation periods.

This system too does not aim to produce a painless labour only. The question of future pains in labour do not concern women in the early stages of pregnancy. This system of psychoprophylaxis embraces all neuro-dynamical functional nervous disturbances during pregnancy and future labour, and it takes into consideration the post-natal period too. Of course, the system includes prophylaxis of pains during the last stages of pregnancy. But the system, applied from the first weeks of pregnancy is a system not only of psychoprophylaxis, but also of psycho-hygiene and psychotherapy. We speak of psychotherapy, when during the process of pregnancy some neuro-dynamical and functional and nervous disorders demands treatment. As such disorders are treated by psychotherapy, we are also at the same time able to obtain psychoprophylaxis of pains and psychoprophylaxis of many other disorders.

In this much more important system, as the first step in the preparation of a pregnant woman we have already initiated a complex of twenty-two lessons conducted during the whole term of pregnancy. These lessons, depending on the stage of the pregnancy, are divided into groups. As we are not able to describe fully the structure and contents of this new complete system here, we refer our readers to our already published works.[4]

In this system all the elements of hygiene of pregnant women are initiated and potentiated by it. This system also includes broadly developed physical exercises, as well as paying attention to aspects of obstetric importance (diet, regime, clothing, etc.).

Furthermore, on the basis of our neuro-dynamical conceptions of functional disorders during pregnancy, we try to correct from the beginning even the slightest hint of disorder by using psychotherapeutic methods. In this way, by psychotherapy we are able to relieve general weakness, proneness to irritation, bad appetite, sleep disorders, tachycardia, hyperthyroidism, excessive salivation, aversion to certain foods and smells, and especially nausea and vomiting. In many cases this is a real psychoprophylaxis of the toxaemia of pregnancy in its first stage, but not so often in the second stage of pregnancy; we have quite often succeeded in producing prophylaxis of eclampsia by the same methods. Considerable success has also been obtained in the treatment of miscarriage, habitual abortions, premature and post-mature births, whenever their aetiology was neuro-dynamical or psychological, but not of an organic nature. In such cases we apply extensively not only didactic, but especially psychotherapeutic, methods of treatment, not only in the alert state of the cortex, but also in hypnotic states, as we deal here with occurrences of a patho-physiological nature.

5

Conclusion

Summing up all the foregoing, we wish to emphasize once again that the system of psychoprophylaxis of labour pain is based on social-organizational and individual measures.

The *social-organizational measures* are based on mass educational work aimed at combating the erroneous ideas of labour as a tormenting, dangerous and traumatic process, and of the inevitability of labour pain. Proper ideas of labour should be inculcated in the masses.

At the same time, it is necessary to organize obstetrical aid properly, and to ensure unity and continuity in the work of the maternity health centres, patronage and maternity homes.

The following must be taken into consideration in carrying out the *individual measures*:

(i) the dynamics of the intracortical and the cortico-subcortical induction relations;

(ii) the regularity in the irradiation and concentration of the excitatory and inhibitory processes;

(iii) the relations between the first and second signal systems of reality;

(iv) the possibility of influencing the pregnant and parturient woman through the first signal system (mobilization of the motor activity and influence of light sensory stimulations) and the second signal system (the word, education and preparation);

(v) the expediency of using pedagogical and educational forms of work, which are the principal forms in the system; this does not exclude elements of suggestion, although their role is considered secondary;

(vi) the possibility of managing labour by the personnel by means of directed activation of the parturient woman's higher nervous activity, i.e. by purposeful influence exerted on her through her second signal system;

(vii) the necessity of constantly watching the parturient woman to ensure that labour proceeds normally and of rendering timely aid in order to prevent any possibility of deviations from the normal course of labour and to preclude labour complications.

The attention of the obstetrician using our general neuro-dynamical conceptions was first caught by the use of them in the sensorial stage of labour, when pain occurs; but the main issues, in spite of the fact that they were widely published, remained ignored. During the last few years, as a result of our neuro-dynamical conceptions, new work has started on deeper and wider development of the bordering field between obstetrics and gynaecology on the one hand, and neurology, psychology, psychiatry, neuro-surgery, psycho-hygiene, psychoprophylaxis and psychotherapy on the other hand. This new field we call "Women's Psycho-neurology", but our colleagues in obstetrics prefer to call it "neuro-gynaecology and neuro-obstetrics". Work in this direction is growing daily with the co-operation between obstetricians, gynaecologists, endocrinologists and neuro-pathologists, psychiatrists, neuro-surgeons, psychologists, psycho-physiologists, hygienists, psychoprophy-lacticians and psychotherapists, at the central psychoneurological and neuro-surgical hospital of the Ministry of Transport in Kharkov. There are special consultants for women, a maternity home, and departments of neurosis and psychotherapy. The results of this great work by many institutions throughout the U.S.S.R. have found their exposition at a large all-union conference in Kharkov in 1964, and are reflected in a book published in 1967.[1]

REFERENCES

1. A synopsis of Psychoprophylaxis in Obstetrics and Gynecology. *Transactions of the Conference in Kiev, 1967.*
2. VELVOVSKY, I. Z. 1963. *The system of psychoprophylactic painless childbirth.* Moscow.
3 VELVOVSKY, I. Z., PLATONOV, K., PLOTICHER, V. and SHUGOM, E. 1954. *Painless childbirth through psychoprophylaxis,* Leningrad.
4. VELVOVSKY, I. Z., PLATONOV, K., PLOTICHER, V. and SHUGOM, E. 1960. *Painless childbirth through psychoprophylaxis.* Moscow.
5. VELVOVSKY, I. Z., PLATONOV, K., PLOTICHER, V. and SHUGOM, E. 1963. *Psicopro-filaxis de los dolores del parto.* Moscow.

XVII

PAINLESS LABOUR: A FRENCH METHOD

PIERRE VELLAY

M.D.

Secretary General of the International
Society for Psychoprophylaxis in Obstetrics
Paris, France

1

Introduction

Psychoprophylaxis and anaesthesia are two terms and two conceptions which, to the uninitiated or to persons having preconceptions, may appear incompatible, or even wholly opposed. We shall endeavour to demonstrate here that this is not our view after seventeen years of intensive and methodical experimentation in psychoprophylaxis.

Our opinion is based on the following three main ideas.

(1) Childbirth is, in the great majority of cases, a normal physiological process, for which recourse to anaesthesia does not seem necessary, or even useful.

(2) The mother's and the child's safety constitute the prime imperative, ruling out any preconceived or facile attitude on the part of the obstetrician.

(3) Any idea of a routine, any preconceived attitude is false, whatever the technique used in the course of labour.

There are always cases to which the obstetrician must be able to adapt his personal conceptions and his talent.

2

Psychoprophylaxis

Our experience is based on a close clinical study, in the course of which our successes have not allowed us to forget our failures. What follows is based on both. We also offer the statistics of a number of obstetricians belonging to the Société Française de Psycho-prophylaxie, or to the International Society, Prof. Müller (Strasburg), Dr. Bazelaire (Reims), Dr. Blum (Strasburg), Prof. Cotteel (Lille), Dr. Guillaumin (Saint-Denis), Dr. Gutherz

(Nîmes), Dr. Hersilie (Paris), Drs. Vellay and Randon (Paris), Dr. Vittoz (Maisons-Laffitte). Not to burden the text with tedious figures these are shown in Table I.

TABLE I

Based on 40,000 Deliveries

Good results	70–75%
Medium	10–20%
Failures	3–8 %
Forceps without anaesthesia or vacuum extractors	6–8 %
Forceps with anaesthesia	2 %
Caesarians	2 %
Deaths	9 %

On the basis of these combined statistics covering several of thousands of cases, we find:

(1) that the number of patients benefiting by the method and without recourse to anaesthesia amounts to at least 75%;

(2) that the number of forceps or vacuum extractor deliveries not requiring anaesthesia is ten times greater than the number in which anaesthesia proves necessary;

(3) that the number of caesarians is extremely reduced and does not exceed 2%—according to our statistics we find that the only indications are:

psychoprophylaxis;

foeto-pelvic dystocia;

procidence of the cord;

modifications of the foetal-heart beats (exceptional);

cervical dystocia after cauterization, but not a single case for oedema of the cervix.

(4) that the number of delivery haemorrhages is much smaller, this being due to the very simple fact, readily understood, that a uterus which contracts physiologically without "forcing" and without analgesic depressors reacts more effectively. By way of proof we need only point to the rapidity of expulsion of placentae, which occurs in three to eight minutes. We can say that a delivery that is not effected after ten minutes will be an artificial delivery, by reason of an incarceratic placenta, especially in the right horn. We resort to an artificial delivery only for one out of seventy births.

3

Anaesthesia

On consulting other statistics, we must confess that we are rather startled, and we wonder if sometimes the true motivations are not to be found in a field different from pure obstetrics. The number of caesarians, of surgical operations, is considerable. We are entitled to raise two questions.

(1) Are these obstetricians in the unfortunate position of encountering obstetrical pathology only?

(2) Do they perhaps consider obstetrics as being essentially pathological?

This reminds me of the humorous comment of an American obstetrician, widely known in France, who, speaking of certain colleagues, said: "Childbirth occurs naturally only when the obstetrician isn't there, or doesn't get there in time!"

It would be interesting if, in a learned society meeting, each of the participants were to present his results and his failures quite honestly; some startling revelations would come to light!

In the course of the study that we have carried out in various countries, we wonder whether anaesthesia, to which a surgical operation is reciprocally linked (forceps—vacuum extractor and caesarian), is not an easy way out and a comfort for the obstetrician rather than for the patient herself.

I have been struck to see in certain American services (whose influence is great in the Latin-American countries) the use of anaesthesia in a well-nigh routine way. With primipara—and very often multipara—70-80% of forceps with routine episiotomy under anaesthetic are the perquisite of numerous large services in the U.S.A., in Venezuela, in Argentina, etc.

I have been told by a New York obstetrician: "In my practice, all the women are delivered without pain, for I use anaesthesia one hundred per cent and I deliver according to convenience." I told him that I found it surprising to hold "obstetrical sessions", as surgeons hold operative sessions.

In an American Hospital I attended the delivery of a woman having her second baby. Everything was proceeding normally, the patient was beginning to bear down, when I witnessed something unforgettable: a specialized anaesthetist began by making a "saddle block" (while the head of the child was already appearing), then another anaesthetist, assisted by an aide, made a closed-circuit anaesthesia, after which, with wide episiotomy, the child emerged without effort, although rather drugged.

In spite of this, in the U.S.A. a good number of obstetricians and patients react against this routine and are becoming aware of its risks, both from a physical and a psychological point of view. Proof of this is given by numerous articles in magazines like *Time*, *Psychology today*, etc.

The statistics of the U.S.A. Department of Public Health reveal that the greatest percentage of mortality is due to anaesthesia. Grandell, Creiss Jr., J. F. Donnelly and Winston-Jalem,[5] analysing cases of maternal mortality in North Carolina, have concluded that 3% of these were caused by anaesthesia. Between August 1945 and December 1954, 45 deaths were due to anaesthesia. The most serious complications were due to breathing, spinal shock, and heart stoppage; and two cases were due to reactions to medication (cocaine, trichlorethylene). J. F. Jewett,[6] from Boston, Mass. (U.S.A.) reviewing the reasons for maternal mortality in Massachusetts, for the years

1954–55, writes: "The main causes of maternal mortality in Mass. are: infection, haemorrhage, toxemia, with anaesthesia closely following."

To summarize, through the study of methods of routine anaesthesia, we can raise questions on two points:

(1) Is routine, in all its forms, more harmful than beneficial?
(2) Have we the right to deprive our patients of consciousness to the point where they become automatons, wholly left to the will of a hurried or self-indulgent obstetrician?

I recall the cry of alarm uttered by Professor Dixon[4] (U.S.A.) at the meeting of the *Journées Thérapeutiques* held in Paris, in September 1958: "Is it inconceivable for medicine to lend itself to this chemical conquest of freedom? No sane individual, no knowledgeable doctor, no philosopher, can accept this monstrous neutralization of human forces."

4

Benefits for the Mother

We must examine three essential points:

(1) childbirth and its consequences from the point of view of the child;
(2) childbirth as a phenomenon of the sexual life of the woman;
(3) childbirth and its impact on the mother-child relationship, as well as on the relations of the couple.

Childbirth and Fears for the Child

We want to emphasize this essential aspect of childbirth, which is too often neglected or made secondary to the elimination of pain.

The fundamental motivation of the woman in having a successful delivery must be the health of her child; hearing its first spontaneous cry, and seeing immediately that he is perfect.

The pregnant woman, as many studies show, particularly those of Mrs. Hélène Deutsch,[3] has many fears during her confinement concerning her child. Those concerning herself have become greatly attenuated with the progress made in obstetrics in the past fifty years; she no longer feels that her life is in danger. On the other hand, she is afraid of a malformation in her child, of any kind of anomaly; and in this field the public tends to perpetuate these dramatic forebodings. Her frequent dreams on this subject are sufficient evidence to warrant attaching the greatest importance to her anxiety, which often results in poor sleep. The approach of delivery further aggravates her fears and anguish about her child.

Anaesthesia, used unnecessarily or as routine, does not enable the woman to absorb the birth of her child immediately. The umbilical cord is cut without her seeing it. There is a break between the fact of having her child in her

uterus, a part of herself, and that of finding it in a crib, so that she sometimes wonders if it is really her own. This is a situation that we have encountered in prepared women, who had to be anaesthetized for obstetrical
reasons. In such cases the reasons for anaesthesia must be explained, in
order to preclude any guilt-feeling on the part of the woman in relation to
herself or to her own child.

In the U.S.A., thanks to psychiatrists and paediatricians, women are
better appreciating the benefit of remaining conscious and are beginning to
react against routine anaesthesia, which explains the good start made by
psychoprophylaxis there.

Childbirth as a Phenomenon of the Woman's Sexual Life

We cannot forget the importance that childbirth assumes in the sexual
and emotional life of the woman. We owe it to ourselves to facilitate this
experience, without making her blot it out or making it unendurable for
her. Many women have been traumatized in an indelible way by a bad first
delivery, which has remained an ugly memory the importance of which
found expression in aggression toward the husband, in revolt against the
condition of being a woman, and sometimes even—though more exception-
ally—in aggression toward the child itself. It is all very well to say that a
painful delivery is an evil that the woman soon forgets; it does not prevent
the notion of danger, aggravated by the memory of the first experience,
from reappearing.

The woman can and must be able to integrate her delivery in full
consciousness, barring major difficulties, which anaesthesia prevents. We
agree with Mrs. Hélène Deutsch[3] when she writes: "The only effect of
general anaesthesia is that the woman is impoverished by it; she is deprived
of a great experience".

Childbirth and its Effects on the Mother-Child Relationship

This aspect of the problem follows what has been said above. The conscious woman who experiences her delivery to the full offers her effort, in a
sense, for the health of her child. She feels her responsibility acutely, and
her maternal feelings have an early satisfaction in the success of her
delivery. The indescribable joy that she manifests when she sees her child
emerge is an expression of her attachment to this child that springs from
herself and is at the same time her recompense.

This is expressed in the spontaneous words that she utters at this moment
of victory: "My child; my little one; how beautiful he is. Isn't it wonder-
ful?" We often find the same feeling expressed in simple sentences, like
"I have lived the, or one of the, most beautiful moments in my life."

Moreover, the mothers communicate this satisfaction, this happiness, to
their husbands, thus creating that moment of extraordinary human intensity
that so strikes witnesses.

Anaesthesia is responsible for frustrating any such manifestation. We find this frustration in women who have had a caesarian delivery, who sometimes take several days to get used to the idea of the child that cries in the crib next to them. How many women, who have had anaesthesia during a previous delivery, say that they felt less close, less immediately attached to their children! They lacked the link of *continuity*. Depending on the case, they would emerge from a nightmare that disturbed their balance and their affective reactions to the child, with a very strong feeling of frustration. Thus they say in their reports: "I have been deprived of the moment I was looking forward to; I was unable to witness the birth of my child."

However, it is worth noting that prepared women, according to our anaesthetists, are much calmer than the non-prepared ones, and this calmness simplifies the anaesthetist's task and diminishes the risks for the mother and child.

Another aspect that deserves to be noted is that the decision to operate is always more readily accepted by prepared women. Before psychoprophylaxis, when surgery was decided upon it was sometimes necessary to have long consultations, at the risk of losing the child, with the family doctor, or with doctors plus the family itself. But now it is only necessary to explain to the educated and now "adult" couple the reasons that dictate a caesarian, for acceptance to be immediate. This means less waste of time, better operative conditions and having the child in a better state.

We have also had occasion to note—and this must be gratifying to paediatricians—that the number of women who spontaneously breast feed, or are willing to breast feed their children, has increased by 50% and this, as Niles Newton[11, 12] of Jackson, Mississippi, has clearly shown, is of the highest importance for the development of the mother-child relationship.

Moreover, as some authors have pointed out, I believe that anaesthesia is not wholly harmless to lactation and that it has an inhibitory effect, as well as accentuating the depressive syndrome of the third-to-fifth day.

5

Benefit to the Child

A. T. McNeil[10] had this to say about the possible effects of analgesics on the child: "The use of analgesics during labour plays a much more important part than is generally thought in neo-natal asphyxias. According to Schreiber,[13] apneas were seven times less frequent in the case of normal spontaneous deliveries. Bobath[1] notes that neo-natal asphyxia comes second among the aetiological factors in cerebral disturbances at birth."

Professor Varangot with J. Chabrun and P. Parent,[15] in an article entitled 'The prevention of cranio-encephalic trauma of the newborn during delivery', writes: "I think that the more useful and necessary anaesthesia is in certain cases, the more the inconsiderate use of ocytocics or anti-spasmodics, with a too often unavowed view to hurrying things up, should be prohibited and condemned".

We would agree with the above, as we are not systematically hostile to anaesthesia; but with one reservation, namely that anaesthesia coming after an untimely and excessive use of anti-spasmodics and ocytocics will in no way improve the situation of the foetus *in utero*.

Wishing to be wholly on the safe side, we approached a number of paediatricans for their views—Messrs. Attal, J. Weill, Guy Vermeil, Caron, Prof. Rossier, Prof. Schneegans, Minkowsky, Sacrez—to whom we sent the following questionnaire.

(1) Do you consider that obstetrical psychoprophylaxis, which, by a precise pre-natal education, endeavours to allow the woman to give birth under the most physiological conditions and independently of any anaesthesia, is beneficial for the child?

(2) Do you believe that anaesthesia, even when given under the best conditions, has no repercussions on the foetus?

(3) What in your opinion are the obvious risks to which anaesthesia exposes the child?

(4) Do you think that the often untimely use of medication is more dangerous for the child than anaesthesia itself?

(5) Do you believe that on the psychic level anaesthesia is used to the detriment of the mother-child relationship?

The answers were as follows.

To the first question: All agree in considering psychoprophylaxis as beneficial on the foetus.

To the second question: They believe it is well to avoid anaesthesia, as the risk to the foetus is undeniable.

To the third question: It was felt that there were risks of anoxia and neurological risks. The hepatic immaturity peculiar to the newborn makes the elimination of all toxic substances difficult.

Professor Rossier replied to this third question:

(a) delayed initiation of the first respiration;
(b) disturbances of the respiratory rhythm after the first inspiration;
(c) at times apparent death; in any case increased risks of anoxia.

To the fourth question: "Minimal" use of drugs, which psychoprophylaxis advocates, as we have often stated.

To the fifth question: The responses are not very definite, but refer the question to psychologists.

The study by Irene Lezine and G. Raimbault[9] is significant in this connection: "It can therefore be said that any method making it possible to reduce or to eliminate surgical and medical interventions is beneficial for the development of the child".

Thus there is agreement in giving priority to preparation and instruction, not without observing, however, that anaesthesia, with recent progress, is *less dangerous* than medicines given at the wrong time and in exaggerated doses.

The obstetricians both in France and abroad, who practise psychoprophylaxis have stated that the need for resuscitation has greatly diminished in their practice; this is confirmed by Professor Lacomme:[7] "The number of children who have been resuscitated (I use 'resuscitated' in the lightest sense of the term) is less among the children of prepared women than among the others."

In conclusion, as far as the child is concerned, we may say that we have more to fear from analgesics and acytocics administered to excess than of an anaesthesia administered by a competent anaesthetist, but that the maximum safety is to be found in those cases in which the delivery has proceeded normally, physiologically speaking.

6

The Technique of Psychoprophylaxis

This, then, leads us to our *present concept*:

First of all, the pregnant woman must be prepared and instructed as soon as possible. This is a very old idea, since Dr. Alice Stockman,[14] in 1893, in her book *Tocology*, indicated in the first chapter entitled "Painless childbirth" that it was her opinion that a wrong education was responsible for the sufferings of modern woman. This could be remedied by instruction in pre-natal relaxation and by simple explanations of the physiology of labour, which would eliminate fear.

In order to obtain the best results it would be essential for the medical profession to make every effort to introduce this approach, and for opposition, through ignorance, gratuitous hostility and sabotage, to disappear.

Secondly, we need to move with the progress achieved by modern obstetrics, hence to have a perfect knowledge of the physiology of the Cu and, more generally, of labour; and to adapt the therapeutic applications to the necessities of the moment, but at the same time realizing that in order to be effective medicines need not be prescribed in large doses in the case of a prepared woman. We are neither for *routine abstentionism nor for all-out interventionism*. To know how to educate, how to observe and act advisedly, such should be the motto of the modern obstetrician.

Thus we are in favour of a psychological and physical, and even medical, preparation for labour, as we recently stated in Milan (October 29, 1969) at the Congress in Lombardy.

We have demonstrated that the use of Thiomucase in suppositories, in the twenty days preceding delivery, produces very supple cervices; maximum dilation was obtained when, in the course of labour, was added a perfusion containing:

500 ml. 10% glucose solution,
Spasmaverine: 2 ampules,
Hypo 5 or Syntocinon 5 U (as the case may dictate),
Calcibronate,

of which, most of the time, we use only 100 to 200 ml, or one or two units of Hypo or of Syntocinon.

We think we have in large part removed the "cervix and inferior segment" obstacle, mentioned by all the textbooks.

Thirdly, we believe that anaesthesia is to be used in cases of real necessity, but it should be left to expert hands and used before it is too late. We, for our part, limit ourselves to two formulae: in cases of extreme urgency, after atropine medication and reassuring the patient, we remain faithful to *chloroform* administered slowly. In cases of foreseeable surgery or a too painful labour, our choice goes to *Gamma OH*, with which we have never had trouble either for the mother or for the child.

To conclude, we have chosen psychoprophylaxis because of its safety for both mother and child. We have chosen it because it respected the woman's personality and choice. Because we consider it more human. It can be objected that it is not an easy approach, but then it is up to us to systemize and improve it so that this limiting aspect will be overcome.

We consider, moreover, that a skilled anaesthetist has his place in a psychoprophylactic service. He brings an added and undeniable element of safety. There should be no opposition between obstetrician and anaesthetist, either of person or of theory, but simply a hierarchy to be respected in order that the team may work effectively together. The competent anaesthetists who have worked with us have made it possible for us to do the right thing in difficult cases and save children under conditions which, twenty-five years ago, would have doomed them.

We might therefore briefly summarize our ideas thus:

Education-preparation in all cases and at the very onset;
Anaesthesia; yes, but not as an easy way out, and only when it is necessary and entrusted to competent clinicians.

We prefer, however, controlled anaesthesia, rather than routine anaesthesia practised on women who are supposedly prepared, in the phase of expulsion, with the unavowed aim of making the task easier. We consider this formula to be antiprophylactic, and, what is more, a kind of trickery of which women are more and more conscious.

7

Resistance to Psychoprophylaxis

Resistance to painless childbirth may stem from a variety of causes and manifest itself consciously or unconsciously. The listing below is an attempt to schematize them.

(1) Resistance by the Patient

(*a*) The subject has no faith in the worthwhileness of the painlessness of the method; this lack of faith is encouraged by a number of doctors.

(*b*) Fear of the act of giving birth outweighs all other considerations. The subject consequently opts for anaesthesia, which amounts to actual withdrawal from fear and pain.

(*c*) The easiest way out: it is easier to have anaesthesia than to expend preparatory effort.

(*d*) Lack of time: this can be a justifiable reason for women who have other children to look after.

(*e*) Refusal to be part of a group with other women from different social classes (collective group preparation is beneficial, as it develops group dynamics, which are psychologically beneficial).

(f) Like sexuality, pregnancy is "taboo": it is not something to be talked about. (Total withdrawal from all expression of sexuality).

(*g*) Complete selfishness: the woman gives no consideration to the child she is bearing, but assigns importance to herself alone.

(*h*) Masochistic behaviour: pain is necessary and beneficial, to make the mother love the child more.

(*i*) Unhappy couple, rejection of child, desire to assign guilt to the husband or simply to men in general.

(*j*) Mistrust of new, dangerous, or unproven methods.

(*k*) Erroneous interpretation of the method because the subject has been misinformed.

(*l*) The desire not to be different from a group that is, without reason, against painless childbirth: a subject who is easily influenced and impressionable.

(*m*) The passive, submissive woman, who does not avail herself of the freedom and independence that painless childbirth affords.

(*n*) Erroneous self-judgement: "I'm too nervous, too emotional to do it successfully, so why make the effort?"

(*o*) Fear that the child may be born abnormal: "I don't want to see it being born."

(*p*) Complete refusal of femininity.

(*q*) Refusal of giving birth as a distasteful act, the conscious experience of which is not worthwhile.

It should be noted that some negative or restrictive motivations listed above may occur in reverse, becoming basic reasons for preparing for painless childbirth.

(2) Environment

(a) Family Environment:

(1) *The patient's mother*, because of either tradition or lack of enlightenment, is opposed to painless childbirth: "In my day there wasn't so much fuss. . . I've had three or four children and I didn't bother with painless childbirth."

(2) *The patient's mother-in-law* is opposed to it: this can be an even stronger influence. In this case, the psychological motivations are particularly clear.

(3) *The patient's husband* shows unjustified opposition: this is the principle of authority. (Such situations are very rare; generally the contrary prevails). Or he shows excessive protectiveness: "I don't want my wife to suffer."

(b) Social Class

Groups that exert either a positive and stimulating influence, or a negative and deleterious influence.

(3) Obstetricians and Doctors in General

(a) *The Doctor:* Attitude negative in principle, coupled with complete ignorance. Because of the family physician's importance, his opinion is the determining factor. Since he is, *a priori*, the Man of Science, the possessor of knowledge, his opinion is definitive. He is one of the last bastions of resistance to painless childbirth. The myth of the omniscient doctor has preserved all its power. This absurd form of obscurantism must be combated.

(b) *The Obstetrician:* In this field, and especially in Europe, immense progress has been achieved. Most obstetricians accept both the principle and the reality of painless childbirth. The reluctance and resistance of those who do not accept it have several causes, either conscious or unconscious. They include the following.

(1) Fear of lessened prestige, of diminished authority. They are regarded as "saviours", and are reluctant to relinquish any part of their enviable position.

(2) Reluctance to make the effort: it requires long training and preparation to become a teacher of psychoprophylaxis.

(3) Reluctance to make a break with the past, to discard their habits and change their routine, all of which involves changing one's own personality.

(4) Preparing a woman for painless childbirth and assisting her during labour are further duties to be added to the onus of one's profession, which is already harassing enough. Anaesthesia is so much simpler and easier to handle!

(5) Reluctance to have witnesses (especially the husband) who thus have the opportunity to judge for themselves, thereby doing away with the atmosphere of privacy and mystery that has traditionally prevailed in a delivery room.

(6) Reluctance to engage in a dialogue, which involves placing oneself on the same level as one's collocutor and stepping down from the pedestal.

(7) Practising painless childbirth requires constant study, keeping up with the latest developments, investigating fields that formerly lay outside the province of obstetricians (physiology, psychology, sociology, etc.). It means that one is no longer a mere machine for bringing children into the world. As Mr. Lamaze[8] has pointed out, it also means humbly returning to school and accepting an awareness of the importance of the reciprocal relationships between doctors and patients.

There are several ways in which such resistances might be overcome.

(1) General and advance releasing of information to the public, with the method being emphasized from the standpoint of the foetus, the psychology of the mother, and the psychology of the couple.

(2) Radical change in the prevailing attitudes about the act of childbirth.

(3) The re-education in all fields of the personnel of maternity departments and maternity hospitals.

(4) A mutation in the obstetrician so as to provide him with awareness of his true role, which is no longer that of an excellent technician, but also that of a physio-psychologist prepared to make use of all the elements that govern the bringing into the world of a baby with the least number of risks and the greatest chances for the child's eventual development.

As Hans Selye stated: "Neither the prestige of your field and the power of your instruments, nor the scope of your knowledge and the accuracy of your plans can ever replace the originality of your thinking and the astuteness of your observation."

8

Summary

In concluding, we should like to summarize and define our idea and our position about anaesthesia and psychoprophylaxis.

(1) We consider that prenatal preparation enables us to obtain a minimum of 80% of spontaneous deliveries without recourse to anaesthesia. It makes it possible, moreover, in all the other cases, to prepare the woman for good anaesthesia.

(2) We consider the use of antispasmodic or ocytocic medications, in haphazard doses and in the hands of inexperienced persons, as particularly dangerous, both for the mother and for the child.

(3) We believe that anaesthesia, properly handled by competent special-

ists, and not consecutive upon untimely therapies, is a valuable aid and an unquestioned safety factor.

As a final conclusion, I wish to quote John J. Bonica, M.D.[2] who expresses himself as follows: "Hypnosis, natural childbirth, and the psychoprophylactic method of analgesia, when properly used, are of great value to mother, infant, and obstetrician."

REFERENCES

1. BOBATH. 1956. Cited by McNEIL, A. T. (reference 10 below).
2. BONICA, J. J. 1967. *Principles and practice of obstetric analgesia and anesthesia*, Oxford: Blackwell Scientific Publications, Vol. I.
3. DEUTSCH, H., 1946–7. *La psychologie des femmes, Vol. II—Maternité*. Presses Universitaires.
4. DIXON. 1958. *Journées thérapeutiques de Paris*. September.
5. GRANDELL, D. L., CREISS, J. C., JR., DONNELLY, J. F. and WINSTON-JALEM, N. C. 1956. Analyse de la mortalité maternelle provoquée par l'anesthésie en Caroline du Sud. *Med. J.*, **17** (3), 109–115.
6. JEWETT, J. F. 1957. Modifications de la mortalité maternelle dans le Massachusetts. *Med. J.*, **256**, (9), 395–400.
7. LACOMME, M. 1963. Quoted by *Constellation méd.*, **26**, April.
8. LAMAZE, F. 1956. Introduction au dernier stage. *Encyclopedie médico-Chirurgicale*. Paris.
9. LEZINE, I. and RAIMBAULT, G. 1960. Problems of development of a group of children born by the painless childbirth method observed through the first year of their lives. *Arch. franç. Pédiat.*, **18** (6).
10. McNEIL, A. T. 1961. The Soviet or psychoprophylactic method of painless childbirth. *Cerebr. Palsy Bull.*, **3**, 159–166.
11. NEWTON, N. 1958. The influence of the let-down reflex in breast feeding on the mother-child relationship. *Marriage and Family Living*, **20** (1), 18–20.
12. NEWTON, M. and NEWTON, N. 1962. The normal course and management of lactation. *Clin. Obstet. Gynec.*, **5**, 44–63.
13. SCHREIBER. 1938. Cited by McNEIL, A. T. (reference 10 above).
14. STOCKMAN, A. 1893. *Tocology* (Chapter I—Painless childbirth).
15. VARANGOT, CHABRUN, J. and PARENT, P. 1962. The prevention of cranioencephalic traumatism of the new-born in the course of delivery. *Sem. Thér.*

XVIII

MANAGEMENT OF THE HOME CONFINEMENT

PHILIP HOPKINS

F.R.C.G.P., M.R.C.S., L.R.C.P.

and

MAX B. CLYNE

M.D., F.R.C.G.P.

London, England

1

Incidence of Home Confinements

In Great Britain home (domiciliary) confinements are still fairly common. In 1957 64·6% of all births took place in institutions in England and Wales, i.e. 476,783 out of a total of 737,704 notified births. The proportion of births taking place in institutions varies in different areas, from nearly 100% in the Isles of Scilly to 33% in the City of Middlesbrough. In the Greater London area approximately 80% of confinements took place in institutions in 1957 (Report of the Maternity Services Committee, 1959[8]). The latest report (Baird and Thomson, 1969[1]) claims that 41% of pregnant women (ranging from 20% of primigravidae to 60% of multigravidae 4+) booked for domiciliary confinements with their general practitioners, local authority midwives, or both. The advent of the National Health Service in 1948 freed expectant mothers from the burden of direct payments and enabled them to contract for maternity services with their general practitioners, whereas previously they would have sought the services of the midwife only.

Not every general practitioner may wish to include in his work the practice of obstetrics, although "every family doctor is responsible for securing for his patients the best supervision and management of pregnancy, delivery and puerperium" (*The field of work of the family doctor*[2]). Although most home deliveries are carried out by midwives, the general practitioner-obstetrician will frequently be present during the second and third stages and will usually attend at some time during the first stage of labour. He will carry out the actual delivery in a minority of cases only.

In Great Britain, many specialist-obstetricians, as well as a number of family doctors, think that home confinements are out-dated in the same way that it is no longer thought proper to remove an acute appendix on the kitchen table! In their view, a properly equipped hospital, with every modern facility, is by far the safest place in which to have a baby—with the general practitioner-obstetrician still in attendance. In many other developed countries there is an almost 100% institutional confinement rate.

Of women who had booked for domiciliary confinements 13% were eventually transferred to hospital, most on medical grounds, and some for social reasons, as reported by Baird and Thomson.[1] In addition, in 1–2% of home confinements there is need for the emergency obstetric service ("Flying Squad") to be called.

2

Advantages of Home Confinements

In spite of the above, a fairly large number of women prefer to have their babies at home, so that altogether about 184,000 babies are born at home in England and Wales each year. This is in agreement with the findings of a committee[8] of distinguished obstetricians, psychiatrists, physicians and lay-men, who found that the advantages of home confinements for apparently normal cases outweighed the risk of unforeseen complications.

Much has been written about the physical aspects of obstetric care since the maternal mortality rate was dramatically reduced by the simple sugges-tion made by Semmelweis in the mid-nineteenth century that medical students should not go directly from the dissecting room to the lying-in wards without first washing their hands in chlorinated water before conduct-ing the delivery, and the even more dramatic changes that followed the work of Louis Pasteur and Joseph Lister. The maternal mortality rate was 4·4 per 1,000 in 1928, and was reduced by the introduction of penicillin to little over 1 per 1,000 by 1945.

Even with a maternal mortality rate as low as 0·2 per 1,000, ". . . there is still an avoidable factor of approximately 40% ",[6] so that much remains to be done to improve the physical care of the expectant mother. But another challenge faces us, as Professor Norman Morris[5] asked: ". . . are we to measure success simply in terms of life and death?" He goes on to suggest that there are serious gaps in our knowledge and understanding of the patient's emotional condition in pregnancy, labour and the puerperium.

It might be possible to combine the safety of hospital confinement with the friendlier and psychologically happier atmosphere of the home by a move towards the short stay in hospital, i.e. home within forty-eight hours, provided all is normal with mother and baby.

The actual delivery of the baby (second stage of labour) and the delivery of the placenta (third stage of labour) demand a great degree of technical skill and those general practitioner-obstetricians, who provide something like 75% of the maternity services, are required to have held a six months' residential appointment in an obstetric unit, or to have had equivalent obstetric experience, before they are allowed to join the "Obstetric List".

Midwives are qualified nurses with additional qualifications for maternity work, for which they are highly trained, strictly supervised and required to attend regular frequent refresher courses.

3

Psychological Aspects of Family Practice

Ante-natal Care

Essentially, good obstetric care means good ante-natal care, since reports of detailed and searching official enquiries[4] into maternal deaths, which are published every three to four years, have shown that the most serious and frequent avoidable factor of maternal deaths is inadequate ante-natal care. Thus, the success or failure of the management of home confinements depends largely on the quality of the preceding ante-natal care.

Nevertheless, although there has been a great improvement in the standards of ante-natal care with the resultant improvement of maternal, foetal and infantile deaths and morbidity rates, some aspects of peri-natal morbidity have gained far less recognition and are still common.

Good clinicians and clinical observers as well as, not least, patients have always had the impression that a woman who had suffered an emotional upset during pregnancy was more likely to have a complicated pregnancy or delivery, or to abort, or deliver a still-born or handicapped child. Little progress was made in the scientific assessment of this subject and in the practical application of its implications until Grantley Dick Read[7] published his findings about the influence of the emotions upon pregnancy and parturition. His books were the first milestones towards the recognition that the emotional state of the mother may deeply influence her own and her infant's life, health and happiness.

It is now commonly accepted that emotional "shocks" and upsets are not likely to cause foetal or maternal injury; but the emotional factors likely to influence foetus and mother are expressed by the mother's expectations of, and her attitudes and behaviour towards, the foetus; and there is evidence[3] that these may determine the outcome of pregnancy.

Emotional Attitudes in Pregnancy

One of the most decisive changes brought about by pregnancy is the re-definition of the woman's role. The woman may have been her husband's little girl, or his mother-substitute, or she may have been an efficient career girl. When expecting her first baby, she will have to re-adjust her role, perhaps towards her husband or her job, as she will now have to become a mother to her baby, or, if she already has children, instead of having to mother one or two children, she will now have to be mother to two or three children. Sometimes, this re-definition of her role brings out old, and possibly long-forgotten, conflict relationships, for example with her own mother, and the woman desperately tries to become a better mother than her own mother; or she resignedly feels that she can never be as good a mother as her own mother was. Old sibling rivalry, conflicts with her sisters or brothers, may be aroused when the baby is born, and the new mother may feel that she is placed in the role of a very much older sibling in relationship to her baby.

There are other fields in which some pregnant women have difficulties. Sexually inhibited women often feel that pregnancy is a prominent manifestation to all and sundry that they have had sexual intercourse. Any feelings of shame, disgust, or anxiety about sexual intercourse can then no longer be hidden from the world and may be reflected in similar feelings about the pregnancy. This is expressed by feelings of shame or disgust about "being big", or by their expressing satisfaction about the fact that their pregnant abdomen is "really quite small". Moreover, a woman who has felt guilty about her sexuality may indeed punish herself by becoming pregnant with all the "pain" ("labour pains" = uterine contractions) that this implies.

There is a danger that the mother may try to solve her problems, whether they are about sexual damage, guilt about her relationship to her own mother, jealousy about her sister, by involving the future baby in the solution. If this happens, the baby comes to mean to her a damaged part of herself and this fear remains with her, even if the baby is perfectly normal when born. This often underlies frequent attendances by young mothers at the doctor's consulting room or baby clinic, where they come with their babies because they fear there is something wrong with them. Some mothers present their well-nourished, fat babies, saying that the baby has taken no food for days and is losing weight. Others ask over and over again for the baby to be examined because of vague fears that the baby is not all right.

Another interesting phenomenon is the overwhelming desire of some women to become pregnant repeatedly and to have many babies. This might be called an "addiction" to pregnancy or to having babies. These women use pregnancy to calm their doubts about their womanliness or about the integrity of their sexual organs. It is often for this reason that women want to be examined vaginally by their doctors, because, quite apart from any realistic reasons, many women suffer from a gnawing fear that something is wrong with their genital organs, in other words, with their femininity. Becoming pregnant and having a large family means to such women a confirmation of their being "proper women".

Some women have a feeling of emptiness inside, a symptom not uncommon in depressives. This feeling of being empty, often expressed openly in so many words, is very painful, and some women become pregnant to fill this psychic void that they are experiencing, and they perceive the swelling of their abdomens as something very pleasurable and satisfactory. Such women sometimes swell up without really being pregnant—pseudocyesis.

In addition to these inner emotional problems, there are also some external or environmental factors that may lead to emotional disorders during pregnancy. One of the factors that arouses anxiety in pregnancy is the need to enter hospital for childbirth, and some doubt may be expressed as to the advisability of this for some women who apparently are likely to have normal labours, so that, if it could be arranged, their confinements should be carried out at home.

There is little doubt that the incidence of post-puerperal depression, of emotional disorder generally, and of disturbances in the mother-baby relationship, are less frequent in home confinements than in hospital confinements.

What is the pathological significance of the emotional and relationship factors described? We have already given some examples of the difficulties arising from the mother's unrealistic feelings towards the foetus or baby. Even "addiction to pregnancy", which seems such a charming weakness, may bring difficulties. One of us (M.B.C.) had a patient who was a pregnancy addict. She was a depressed woman, who may well have felt the void within herself, but she always felt very well, somewhat hypomanic, when she was pregnant, and she could hardly wait for the next pregnancy after she had given birth to a child. Unfortunately, her children, once born, were no longer important to her; it was the pregnancy that she wanted. She had ten live children altogether and between these live births she always had two or three self-induced abortions. When she came near the climacteric and when her husband definitely wanted no more children, she left the whole family, including the youngest baby. Several of the children have become law-breakers, although they are all pleasant, but rather unfeeling and detached people. One girl, who is also a depressive like her mother, joined a gang of drug addicts and became a drug addict herself, perhaps also to fill her inner void. She went to an approved school and when she came out promptly became pregnant. Like her mother, she liked to be pregnant but did not want her baby.

Emotional disorders during pregnancy have long-term effects not only on the mother-child relationship, but also on the future of the children. Many women who suffer from toxaemia of pregnancy have been described as having a low ability to accept emotional strains and stresses. Few cases of toxaemia or hypertension have been recorded in women of emotional stability. Hyperemesis gravidarum is doubtlessly a psychogenic disorder, and women with very disturbed personalities are commonly found among hyperemetics.

Women who are depressed during pregnancy are likely to suffer from deep post-puerperal depression of long duration, so depriving the child of proper maternal care, with consequences that may reach well into adulthood. It is not uncommon for patients suffering from depression to report that their mothers suffered from depression after childbirth. Women who are very tense and anxious during pregnancy are more apt than women who are relaxed and calm to have extensive perineal tears.

If we accept the reality of psychic and somatic interaction in the pregnant woman, we must attempt to answer the question how we can diagnose those conditions that will adversely affect the outcome of pregnancy or the future of the child. The pathological conditions of pregnancy are not simply related to the presence of some well-defined psychiatric syndrome. Pregnancy is a time of emotional turbulence, so that not every show of anxiety, depression, or irritability is necessarily pathognomonic. But excessive degrees of these, and particularly any odd attitude, whether it is excessive love, excessive hatred, excessive dependency, or excessive depression, should draw the doctor's attention to a possible emotional instability of pathological significance. Such findings in the emotional field, and the reactions aroused by them within the doctor, are as important as the observations of the woman's physical state. The pre-condition of such observations is, of course, that a woman during ante-natal care must be given the opportunity to vent her feelings and to voice her fears and anxieties, without risk that the doctor might laugh at her, scold her, or refuse to understand her. This care also needs a doctor who is perceptive of such feelings so that he can understand what the woman is trying to convey to him. This is not an easy task—it is easier for some than others—but it can be learned.

Mother's Attitudes to the Child

The attitudes and feelings of the mother towards the foetus vary greatly, some mothers think of the foetus as an inanimate asexual object which they refer to as "it". Others in their phantasies will give the foetus a name and sex at a very early stage and talk about the foetus as "he" or "she". Some women go even farther in their phantasies and talk about the foetus as if it were endowed with human characteristics even at a very early stage of pregnancy, as if they were unable to think of their foetus as a foetus at all, but could only think of it in terms of the baby it will become. Sometimes their references to the foetus suggest that they regard it not as a baby yet unborn, but as an infant, an adolescent, or even as an adult, for whom they are mapping out certain roles and careers well in advance.

Maternal feelings may vary to the greatest extent in pregnant women, some of whom express intense feelings of love for their baby even during the earliest stages of pregnancy, and a miscarriage means a major loss and emotional catastrophe to them. The feelings of others are more temperate, while others violently hate the foetus and the baby.

One of us (M.B.C.) recently saw a woman who, at the age of forty, hated her husband for having made her pregnant against her wishes. She also hated the unborn baby, which turned out to be a Mongol. The mother, at first, hated the new-born baby even more; but at the same time she felt very guilty, as though her hatred had caused the baby to be a Mongol. When she was seen six weeks after delivery, she had apparently come to terms with her baby and was no longer bothered that he was a Mongol. She now found him to be beautiful, with many features which she had not seen in her previous children, such as peacefulness and good-naturedness; and he never woke up and disturbed her in the night. He seemed to be a very happy child, so that the pendulum of her feelings had swung to the other extreme and she now idealized this Mongol child, a feeling that will make it impossible for her to assess realistically the child, his influence on the family, and his own future and interests. Consequently, she might not be able to accept certain actions that might later be in the best interests of the child and indeed of the whole family, for example admission to boarding school, or placement in a special home or hospital.

Another patient, at the age of forty-four, came to one of us (P.H.) with an unwanted pregnancy, which later was found to be triplets—and she so hated these babies that she arranged for their immediate adoption at birth, several weeks before their arrival.

Usually, however, the feelings of a woman towards her unborn baby are mixed; there are both positive and negative, and these ambivalent feelings that arise normally during pregnancy make this time a period of heightened sensitivity leading to an increased sensation of anxiety and tension. It may well be expected that these tensions will weaken the established structure of the woman's personality so that she is no longer able to solve problems easily. Most women during pregnancy, especially in the early stages, need a considerable amount of attention from their husbands, their families and their doctors. Some of this emotional support is required to counteract the fear of the unknown event, the effects of old wives' tales, together with their doubts about their ability to handle the new-born baby. If these anxieties aroused by the pregnancy are ridiculed by the husband, family, friends or the doctor, they will be suppressed by the woman, who may become unable to deal with them, and thus show signs of emotional or physical illness.

It is part of the general practitioner-obstetrician's functions during the antenatal examinations to allow adequate time for discussion of these problems.

Sequence of Symptomatology

There is an orderly sequence of certain emotional states in pregnancy. During the first trimester considerable mood-swings appear, with depression and irritability, and a great need for dependency on others, including the doctor.

Around the fourth month of pregnancy, the beginning of the second trimester, women become more passive. The Victorian picture of the expectant mother sitting in passive contemplation, or knitting baby clothes, comes to mind. Some women resent this passivity and feel it as an enforced and unpleasant inhibition of their normal functioning. These women have difficulty in establishing their earliest relationship with their baby. Women usually become more self-confident during this period and have less need to lean on the doctor.

The last trimester of pregnancy is characterized by an increase in lethargy.

In the last trimester the need for dependency decreases, and the affects of the expectant mother become centred on the baby to the exclusion of other people.

During the first stage of labour there is little need for dependency, but a great deal of anxiety and restlessness. If ante-natal care has been good in the emotional field, contact with the doctor during the first half of the first stage need not be prolonged or intensive. His mere presence is often quite sufficient to reassure the expectant mother.

As the second stage comes nearer and during it, the woman usually regresses deeply and becomes very dependent. The typical scene is that of the woman with closed eyes following the commands of the midwife or doctor to push or to relax, and firmly holding and often fondling the hand of the attendant who is not actually carrying out the delivery.

As soon as the baby is born, the dependency completely disappears. The woman usually withdraws into herself, with no particular desire to either see or cuddle the baby. This state of withdrawal may continue till an hour or so after the third stage. Then the mother usually wants to see and cuddle her baby, on whom she then concentrates, without fully excluding the rest of the family.

4

Diagnosis and Management

Once a diagnosis has been made in a pregnant woman of an emotional disturbance, how can the condition be treated? Talking about disturbing feelings, especially if these are of an ambivalent nature, sometimes brings relief. But this in itself is often not enough. It is necessary to understand and to convey the doctor's understanding to the patient. Quick reassurance, such as "you, or your baby, will be all right', will only succeed in silencing the woman without relieving her anxiety. Perhaps the most important feature of antenatal care is the woman's feeling that the doctor does care; this requires an attitude of warmth, sympathy and empathy that can only arise out of understanding. It may require a greater flexibility of ante-natal care than is usual; some women may need more frequent attendances than others, or different degrees of privacy with the doctor, without the presence of the practice-nurse, the midwife, or secretaries. It may also be necessary to convince the woman that problems that existed between her and her mother or her sister when she was a child are no longer current, and that her baby is not the embodiment of her sister or of her mother. She may also have to be convinced that the baby is not a symbol of sex, or an indication of a damaged sexual apparatus, and that it is not a punishment for her supposed sexual sins. To demonstrate this to a woman requires knowledge of, and skill in, certain psychiatric techniques that can be acquired without too much difficulty; and, if ante-natal care means not only the simple detection of abnormalities, but also the important preparation of the expectant mother for her labour and forthcoming motherhood, these techniques are of great importance.

Throughout the ante-natal examinations the important relationships between the patient and the doctor should develop, and the doctor should help the patient to build up her confidence in herself as well as in her doctor.

The question of relationships is of considerable importance, particularly when the labour is to be conducted in the home. Indeed, one of the main advantages of the family doctor looking after his own patient during this important episode in her life is that the expectant mother can expect to see the same doctor each time she attends for ante-natal examination. It is also helpful if the same local midwife will see the patient for alternate ante-natal examinations, as well as being present at the actual delivery. This practice would obviate one of the commonly heard complaint that "I never see the same doctor twice when I go to the hospital".

It is equally important that the doctor builds up a relationship with the husband and other members of the family who might be present during the time of the labour. Discussions should take place between the doctor and the prospective father and suitable arrangements made if he wishes to be present at the time of his child's birth.

The relationship between the doctor and the midwife also is of great importance. The days when there was actual antagonism between the midwife and the doctor are past, since the present arrangements allow for both to play their respective roles during the pregnancy and labour. The family doctor-obstetrician should also establish a sound relationship with his local consultant obstetric colleagues so that, should the need arise, he feels no hesitation about consulting them.

This is not the place for a detailed description of the actual obstetric techniques of handling the labour; suffice it to say that it is part of the family doctor's function to ensure that the conditions are suitable for a home confinement and that there is a satisfactory room for the delivery, with a good light in the right position. And, once labour has started, it is essential that somebody is constantly present with the expectant mother. The doctor should visit at some point during the first stage to check the arrangements, to encourage the patient and the family, and, of course, to check the lie of the baby and to make sure that the foetal heart is satisfactory. He will have discussed with his patient his choice of drugs for her comfort, and when the os is dilating he might start analgesia with an intramuscular injection of pethidine hydrochloride.

During the ante-natal consultations he will have explained how the mother will experience a change in the type of contractions, which indicates the onset of the second stage. The mother will have attended relaxation or antenatal exercise classes, so that she will know how to play her part most efficiently and with a minimum of anxiety.

Unfortunately, the recently developed epidural analgesia is not yet available to all hospital patients, so it is highly unlikely that many women having their babies at home will be able to benefit from this excellent procedure. Nevertheless, it is highly important that the woman should suffer the minimum of discomfort and pain during labour, so that when it is all over she can look back over her labour and be pleased with her achievement, rather than overwhelmed by memories of her suffering.

Once the baby is born and the cord cut, the baby should be given to the mother to cuddle—not wrapped up in towels or napkins, but naked, even if the skin is greasy and dirty. Lastly, the doctor should always give the mother all the credit for giving birth to her baby and should not talk about the way he "brought her baby into the world". She should be told that she did it and that she did it well, so that she can feel the satisfaction and pride in knowing that having her baby was her achievement.

The doctor cannot expect to see the successful results of his work until he has made his post-natal visits, and has confirmed that the breast-feeding is progressing satisfactorily and that the relationship developing between the mother and her baby is satisfactory.

REFERENCES

1. BAIRD, D. and THOMSON, A. M. 1969. In *Perinatal problems. The Second Report of the 1958 British Perinatal Mortality Survey* (N. R. Butler and E. D. Alberman, eds.). Edinburgh and London: Livingstone.
2. Central Health Services Council. 1963. *The field of work of the family doctor.* London: H.M.S.O.
3. CLYNE, M. B. 1967. Habitual abortion: a psychosomatic disorder. *Practitioner*, **199,** 83–90.
4. *Maternal Mortality.* 1964. Summary of Report of Confidential Enquiries into Maternal Deaths in England and Wales 1958/60. London: H.M.S..O.
5. MORRIS, N. 1960. Human relations in obstetric practice. *Lancet*, i, 913–5.
6. PEEL, J. 1968. A century of obstetrics. *Practitioner*, **201,** 85–93.
7. READ, G. D. 1933. *Natural childbirth.* London: Heinemann.
8. *Report of the Maternity Services Committee.* 1959. London: H.M.S.O.

XIX

MANAGEMENT OF THE HOSPITAL CONFINEMENT

J. STALLWORTHY

F.R.C.S., F.R.C.O.G.

The Churchill Hospital
Headington, Oxford
England

1

Introduction

Attitudes to delivery in hospitals are changing rapidly and are relevant to any detailed consideration of the management of labour, wherever it is conducted. Certain of these changes and their implications deserve mention if the following concept of how an institutional confinement should be conducted is to be seen in perspective.

Gone are the days when the mechanics of delivery were the main concern of the doctor attending a confinement. He would confirm the presence of an early pregnancy, calculate the expected date of delivery, advise engaging a midwife, and tell the patient to send for him when labour started. It was expected that the confinement would take place at home and the midwife would make the necessary arrangements for this. Some of us still practising remember those days but without much enthusiasm. Mortality and morbidity, both maternal and foetal, were high and, unless the doctor was "kind" and administered chloroform with a rag and bottle, there was little prospect of help for the labouring mother. Many women knew of friends or relatives who had died in labour or been impaired permanently in health by it; and it is not surprising that fear was a frequent visitor during pregnancy and was often present during labour.

Transfer to hospital, or delivery in hospital, usually meant that serious complications had developed and it was inevitable that mention of a hospital confinement increased the anxieties of a patient and her family. Traditions die hard, and as far as England and Wales are concerned it is only in recent years that there has been a rapidly increasing demand from the public for institutional confinements.

2

Institutional v. Domiciliary Delivery

In 1959, in its report to the Minister of Health, the Committee on Maternity Services (H.M.S.O. 1969) stated "we have come to the conclusion that taking the country as a whole the provision of maternity lying-in beds for 70% of all confinements would be adequate. . . . We have assumed that the remaining 30% of confinements would take place at home." Within ten years of this official assessment the demand for hospital beds has been such that the national pattern of maternity service has changed, until in many areas of the country there is virtually no domiciliary midwifery. In England and Wales the incidence of institutional confinements has risen to 80% and still rises. In Scotland it is higher. A concurrent dramatic increase in the number of early discharges after delivery has made it possible for the hospitals to meet this accelerating demand without any appreciable increase in the number of beds.

Associated with these changes there has developed a more widely accepted human understanding of what the management of a confinement should involve. The mother should be enriched physically and emotionally by the experience of bringing her baby into the world. This means that not only must she survive the process but be the better for it. If this is the standard by which achievements are to be measured, attention must be paid to morbidity in its widest aspects, namely morbidity of both body and mind. Moreover, with this goal of perfection we are not satisfied when the infant has been placed in its cot unless we know that it has not suffered in the process of birth. A reduction in stillbirth rate is important, but not if it is achieved at the cost of a rise in neonatal death rate or—possibly even worse—an increase in severe neonatal morbidity and subsequent impairment of the child.

3

Maternal Mortality

An obvious basic yardstick for assessing a maternity service is the standard of safety achieved for mothers and babies. When 44 in every 10,000 women in England and Wales died during pregnancy or childbirth, as was the case in 1928, maternal mortality was a matter of such national concern that a Departmental Committee of the Ministry of Health initiated procedures which, though not dramatic in their immediate contribution, led ultimately to the institution of the Confidential Enquiry into Maternal Deaths. This created progressively higher standards of safety since 1952. The risk to a mother of dying in pregnancy or childbirth is now 2·5 per 10,000 (1946–66).

a figure which is an encouragement to all working in the service and the envy of many countries. Both maternal and perinatal mortality rates are certain to be reduced still further. Paradoxically, this increasing safety introduces new dangers, one of which is related to ill-founded claims for, or misunderstanding of, the role of psychoprophylaxis in obstetrics.

The birth of a stillborn child, or the death of a neonate, can be a tragedy from which some women never recover, just as the death of a woman in labour may destroy a home and may embitter a man for life. These issues of life and death are of fundamental importance and must not be forgotten when discussing other important aspects of childbirth such as the emotional and physical quality of labour.

Difficulties may arise if it is forgotten that, however natural the processes of pregnancy, delivery and the puerperium should be in an ideal world, the fact remains that in no aspect of life is the dividing line between the normal and the abnormal narrower than in obstetrics. Seconds of time, an ill-judged decision, or lack of facilities, experience, or skill can separate joy from disaster. The safety and efficiency of a maternity service depends largely on recognition of these facts. All pregnant women cannot be treated alike. There are high-risk categories, and those included in them require special and skilled consideration and supervision. This often means that, however normal and satisfying their labour proves to be, it should be conducted in an institution designed with the requirements necessary for the protection of both mother and baby. The fact that safety exits on an aircraft or in a theatre are seldom used does not justify their abolition. From time to time loss of life reminds us that existing ones may be inadequate.

4

Ante-natal Care

Some women will require more time, encouragement and patience from their doctor than will others. For this reason the programme of appointments must be flexible. The accepted routine of one a month until the 28th week, once a fortnight until the 36th week, and weekly until delivery is in most cases only a reasonable minimum, but no more. Skilled attention at these visits will usually detect departures from normal in time for appropriate action to be taken, but in some high-risk categories visits will need to be much more frequent, and the patient may require to spend intervals under supervision in hospital. For her peace of mind she must understand why the usually accepted routine is altered, because she will be well aware from friends what arrangements are normally made.

It is also important that, whenever possible, the husband should be interviewed, preferably early in the ante-natal period and as often afterwards as necessary, so that he may have a better understanding of those changes inevitable during pregnancy which, if misunderstood, may create tension and unhappiness. His understanding and sympathy can prove a source of great strength and comfort to his wife.

In an ideal service, in addition to routine antenatal visits, there will be classes for instruction of both the patient and her husband. An important practical point arising from this concept is the need for coordinated team-work so that the patient will not be told one thing at one clinic and some-thing different at another. It is obviously important that instruction in preparation for childbirth should be given by someone who is aware of any special physical problem which may complicate the particular case.

In large and busy antenatal clinics it is difficult, though not impossible, to establish the necessary degree of cooperation and personal supervision. For example, after their initial interview and assessment by a senior clinician, problem patients can be seconded to medical members of the staff who will be personally responsible for their subsequent care, both in the ante-natal period and on admission to hospital. This arrangement also makes it possible for the doctor to arrange antenatal visits at times mutually suitable to the patient and himself and in this way reduce the workload at the routine clinic. It also ensures that the patient will see the same doctor each time.

5

The Importance of Confidence

The labour ward should no longer be a place of suffering, but a room of peace, quiet and achievement. For this to be possible, the management of labour should commence, at the latest, with the first ante-natal visit. This is when the beginnings of mutual confidence are established between patient and doctor or midwife. At the best, management of labour will begin in childhood with a mother who answers with truth and understanding ques-tions from her enquiring daughter. Many an unsatisfactory labour has been feared in advance for as long as the patient can remember because of terri-fying stories heard in childhood.

6

Preparation for Labour

Patient devotees of psychoprophylactic preparation for childbirth, according to various gospels including those of Read, Lamaze, Nikolayev and Vellay, have been delivered under my care. The experience of some was obviously satisfying to them and impressive to the observer, while others were either ill-prepared for what proved to be an ordeal or were victims of a delusion. Some became resentful as labour progressed and felt they had been be-trayed. One who held this view with great vehemence subsequently committed suicide several years later. The psychological trauma of her obstetrical experience may or may not have been relevant to the final tragedy.

In spite of these disappointments, or because of the many encouragements, all women delivered in the maternity unit of the United Oxford Hospitals are encouraged to attend classes of preparation for childbirth. These are provided as part of the maternity service and will be expanded in number and scope in the new teaching hospital.

Forty years of concentrated experience in delivery rooms at home and at hospital, in general practitioner units for normal midwifery, and in specialist departments for emergency and complicated cases, have convinced me that three things are of major importance to the patient in pregnancy and labour. They are:

1. The therapeutic value of patient confidence, confidence in her doctor and herself.
2. The need for a broad and flexible concept of ante-natal and intrapartum care.
3. The importance of providing standards of obstetric skill of the highest quality.

If all three are to be achieved, skilled teamwork is necessary and, for any team to succeed, its members must be selected, trained and experienced.

The comments and suggestions which follow will not be endorsed by all obstetricians, but they are based on extensive experience which for many years has been in a region of England in which a resolute attempt has been made to establish an efficient comprehensive maternity service. Moreover, it is a region, which, as measured by maternal and perinatal mortality rates, has the proud double record of now being the safest place in Britain in which woman can be delivered, and the safest in which infants can be born. There are many reasons for this, not excluding the health and physique of women themselves and the conditions under which they live; but a major sphere of the credit must be given to the local doctors and midwives, who recognize and accept the three requirements already mentioned.

7

The Effects of Fear on Labour

The effects of fear and tension on labour were stressed by the late Grantley Dick Read, in whose ideas I was critically interested. He was no stranger to the department at Oxford; on several occasions of important decisions in his life he visited it to discuss his problems and ask advice. It was seldom accepted. Because he was not a consultant, the advent of the National Health Service resulted in his exclusion from hospitals in which he had worked. This seemed so unfair that with the help of the late Sir William Fletcher Shaw, a former President of the Royal College of Obstetricians and Gynaecologists, we planned and organized a clinical and research unit in which he could continue his practice and teaching. Acceptance of controls for comparative assessment of results was stipulated, but the offer of this unit was rejected and Mr. Read went to South Africa. He had, however, made a great contribution by explaining that childbirth could be an exhilarating experience for a woman and by demonstrating one way of achieving this. His success, which was considerable and international, depended upon winning the confidence of the patient and preparing her during pregnancy for the hours of labour, but his methods were not always successful. Many women fear labour, particularly with the first pregnancy, because of their dread of the unknown and their belief that it will be a terrifying and painful process. In this view they are often encouraged by their friends and sometimes even by their mothers. Once again, if the relationship between the doctor and patient, or midwife and patient, is what it should be, these fears will have been uncovered during the ante-natal period and appropriate action will have been taken to dispel them.

There are other women who dread labour, not because they fear its probable pain, but because they believe they will be given drugs and anaesthetics whether they want them or not. Their terror is caused more by what they believe will be the effect of these in the possible resultant loss of self-control than of pain itself. Adequate preparation during the months of pregnancy can so build up the confidence of the patient that these fears will be dispelled.

In an enlightened, well-equipped and well-staffed labour suite each patient and her requirements will be assessed carefully and dealt with accordingly. There will be no standard routine procedure for administering analgesics or anaesthetics, because it will be known that what is required for one will be inadequate for another and unnecessary for a third. Attention to these matters can be a great contribution to the happiness of the labouring woman.

8

Labour-room Priorities

The following two case histories demonstrate that, when measured in the terms of the life or death of the mother or baby (and both can be at risk), comfort, personal whims, and even pain are sometimes of secondary importance. Essential priorities must be assessed and professional conduct planned accordingly.

Case One. A highly intelligent university couple were deeply distressed because they were infertile. After investigation they were informed that they were sterile with no prospect of cure, a verdict which they accepted. Years later, with little hope of success, a second opinion was requested from a specialist interested in these problems. Further investigation was followed by an abdominal operation and pregnancy.

Arrangements were made for supervision of ante-natal care, including instruction in preparation for childbirth, and for delivery in a well-equipped and well-staffed consultant unit. The relationship between husband and wife was excellent. All went well until, at the 28th week of pregnancy, both patient and husband decided that the baby should be born at home. Preparation for childbirth classes had been found so helpful that both parents were convinced that natural childbirth was a woman's right and that home was the place in which to enjoy it. They both knew that the original plans for delivery in hospital included the assurance that the husband could be with his wife during labour; so there was no anxiety on this point to explain their sudden change of plan. Only after a long discussion on the issues involved did they agree reluctantly on hospital delivery.

At term a large baby was not lying favourably either for ease of delivery or for its own safety; but considerable pressure was necessary before the patient agreed to come into hospital a week after labour was due, for supervision and induction of labour. She was reassured in hospital at 7 p.m. by her consultant who had operated for her infertility and cared for her and her husband during the pregnancy. Just before midnight she got out of bed, dressed and went home without saying anything to the medical staff. At 3 a.m. she was re-admitted in labour with acute complications which had developed an hour before and were threatening the immediate death of the infant and grave danger to the mother. Fortunately immediate Caesarean section saved both.

Case Two. A woman with a rare multiple congenital heart deformity was referred for specialist obstetric care by her consultant cardiologist. Not only was he responsible for the supervision of her heart, but he had become a valued and trusted friend to the patient and her husband because of the great help he had given in enabling her to adjust herself to the demands of daily life. Much to her distress, on two previous occasions pregnancy terminated spontaneously by abortion in the early weeks. No case has been reported in the world literature of succesful pregnancy associated with this particular serious form of congenital heart disease.

The patient herself was aware of the position. The cardiologist worked in such close association with the obstetrical team that, when the patient was admitted to the Maternity Home many weeks before the baby was due, it was agreed that every day he and the obstetrician would meet together with her so as to encourage and advise. In order that in an emergency she would not be terrified by it, she was introduced to the elaborate electronic equipment which at any stage might be required for her safety if her condition deteriorated. She knew that it was always available in a room nearby and that it would be in the labour ward when her child was born. As far as a lay person could do so, she understood the problems associated with the remaining weeks of her pregnancy and with her delivery.

In spite of all this extra care, the patient decided that she would not stay in hospital. She maintained that she could see no reason why this was necessary and why she could not manage at home, where she was alone all day while her husband was at work. Although she realized that the necessary facilities could not be provided at home, she was determined to return there. The explanations, encouragement and firmness to bring about a change of attitude took many hours over many days but finally were successful. The result was the safe delivery of a healthy child and the joy of a mother who had almost given up hope.

The above illustrations also demonstrate the failure in one case and success in the other of efforts to maintain the patient's confidence in the doctor. This is particularly important in obstetrics for the following reason. Whereas most doctors are consulted because a patient feels ill and is anxious for a speedy return to health, the relationship between the pregnant woman and the physician is different.

The care of the pregnant woman involves preparation for an event which may not take place for many months. If it is her first pregnancy these months will be filled with new experiences which should be exciting and satisfying, but can be disturbing and terrifying. Even awareness of the movement of her child within her body may give rise to conflicting emotions; but if she is prepared and expecting the experience, she should welcome it as a sign that all is well. Minor disturbances due to skeletal changes affecting particularly the back and the pelvis, with possibly tenderness and even pain over the symphysis pubis, may cause unwarranted concern if the reason for them is not understood and no assurance has been given that this is nature's way of making the pelvis larger and the delivery easier. The knowledge that her figure can be restored afterwards will encourage care over posture and exercises and the reasons for each of these should be explained. Similarly, circulatory changes in early pregnancy and again in the later weeks may cause dyspnoea and anxiety if the reason for them is not understood so that they are recognized as usual features in a normal pregnancy.

Awareness of the first uterine contractions provides an important opportunity of giving a simple explanation of labour itself. The great enemy is fear; and if this is still present when labour begins, ante-natal care has been inadequate and the course of labour is likely to be affected adversely. Obstetrics is no longer an exercise in mechanics but an opportunity for practising preventive medicine at its best.

9

Role of Husband

The third member of the family, namely the husband, is also of much greater importance than has hitherto been acknowledged in relation to the maternity service. A husband's obstetric responsibility to his wife does not end when she conceives. It has only just begun. He should neither be disregarded, nor treated as a necessary nuisance. If his sense of responsibility was encouraged, and this attitude spread throughout the community, there would be fewer concealed pregnancies, fewer uncooperative ante-natal patients, and fewer maternal and foetal disasters. Such a change of attitude would require a great deal of re-thinking by both the profession and the public. It would require a certain amount of re-designing even in the architecture of future maternity hospitals so that husbands and wives could spend more time together.

When a husband and wife share the joys as well as the trials of a pregnancy there is much less chance that the woman will default in her ante-natal care, and a much greater chance that when the time for labour comes it will provide the experience which she herself would desire and which her husband can share. For this experience to achieve its potential the husband must be brought actively into participation during the ante-natal period. If the mother is interested in relaxation, it is a help to her and to him if he becomes interested in it too.

Should a wife want her husband to be present during her labour, nothing but good can be done by granting her request, subject to reservations which will be defined later. The salutary effect on him of seeing what his wife has experienced in bringing his child into the world is important to him as well as to her. Not only does a husband lack understanding, but his wife's labour may be influenced unfavourably when he brings her into hospital in the early stages of labour and departs immediately for a drink or a dinner, or goes home to bed and to sleep. When at 3 a.m. the telephone call to tell him that his child has arrived safely remains unanswered, his wife may conceal her sadness, but it will be present and in some cases will be the beginning of much subsequent unhappiness and disharmony. When he ought to have been present to share her triumph she has experienced a feeling of unnecessary loneliness and even rejection which she may never forget. There are conflicting views concerning the wisdom of having a father in the labour ward while his child is born. In my opinion this is a practice to be encouraged.

Another side of the problem is seen when the husband is invited to be with his wife during labour but refuses the invitation, and her disappointment at his refusal is obvious. Occasionally she does not wish him to be present, although the knowledge that he is waiting nearby can help her. These are matters which should be settled by discussion between the doctor, patient and husband during pregnancy and not at the last minute when labour begins.

The more interest the husband is encouraged to take in the pregnancy, the more likely it is that he will welcome the opportunity of being with his wife during labour. From the experience of many years of having husbands present with their wives, often in opposition to the wishes of attending midwives in the earlier days of this practice, I can testify that I have seen it do nothing but good; and I am certain that in many cases it helps to establish a deeper relationship of respect and affection between husband and wife. It is important nonetheless to remember that there are many senior and experienced obstetricians who do not share these views. After much thought on why this should be, I believe that the explanation is found in the varying ability of different individuals to control a potentially difficult situation.

Returning to the three requirements essential for an efficient service, as outlined earlier, there is the basic need for safety of both mother and infant. The fact that an obstetrician either welcomes a husband to the Labour Ward or refuses to admit him has no correlation with his obstetric skill. If he feels he is in better command of the situation and more able to deal with an emergency should it arise if the husband is not present, it is surely his duty to act accordingly. The disappointment or frustration of wife or husband is to be regretted, but is likely to be forgotten in most cases with the safe arrival of the baby.

On the other hand, whether the doctor is right or not in the attitude he adopts, the fact remains that if an infant is lost the emotional repercussions on both mother and husband could well be permanent. A reasonable analogy would be the pilot of an aircraft who preferred not to have as an observer on the flight deck a layman, however intelligent he might be, or however interested in the problems of flying. Another pilot of comparable experience might be willing to have him there and if necessary explain things to him. Even so, he might request him to leave the cabin when preparing to land, or in an emergency, whereas another pilot under the same circumstances would carry out his duties apparently unaware of the presence of an observer. Each must decide for himself, subject to the one overriding factor —the safety of the aircraft and its passengers.

In the same way, it would not be in the best interest of a patient for her husband to be in the labour ward if his presence was likely to impair the efficiency of the obstetrician. It follows that attitudes to this controversial problem must inevitably vary. There is, however, one important point which should apply to all, namely that if a patient is adequately prepared for her labour, she will know beforehand the conditions under which that labour will be conducted, and if her wishes cannot be met, she will know the reason why.

There is a relevant associated issue and one which ultimately was responsible years ago for winning the support of midwives at Oxford to the practice of husbands being present with their wives during labour. It concerns the all too frequent habit of women being left alone, sometimes for long periods, particularly during the first stage of labour. This is not only cruel, it can be dangerous for both mother and unborn child.

However short of staff a maternity unit may be, the arrangement of duty should be such that when help is needed in the labour ward it should be available immediately, but few units can be staffed so generously that every mother has a nurse or midwife in attendance throughout a normal labour. This is why a husband, properly briefed, can be a comfort to his wife and a help to the nursing and medical staff. When suspicion is replaced by good-will, midwives will welcome him. If properly prepared, he will take an intelligent interest in the progress of labour and when in doubt will know how to summon immediate help.

10

Conduction Anaesthesia

An outstanding advance in this aspect of labour has been the development of conduction anaesthesia. The carefully controlled and supervised injection of local anaesthetic into the extradural space in the caudal canal, or into the thoraco-lumbar epidural area, can produce within a few minutes one of the most dramatic changes seen in medicine. A woman who is tired, dehydrated, ketotic and greatly distressed, will within five minutes of the injection be relaxed, peaceful and completely free of pain. Her labour will continue, and often accelerate, with complete absence of pain to effect a transformation which she describes as a miracle, as do those who witness it for the first time. Evidence is accumulating to show that the blood supply to the foetus is improved and its safety increased with this technique. Furthermore, if it is necessary to assist delivery by forceps or breech extraction the pelvic floor is completely relaxed and interference becomes correspondingly safer for the infant and less traumatic for the mother.

It is sometimes stated that this form of anaesthesia makes operative interference essential. If it were true, the mother who has needed this relief would consider the price worth paying; but it is not true. Though involuntary expulsive efforts in the second stage no longer take place because the patient is unaware of the fact that the presenting part is pressing on the pelvic floor, her ability to bear down is not impaired; and because of muscle relaxation in the pelvic floor, her guided efforts can be more productive than if they were resisted by contracting levator muscles. If therefore the mother is anxious to deliver the baby by her own efforts, she should be instructed how to bear down and when to do so, as a hand on the abdomen palpates each contraction. It seems unbelievable to both husband and wife when the child is born, either spontaneously or by forceps delivery with no sensation of pain or discomfort.

Advocates of epidural anaesthesia have stated in the press, on radio, and on television, that the only reason why in some hospitals this has been reserved chiefly for private patients is that it requires the skill and constant supervision of a consultant anaesthetist. This claim is not justified. Any doctor can learn the technique of either epidural or caudal anaesthesia, if he is prepared to do so. In some departments, as at Oxford, every new house officer in the maternity hospital learns how to administer caudal anaesthesia, and registrars become so highly skilled by frequent practice that in large consecutive series of patients they succeed in giving complete pain relief to over 90%. Moreover, they teach the technique to visiting specialists who in turn take it back to their own units. Few women who have had the benefit of this advance in labour will contemplate a subsequent delivery without its help, should pain relief be required.

11

Emotion in Labour

A fair criticism of many labour wards is that they are too clinical in some aspects of their work and insufficiently so in others. For the midwife, a delivery can provide just another baby before she goes off duty, and it is easy to forget that its safe arrival marks the culmination of months of planning, hopes and fears for the patient and her husband. They should be allowed to enjoy it to the maximum. Once respiration is established with the airways clear and the cord safely secured, the mother who wishes to hold the child in her arms should be allowed to do so. When the placenta is slow to separate, the stimulus of the babe at the breast will often be all that is needed to bring the third stage to a successful conclusion.

A recurring weakness in labour ward management is unimaginative repair of episiotomies and tears. Many a marriage is exposed to unnecessary tensions and frustrations because of ignorance or carelessness demonstrated at this important moment of a woman's life. Meticulous attention to detail is essential so that the cervix is left intact, the vagina sutured with complete haemostasis, and the perineum repaired so that separated muscles are united and the perineal body restored in such a way that there will not be a skin bridge at the introitus. All these details can contribute to future happiness by preventing dyspareunia, lessening the chance of troublesome discharge and perineal discomfort.

12

Rest after Labour

It is not surprising that for the first twenty-four hours after labour the patient may find it difficult to relax and have the rest which her body demands. Perineal soreness, uterine contractions, possible retention of urine, will all require attention; and the greater the emotional strains have been, the more important it is that sleep should be adequate and undisturbed. After months of waiting with hopes and fears often intermingled and anxieties lest the child should be abnormal or the pain of labour greater than she can bear, the mother must have peace. This can be disturbed all too easily even by relatives and well-meaning friends.

13

Breast-feeding

Finally, a word is necessary concerning breast-feeding. It is true that milk mixtures have been so improved that under most circumstances they are practically as safe as breast milk. To be able to assure a patient of this can be a great comfort if she is either unable or unwilling to feed the baby herself. On the other hand, many women who are desperately anxious to feed their babies fail to do so. This is often due to the unsympathetic way in which they are handled by the nursing and medical staff.

Lactation may be well-established while a patient is in hospital, but shortly after she returns home the supply may diminish and trouble begins. It is sometimes forgotten that energy is required to produce a pint of milk, and when the body works it also needs to rest. Guidance on these matters and on how to plan the day should be given before the patient leaves hospital. Discouragement by a visiting nurse, a relative or the husband can contribute to her failure and in this way to her unhappiness. If, during the ante-natal weeks, she and her husband have had the preparation to which they were entitled, these important details would have been learned by them and the chance of disappointment would have been reduced to a minimum.

14

Planned Pregnancy

In conclusion, in an ideal society every pregnancy would be planned, and obstetricians would accept responsibility for making this possible. Spontaneous abortion would be a personal tragedy. Legal abortion would seldom be required, and only for therapeutic reasons. In such a society, preparation for childbirth would commence, not after the first missed period, but with adolescent understanding of the changes taking place at puberty and the significance of reproductive physiology with its challenges, its hazards, and its implications in terms of personal responsibility. Should that day ever come, the task of the enlightened midwife and doctor would be made easier as they prepare the pregnant woman for a labour which would be conducted with such understanding and skill that it becomes for her and her husband a moment of triumph and achievement.

CLINICAL

Post-Natal

XX

EMOTIONAL AND PSYCHOTIC ILLNESS FOLLOWING CHILDBIRTH

LENNART KAIJ

M.D.

Senior Lecturer in Psychiatry
University of Lund, Sweden

ÅKE NILSSON

M.D.

Psychiatrist
University of Lund,
Sweden

1

Introduction

Psychotic complications to pregnancy occur in 1 or 2 cases per 1,000 deliveries. Four to five per cent of all admissions of females to mental hospitals are due to such illness.[1, 13, 34, 35] Although these figures seem moderate, puerperal psychoses have continued to cause great concern to psychiatrists ever since they were first described by Marcé in 1858.[22] Indeed, these psychoses are often extremely dramatic and they always have a great, often tragic, impact on the patient and her family at a time that should be particularly happy.

Despite being very interesting, the psychoses must be regarded as a small group of diseases from a socio-medical point of view and of substantially less significance than the minor psychiatric illnesses following pregnancy, i.e. neuroses, non-psychotic depressions, asthenic reactions and so on. Recent investigations have indicated that the latter are extremely common during the post-partum year.[8, 9, 11, 26, 29] As many as one woman in four experiences more or less incapacitating neurotic and/or depressive symptoms during this period.[11, 26] This is mirrored in the rapidly increasing interest in para-partum neurotic reactions.

The high frequencies of neurotic reactions associated with childbearing is interesting not only from an obstetrical point of view. It has recently been proposed that the psychiatric over-morbidity in females is related to their reproductive function.[16, 21, 31] If this is so, any measure that could reduce the para-partum psychiatric morbidity would also influence the total female psychiatric morbidity.

The present chapter, after a summary of our knowledge of post-partum psychoses, deals with neurotic reactions and speculates on the relation between the mental health and reproductive functions of women.

2

Psychoses

Post-partum psychosis is generally defined simply as psychosis with onset within six months after delivery. The term "lactation psychoses" is based on superstition. It has no scientific support and should be discarded.

While there is a slight decrease in the incidence of psychoses during pregnancy, at least during the third trimester, there is a sharp rise, starting on the third to sixth day after delivery, with a peak during the first post-partum month.[31]

Symptomatology

In the majority of cases the onset is sudden with an extreme variety of symptoms. Although just over 50% of the patients present with mainly affective symptoms, the most conspicuous feature is clouding of consciousness. The degree of clouding ranges from slight disorientation or derealization—the "oneiroid state" of Mayer-Gross—to violent delirium of extreme severity. The slighter degrees of clouding are easily overlooked, as attention is directed towards other, more colourful symptoms. It may present as general anxiety, apprehension or perplexity. Not until after remission the patient may be able to describe her state as "dreamlike", "like a theatre", "unreality", etc. A strong affective colouring is another characteristic of the post-partum psychoses. It may be nearly pure depressive or manic-depressive, but a considerable number of patients show mixed or rapidly changing affects. The latter is true particularly in patients with a clouded consciousness.

Accessory symptoms, hallucinations of all sensory modalities and a wealth of delusions, may be present. The thought content is naturally primarily concerned with the child, the delivery, the patient's role as a mother and her relation to the father of the child. The child is feared to be dead, malformed or severely ill. One patient was convinced that she had a twin left in her womb and later thought that one of the imaginary twins had been taken away. Hypochondriacal delusions about the genitals being destroyed, amputated etc. are not uncommon.[18] Interpersonal conflicts with husband and/or parents may be reflected in a distorted way. At the same time the patient often exhibits an extreme dependency with a demanding attitude towards her near relatives.

Infanticidal impulses have caused great concern. In recent times actual infanticides seem to be very uncommon. It is generally agreed that the risk is greater in patients with marked depressive features than in others.[1]

Diagnosis

From this brief clinical description it is clear that puerperal psychosis is not a nosological entity. The pictures in the acute stage are also too undifferentiated to permit a formal diagnosis, unless data on earlier psychiatric history are available. The gross diagnostic disagreement in this field is illustrated in many studies, giving, for example, quite different percentages of the frequency of probable schizophrenic psychoses, ranging from 14 to 65%. [1, 30, 34, 35] This disagreement is due partly to the conceptual confusion in psychiatry, but above all to the confusing pictures the patients present. Therefore, the long-term course of the disease still provides the best basis for differentiation. The duration of the psychoses ranges from a few days to a year, or they may take a chronic course. If all psychoses are taken into account one patient in five recovers within a month. Forty per cent of psychoses last more than six months.[1, 30] Recent investigations suggest that 10–15% of the psychoses take a chronic course, most of them compatible with the European concept of *schizophrenia*.[1] It may be wondered whether these psychoses are actually post-partum psychoses. The alternative explanation is that the schizophrenic psychosis was first noticed when the woman was responsible for the care of the child. Further psychotic episodes after remission of the post-partum psychosis occur in about 30%. The majority of these psychoses have a more or less classical *manic-depressive* course.[1] In 40-50% of the patients the post-partum psychosis is a single, discreet and benign event in their lives.[1] It should be mentioned that post-partum psychoses used to be life-threatening diseases. As much as 25% mortality has been reported during the first decades of this century.[30] After the introduction of modern physical treatment the mortality rate has radically decreased to nearly zero.

The risk of psychoses in subsequent pregnancies is generally estimated to be 1:7 pregnancies, i.e. a more than 100-fold increase compared with the general population. On the other hand Arentsen's data suggest that the risk of recurrence in women who become pregnant again is only slightly and insignificantly increased compared with those who abstain from further pregnancies, again an expression of the non-specificity of the disease.[1]

Etiology

In patients with chronic *schizophrenia and manic-depressive psychoses* the pregnancy is at most a precipitating factor. This is most apparent in the manic-depressive group, where half of the patients had had psychotic episodes before, and 80% after, the post-partum psychosis.[1] In a minority of cases the subsequent psychoses were exclusively related to pregnancy, which suggests a specific vulnerability in some women. In the majority of cases the stress of the pregnancy and delivery is unspecific.

In earlier days *somatic complications* of delivery (sepsis, thrombo-embolism, toxaemia etc.) were also important causes of post-partum psychosis. With increasing possibilities to control obstetric complications, the incidence of gross organic post-partum psychoses is approaching zero.

It is natural to think that *hormonal factors* are responsible for most of the exogenous post-partum psychoses. Intensive search for any endocrinological disturbance specific for psychotic parturient women have failed to prove this. In 1962 Hamilton[10] published a much cited monograph, in which he suggested that thyroid deprivation could be responsible for post-partum mental illness. He based his theory mainly on his apparently successful attempt to cure the psychoses by administration of triiodothyronine. He had no control group, however, and his statement that the course of the psychoses was shortened by the treatment remains to be proved.

There is conflicting evidence as to the relative importance of *age and parity* for the occurrence of psychosis. Thus the frequency of primiparae ranges from 30 to 86% in different materials.[1, 13, 27, 28, 30, 31, 34, 35] Even studies with adequate control groups disagree on this point. These contradictions are partly resolved when nosological categories are regarded separately. Arentsen[1] found chronic schizophrenics to be mostly multiparous, manic-depressives to be equally often primi- and multiparous, while about 80% of the patients with psychoses complicating gross somatic illness were primiparae. In the residual group—in Arentsen's material labelled "psychogenic psychosis"—67 % were primiparae.

Age is naturally correlated to parity, which partly explains the conflicting data on this point. On the whole it seems as if higher age implies a slightly increased risk. *Marital status* is unanimously related to risk of psychoses, inasmuch as unmarried mothers are over-represented. In addition, it may be possible that many primiparae have married during the pregnancy, resulting in psychosis.

It remains to discuss the importance of *psychological factors* for the occurrence of psychosis. In chronic schizophrenic, manic-depressive and gross organic psychoses, psychological conflicts are of marginal importance. For the remaining group, on the other hand, they are of great interest. This does not mean that their importance is generally agreed upon, as some authors deny any psychological influence on post-partum psychosis. Much of the data, however, do suggest such influence. The preponderance of primiparae and of unwed women among psychotic mothers is most easily explained if the social and psychological insecurity is taken into consideration.

Furthermore, several authors have noted an increased rate of *infantile and immature trait* in the premorbid personalities of patients with post-partum psychosis.[1, 13, 18] This is particularly illuminated in Arentsen's material. The frequency of immature personality and subnormality among patients with chronic schizophrenic, manic-depressive and gross organic psychosis was 15, 22 and 20% respectively. In contrast, the corresponding frequency among the remaining post-partum psychotic women was 40%. In addition, 35% of the patients in the latter group were judged as neurotic, compared with 7% in the other groups. These personality features may imply a lowered resistance against conflicts. It is evident that pregnancy *per se* implies a deepseated conflict for many women. This is established by an abundance of observations and will be further commented upon in the last part of the present chapter. But there is also a growing number of observations which suggest a high incidence of *actual psychological conflicts* amongst women who become psychotic in connection with pregnancy.[1, 18] The content of the psychotic delusions may be taken as reflections of these conflicts, particularly in the exogenous group. No single environmental factor or specific conflict seems to have been identified; it is rather a question of a combination of untoward circumstances. So far no attempt has been made to compare the psychological situations of psychotic and non-psychotic parturient women. Until such a study is made the final evaluation of the relative importance of the psychological factors must wait.

The influence of *genetic factors*, finally, are evident from what is already said about the endogenous psychoses. So far no genetic study of post-partum psychoses is known.

3

Neuroses

The term "neurosis" covers all mental illness of non-psychotic character. It implies that the wellbeing of the woman is disturbed in various degrees and her normal way of functioning is restricted. The forms it takes include anxiety states, phobias, obsessions, hysteria, hypochondriasis, depression, psychasthenia etc.

Incidence

For a long time psychodynamically orientated authors have pointed out the importance of neurotic reactions accompanying pregnancy and childbirth. They have also suggested several explanations, which, however, for apparent reasons, remain unproved for larger groups of women.[3, 4, 5, 32] Systematic investigations on incidence, etiology, prognosis and symptoms of neurotic reactions, in pregnancy and puerperium are virtually non-existent. One retrospective and two prospective studies have been published recently.[11, 29, 36] The prospective studies are biased by being focused on rather narrow problems. The rather nebulous statements about post-partum neurosis, which are found in current text-books, are made mainly on the basis of observations on post-partum psychosis or on a few non-psychotic patients treated by psychotherapy or admitted to mental hospitals during pregnancy.

One common statement is that neurosis is less common during pregnancy than in the post-partum period (which is true in psychosis) or that para-partum neurotic reactions are less common than psychosis.[27, 28, 29, 33] Our own investigations emphatically reject these views.

Information on the frequency of para-partum neurotic reactions is sparse and varying. Post-partum depression alone occurs in 2–11 % [29, 36] According to Gordon and Gordon,[8, 9] 4–8% of mothers need psychiatric help during the post-partum period. Our own retrospective postal investigation of more than 800 unselected parturient women indicated that 25% of the subjects experienced a considerable number of nervous symptoms during the post-partum year.[11, 12, 14, 24, 25] In a prospective study still in progress, substantial neurotic reactions were found in 17% of the subjects during, and 19% after, the pregnancy. A moderate number of neurotic symptoms were experienced by a further 27% during, and 26% after, the pregnancy. Only 16% were symptom-free during pregnancy and 28% post-partum. 16% reported onset of neurotic symptoms during pregnancy.[26]

These figures clearly show not only that neurotic reactions are a substantial problem in the post-partum period, but also that it is equally great during the pregnancy. In our opinion, the conventional opinion that the pregnant woman is full of bliss and free of problems is unfounded. This opinion is shared by medical men, who seem to have taken it for granted. Probably the relatively healthy period between 20 and 35 weeks of gestation has been taken as supporting evidence.

Symptomatology

The following description of the clinical pictures of para-natal neurotic reactions are based mainly on experience from a prospective investigation of an unselected sample of pregnant women.[26] First the psychological reactions commonly found at different stages of the pregnancy are described, then some of the pathological pictures are dealt with.

The Normal Course. The first trimester is characterized by the familiar nausea and emesis, sometimes regarded as a psychogenetic symptom, a considerable increase of emotional lability, increased irritability and varying degrees of depressive mood, ranging from a slight inhibition of activity to deep melancholy including suicidal thoughts. These mental symptoms are accompanied by a decrease in libido and often an increased aggressiveness towards the father of the foetus. At the same time the woman often shows a paradoxical dependency on the husband and also on other members of her family, particularly her own mother.[2]

Although the pregnancy can hardly be regarded as a physical stress at this early stage, a most outstanding feature is an often dramatically increased need of sleep, and fatiguability. Indeed, some multiparae allege sleepiness to be their first sign of pregnancy. On the other hand insomnia, anxiety, or neurovegetative symptoms are not particularly common during the first phase of the pregnancy.

The second and the very first part of the third trimester are comparatively free from psychological symptoms. Even women who were clearly disturbed during the first months often feel healthy in the middle of the pregnancy. Some women attribute this comparative well-being to the quickening, when they feel "contact" with the foetus, which now is regarded as an individual dependent on the mother, rather than as a part of her. Many women "chat" with their foetus, give it a provisional name etc. Some of those who initially were negative to the pregnancy begin to accept it; but, contrary to early opinion, this is by no means true of all women. It is our impression that some of those who accept the pregnancy at this stage do it reluctantly, and rather as a matter of fact, than enthusiastically. Some of those women who experienced a decrease of sexual desire in the beginning of the pregnancy, regain it during the second trimester. Others report an even better sexual relationship than before the pregnancy. The latter is true particularly of women who have legitimized their relation to the father of the foetus by marriage, and of those with earlier fear of pregnancy. The majority of pregnant women, however, experience both a diminished desire and less satisfaction. A fear that intercourse might hurt the foetus is often encountered and may be the reason for total sexual abstinence throughout the pregnancy.

During the last months of the pregnancy there is again a rise of the frequency of mental symptoms, but the picture, quite different from that during the initial stage, is characterized by symptoms of psychomotor tension, restlessness and anxiety. During the last few weeks panic attacks may appear. There is also increasing physical discomfort: calf cramps, back-aches, orthostatism, disturbed sleep etc., to which practically all women are subjected. During the very last days before delivery many women become increasingly active, busily occupied with more or less unnecessary household work, tidying, sewing etc. often interpreted as a sign of impatience.

Many women are naturally preoccupied with the imminent parturition, although the fear and anxiety are often denied or concealed. Often the child is feared to be malformed or even stillborn; but most of all, the woman has worries about her own fate: possible complications of the partus, pains, or even fear of death. It is interesting to note that primiparae are more concerned about the child, multiparae about themselves.[26, 37] These fears are most pronounced among women with an initially negative attitude towards the pregnancy, indicating a problem of guilt and punishment. More superficially, the women are concerned about being left alone during labour, fear of losing control of themselves, or being awkward patients, etc.

Parturition is of course experienced in many different ways. Some women react with strong anxiety, or panic in their helplessness and pains, and may behave in an extremely primitive and regressive way. Several authors have noticed that anxiety before and during labour is often associated with a lengthy labour.[7, 23] There is, however, no relation between the course of labour and post-partum neurotic reactions; which indicates different mechanisms.[11, 26]

The first 24 hours post-partum is a period of restoration after the trauma of the delivery. The woman is in a drowsy condition, physically and mentally relaxed, with long periods of sleep. Her attitude towards the child is almost always positive; even disappointment with the sex of the child is carefully concealed during the first few days.

The subsequent 3 or 4 days are characterized by extreme emotional lability.[17, 26, 38] To the observer the mother appears slightly euphoric, unrealistic, "whimsical". Many women can later describe these first days as a dreamlike state, with slight derealization and deficient contact with reality. The mother feels an intense need to be on close physical contact with her child. The so-called "maternity blues" or "third day blues" are generally described as depressive states. To the "blues" is also ascribed a prognostic value for later neurotic reactions. On close observation, however, it is found that 70–80% of the women exhibit "blues" symptoms; and this percentage is hardly compatible with any prognostic value. We agree with Yalom et al.[38] that previous investigators have often diagnosed later depression from this early emotional lability, which is so common. But, firstly, tearfulness is not a very characteristic sign of depression,[6] and secondly, the crying of the puerperium is not accompanied by a depressive mood, but is rather a stereotyped reaction to both positive and negative affect. Yalom et al.[38] list a large number of reasons for crying given by their subjects, and they feel that, if any affect is characterisetic for this early post-partum period, it is dysphoria and irritability rather than depression.

The slight euphoria, the irritability, the emotional lability, the stereotyped crying behaviour and the impression of slight confusion are all, in our opinion, characteristic of the early post-partum period. We are inclined to interpret these symptoms as physiological, rather than psychological reaction, perhaps due to an increased secretion of corticosteroids. On the other hand, these reactions may also have the psychological function of protecting the mother from everyday trivialities during the important period when the mother-child imprinting takes place.

The "blue" syndrome is of objective rather than subjective importance and the first post-partum week is, on the whole, free from pathological psychiatric symptoms. Many women, particularly primiparae, who are ignorant of the hardships ahead, are eager to get home and demand to be discharged even against medical advice. There is, however, a small group of women who from the first post-partum week already show signs heralding more serious troubles. These signs are subtle and often difficult to distinguish from the "blues", but we have noticed that actual depressive symptoms, including psychomotor retardation, lack of interest in the child, and concern about practical and emotional problems to be encountered after returning home, may imply the first signs of post-partum neurotic reactions.

In the second half of the first post-partum month the picture changes again. Many of the neurasthenic symptoms experienced during the first trimester of the pregnancy reappear. Thus many women again become more easily fatigued, need much more sleep than usual, feel tired, irritable and complain of a number of psychosomatic symptoms. These complaints are often explained as a consequence of caring for the child. The fact that some overburdened women do not complain, while others who lead an easy life experience an abundance of symptoms, suggests, however, that exogenous factors are relatively unimportant. We feel that the main cause of this post-partum "hang-over" is to be found in physiological factors, perhaps in the hormonal readjustment. Symptoms of clearly psychological nature do, of course, also exist. Manifest anxiety does not belong to the natural course, but increased arousal and concern for the baby, listening to its breathing, crying, observation of its behaviour does, and is of course more common amongst primiparae.

Thoughts of infanticide are generally regarded as very alarming symptoms, particularly by the women themselves. In our two investigations, about 10%, probably a conservative estimate, reported "fear of hurting the child". In the majority of those admitting such fear, it appeared more as a single episode than a lasting or painful obsession. Nevertheless, many women were obviously relieved by reassurance about the nature of the symptoms. According to literature other obsessions are also a conspicuous feature of the post-partum period. Our experience is rather the reverse. Many women, who reported perfectionistic behaviour before the pregnancy, said they had no time for perfectionism after the child's birth. We cannot, however, exclude the possibility that their perfectionism had been transferred to the care of the baby.

The decrease of sexual desire, so common during pregnancy, usually persists; sometimes it decreases even more, and is experienced by more women. Some of them can openly admit their sexual indifference or frigidity, others hide it behind various complaints of genital pains and discomfort following childbirth. When these sexual symptoms are not part of a sexual neurosis, they may be regarded as an expression of the woman's preoccupation with the child.

To summarize; in the first three post-partum months there is a steep rise in the incidence of mental symptoms. Usually, these symptoms are limited to a moderate or mild neurasthenia, lasting only one or two months, although the improvement continues throughout the post-partum year (Fig. 1).

So far we have described the natural course of pregnancy and the post-partum period from a psychiatric point of view, although any delineation of normal reactions is admittedly arbitrary. We feel, however, that for the para-partum neurotic reactions a full description is a necessary background. We want to stress that we are concerned with reactions both during and after the pregnancy; a limitation to the post-partum period, such as could be made with the psychosis, would be artificial. The pathological reactions differ from the "natural" course in respect of intensity, duration, subjective suffering, impairment of functioning and a number of symptoms rather than type of symptoms. In other words, the difference is quantitative rather than qualitative. Furthermore, we are concerned with overt, mainly subjec-

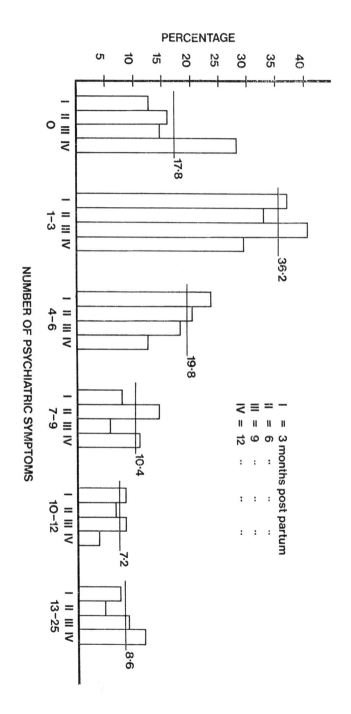

tive symptoms and only in lesser degree with objective signs. This limitation implies that, character neurosis, for instance, has not been counted, although its importance as a fertile soil of symptom neurosis is recognized. In other words we are concerned with *neurotic illnesses* in a conventional sense. These will be described in terms of their history rather than in terms of symptomatology.

The Neurotic Mother

Both in prospective and in retrospective studies a previous history of neurosis was found to be the most important single factor in predicting neurotic reactions during or after pregnancy.[24, 26] Women with a previous history of neurosis often report continuous symptoms throughout the pregnancy and the puerperium, and also that the symptoms are worse than before the pregnancy. As the period preceding the pregnancy is assessed retrospectively, it is not possible to verify if there is a real deterioration due to the stress of the pregnancy, or whether these women generally tend to project their inner difficulties on current life events, and to belittle previous distress. It is clear that single temporary neurotic reactions in the past are of little predictive value, particularly if they are of a reactive nature. On the other hand, repeated neurotic episodes, or continuous neurotic complaints, imply a very high risk of para-partum neurotic reactions. However, a small group of women, about 3–5%, report improvement during pregnancy, but have been unable to identify any factor that would predict this outcome.

Case history no. 1. Twenty-seven-year-old, three-parous woman from the lower middle class. Probably some conflict with her mother. Elementary school, unqualified jobs before marriage at twenty.

When examined during her fourth pregnancy: grossly insufficient, tired, irritable, weeping, depressed, could not manage her household duties, needed much help from husband; refused to seek medical advice.

Three months post-partum, admitted to a neurological unit under dramatic circumstances with suspected epileptic fits. Epilepsy could not be confirmed. Two months later, spontaneous contact with the investigator via a neighbour. Completely unable to manage home and children, extremely tearful, tired; also depressed. Admitted severe neurotic symptoms continuously since delivery, and also some neurotic symptoms before last pregnancy. The six-months follow-up, according to the research plan, revealed a severe life-long neurotic history with symptoms of anxiety neurosis, phobia, earlier attacks of hyperventilation and fits, interpersonal conflict with parents and in-laws, difficulties with at least two of her children, who had been admitted to child-guidance clinic.

Para-partum neurotic reactions proper as defined begin during the pregnancy or thereafter. At least two main groups can be distinguished:

1. Reactions immediately caused by the practical difficulties and stresses of the current situation; 2. reactions based mainly on deep-seated intra-

psychic conflicts, particularly concerning femininity, motherhood, or the sexual and reproductive role in general. This effect befalls women who can be regarded as latent neurotics. Combinations of the two groups do, of course, exist.

Reactive Neurosis

Reactive neurosis is common, at all times, as well as being the most common neurosis during pregnancy. An unintentional pregnancy may imply a severe psychological trauma to some women, without their being neurotic. Many women are insufficiently prepared for a pregnancy both from a practical, social and psychological point of view. Unstable socio-economic conditions, such as unsatisfactory work, housing, education, relation to the male partner etc., are often obvious obstacles to a whole-hearted acceptance of an unplanned pregnancy, particularly in primiparae. The reactions of the family and friends may add to the psychological maladjustment. The woman not only has to cope with her own inner and outer problems, but is also exposed to the pressure of convention. The size of this problem is made clear from the fact that almost 50% of the women in our samples were unmarried at the time of conception. Nearly 40% of the women in our samples stated that the pregnancy was unwelcome and a further 20% that is was unplanned —a total of 60% unplanned pregnancies.

Many women, even in Scandinavia, are grossly ignorant of elementary facts about sex. In our sample 40% of the women had never received adequate information about contraceptive techniques. In many cases this ignorance is the direct explanation of the pregnancy. Unplanned pregnancies are not limited to primiparae; the second pregnancy is usually planned, but amongst the third and subsequent ones the number of unplanned pregnancies rises steeply.[14, 26] In poor families, or those who have adjusted to a certain size, or where the wife has resumed her work etc., an unintentional pregnancy may cause great difficulties and give rise to severe neurotic reactions.

We feel that the desirability of the pregnancy is a central issue and therefore it is important to try to understand why an unwished pregnancy comes about. Neurotic reactions to unwanted conceptions will often appear early in the pregnancy. It is characteristic that these women are conscious of their problems and—what is important—they are less hesitant to admit openly a negative attitude to the pregnancy. Often, they are also conscious of the accompanying guilt feelings and their origin. Usually they are depressed and anxious, but are able to show their grief and concern about their future openly and freely. Although these reactions may be quite alarming, they are in general of benign nature, provided the personality of the woman is reasonably healthy and she can have some help to manage her external difficulties. To offer support is one of the most important tasks of the ante-natal clinics; another important practical matter is to make sure that these women receive information and advice on contraception. They often, and quite unnecessarily, become worried by fear of further pregnancies, with consequent marital and sexual maladjustment.

Case history no. 2. A thirty-three-year-old primi-parous woman of lower middle class. Son, nine years old, healthy. The husband has now and then problems with alcohol; which have been a strain in the marriage. Mostly he has been well adjusted, probably due to the beneficial influence of his wife. She has worked as a clerk, which has given her security. Before the present pregnancy she was very well adjusted, probably a support to her husband. The couple had agreed not to have any more children.

She became pregnant after neglecting contraceptive measures, as she thought herself to be too old (!) to become pregnant. Immediately depressed, weeping, sleepless, tense, much concerned about the future, particularly her job. This lasted for five months; but throughout the pregnancy she had a negative attitude to the child. After a short recurrence of symptoms post-partum, excellent recovery and adjustment.

Latent Neurosis

The second group, which we have called the "latently neurotic" group, is much more difficult to describe. As the women belonging to this group usually are unconscious of their conflict, the clinical picture is often difficult even for specialists to understand and interpret. The symptoms are polymorphic and changing, due to defence mechanisms and secondary gain. Nevertheless some characteristic traits can be discerned.

At a superficial level rapport is often difficult to achieve. These women appear reserved, cool, *"noli me tangere"*, intellectualizing, conventional. When the mental symptoms are not too severe, or do not include too much anxiety, these women are obviously frustrated and tend to project their feelings in a wealth of psychosomatic symptoms, or give somatic explanations for their disorders. They often conceal earlier neurotic symptoms or conflicts; they give conventional answers to questions, often very quickly, even before the question is finished.

Only an indirect approach gives indications of neurotic disturbances, such as subtle signs of disturbed sexuality, psychosomatic gynaecological symptoms, other psychosomatic illnesses, puzzling idiosyncrasies etc. Socially, these women are often careerists, and have good professional training. Since puberty they have shown preference for a professional role, rather than for a conventional role as housewife; but they show signs of ambivalence even in this. In marriage they are mostly the dominant partner and the perfect "organizer" of the house. Closer investigation, e.g. in a therapy situation, may disclose a deep intrapsychic conflict, which can be traced back to childhood, since when the whole spectrum of neurotic mechanisms has developed.

The overt neurotic reactions of these women usually do not appear until the post-partum period. Generally speaking, they run their pregnancies as perfectly as their houses. Probably the very existence of the foetus is sometimes denied or repressed; later in the pregnancy the inevitable difficulties are compensated while waiting for the "parasite" to be expelled. After the child is born, it is no longer possible to deny its existence and to keep the neurotic defence intact. Then a full-fledged neurosis breaks out.

Case history no. 3. Twenty-eight-year-old, nulli-para, research worker. Claimed perfect adjustment denies all mental symptoms, "never shed a tear". Perfectionist. Husband weak, dependent on his mother. Marriage "a dream', but she admits numerous quarrels. Sex life "ideal"— but intercourse only when she "feels like it". After four years of marriage, hesitantly pregnant. Moderately severe morning sickness first month, then again "perfect health". Well until she resumed work after delivery, then sleepless, precordial pains, "heart attacks", fear of heart disease, infectious disease and insanity. Much concerned about the health of the child, numerous visits to several doctors, always specialists, for herself and child. Eventually after severe panic attacks, psychiatric consultation. Gradually numerous neurotic symptoms; phobia, obsessions, constant anxiety etc. were disclosed, as well as severe infantile conflict with mother and an older sister. Later she realized identification with father and his expectations, aggression towards husband, disgust and guilt feelings towards child, conflict between the roles of wife and professional woman. After first year of therapy great relief of symptoms, good adjustment to mother role, but still not reconciled with husband.

Nature of Symptoms

The separate symptoms and syndromes of the neurotic reactions will now be briefly commented upon. The commonest symptom encountered in pregnancy and puerperium is *depression*. This is illustrated by the fact that recent reports of post-partum neurosis mainly deal with the depressive syndrome.[11, 29, 36] Depression is common both during pregnancy and post-partum, and varies from transitory mild reactions to long-lasting deep reactions. Classical deep melancholia with "endogenous" features is comparatively rare, but does exist and must not be overlooked. The clinical picture is seldom clear-cut, as it usually includes asthenic, somatic and sexual symptoms, which make a correct diagnosis difficult. The depression is usually reactive to outer difficulties. The prognosis of the depression is largely determined by the nature of these difficulties. If the depression is caused by the pregnancy being unwanted, e.g. because the woman fears her parents' reaction to it, the depression may be of short duration, but nevertheless of considerable depth. Depression lasting several months during the pregnancy tends to recur in the post-partum period, as mentioned above.

The common *neurasthenic reactions* which we have described as "natural" may become deeper and more protracted. Sometimes extreme fatigue, sleeplessness, emotional lability, irritability and aggressiveness may occur and last for several months or even for a year. The fatigue may be associated with lowered muscular tonicity, impaired or changing alertness and feeling of derealization. These conditions may leave the woman incapacitated for a considerable time.

Anxiety states of a more pronounced degree or attacks of panic are uncommon features, apart from the last weeks before confinement. Post-partum feelings of fear are common when the woman feels abandoned, especially by her husband. Even during short legitimate absence (business travel and the like) in the first post-partum week, a husband should secure adequate company for his wife. Her anxiety easily becomes chronic, but when appropriately handled is relieved at an early stage with equal ease.

Hysteria is no more common para-partum than in other stressful situations.

The characteristic post-partum phobia is the fear of infanticide, usually combined with fear of insanity. This symptom has been discussed above; it remains to note that in a minority of women it may become a chronic obsession, limited to one child only or extending to other persons. When not heralding a schizophrenia, it *never* implies any risk of infanticide.

Sexual difficulties, including decreased libido and incapacity for orgasm, are common features both during and after the pregnancy. When not part of a sexual neurosis, they are usually benign, but may become protracted, or even chronic, under unfavourable circumstances. A forced marriage, a demanding husband, fear of another pregnancy etc., may act as conditioning factors. However, if properly handled, these states have an excellent prognosis.

Etiology

The influence on etiology of *age, social status and parity* is surprisingly small. Age and social status have not proved to have any influence, at least in Scandinavian studies. These findings can probably be applied to other countries as far as age is concerned. The differences between social classes, however, are much greater in many other countries than in Scandinavia, hence caution is needed when generalizing on the absence of social influence.

The influence of *parity* is difficult to elucidate. In our studies we found no direct linear association between the number of children and frequency of neurotic symptoms. In the retrospective sample, about 40% of the women reported no symptoms, or very few symptoms, regardless of the number of pregnancies. In the rest of the sample, however, there was a greater number of women with many symptoms, while those with a moderate number of symptoms became fewer with increasing parity.[14] This finding may imply that some women are comparatively resistant to para-partum neurosis, and others more susceptible to it. In the latter group the degree of the neurotic reaction is a function of parity.

It must be remembered, however, that the parity of a woman is not randomly determined. One of the decisive factors is her health. A woman who has been ill—emotionally or physically—during or after a pregnancy is probably more reluctant to endeavour a new pregnancy than one who has been healthy. This assumption is substantiated in our retrospective study, where the proportion of women who said they had been healthy until their last delivery was greatest among those with four or more children. This selective factor will become more important as more family-planning devices are accepted. Again, our sample is perhaps slightly unusual, as contraception has been generally accepted in Scandinavia for several decades. In a population where the woman has less opportunity to decide whether or not she will have another pregnancy, an investigation would probably yield a different result, i.e. parity would prove to have a much greater influence. This assumption is supported by another of our observations, namely that women who have experienced neurotic symptoms during or after earlier pregnancies are clearly poorer risk during the pregnancy under observation.[26]

Data permitting any conclusion on the importance of *specific* genetic *factors* for the occurrence of para-partum neurosis are lacking. One may venture the hypothesis that such factors, if they do exist, are multiple and hence extremely difficult to ascertain with present methods.

Our knowledge of the importance of *somatic factors* is likewise insufficient. In our samples there is no association between para-partum neurosis and pre-pregnancy somatic illness or somatic complications of pregnancy and parturition. As most of the serious somatic complications can be effectively controlled, their number in our sample is small. In contrast, a number of subjective gynaecological symptoms, such as genital pains, feeling of laxity in the abdominal wall and perineum, temporary increase of the lochia, etc. were associated with a high number of post-partum symptoms. Sign of delayed genital involution post-partum was significantly related both to pre-pregnancy and post-partum neurosis. The causal relationship between such rather subtle gynaecological and psychiatric abnormalities has not yet been clarified, but psychological factors can certainly explain a great deal.

Many unsuccessful attempts have been made to find organic parameters, particularly *endocrinological*, parallelling post-partum mental illness. But we can assume that hormonal changes contribute to the normal neurasthenic reactions described above.[38] This assumption is supported by observations of the psychiatric complications caused by oral contraceptives, the psychic fluctuations during the menstrual cycle, during puberty and during the menopause. Hormonal influence is, however, a poor explanation for frank pathological reactions, e.g. involutional melancholia or post-menopausal paranoid jealousy. We believe that this is also true for the majority of the para-partum mental illnesses.

In contrast to somatic factors, *pre-existing neurosis* is one of the most powerful predicting factors, if not the most powerful one, for post-partum mental health. However, deterioration of an existing neurosis in association with pregnancy should not, as pointed out above, be regarded as para-partum neurosis proper.

Amongst women with apparently normal mental health before the pregnancy we singled out two groups with increased risk of para-partum neurosis: (1) those with "reactive" neurosis and (2) "latent neurotics". The first group, which is easily understood, has been dealt with at length earlier in this chapter. It includes women with current problems, of which they are themselves usually aware. Unmarried status, housing and economic problems, unsatisfactory relations with the male, or desertion by him, open conflict with parents or in-laws, are examples of such problems. We should like to add one more—a rare situation which is only partly understood—namely the presence of a malformed or defective child. Particularly if this is the first child, a second pregnancy is often unwelcome and may produce severe anxiety and depression, often resulting in a desire for termination of the pregnancy. The conscious motive for this desire is that the abnormal child is too great a burden and/or that the woman cannot stand the fear of having a second defective child. Unconsciously there is often severe guilt feelings towards the first child, sometimes originating from hostility towards it while still unborn. This situation is thus an example where both conscious and latent conflicts are present. It is a delicate task to advise these parents, and it is often necessary to grant their intense wish for a termination.

A few comments should be added on the second group, the "latent conflict" group. It is tempting to assume that psychological complications of childbirth are influenced by the mother's attitude towards being a woman—her femininity. Much confusion arises from a failure to distinguish between the social and the psychological (or rather psycho-sexual) gender role. Here we are concerned with the latter. We do recognize, however, that the two kinds of roles are highly correlated, and that they may be in opposition. As Helene Deutsch[5] puts it: "Conflict easily arises between the woman's service for the species and the aims of her ego." We believe, however, that such conflicts are fairly overt and often conscious.

The psycho-sexual gender role is less influenced by social and cultural factors than by the individual's personal infantile experience. We are inclined to adhere to Freud's theory of the Oedipal conflict, and particularly the importance of its resolution; the pre-requisite of a successful functioning as a man or a woman is an identification with the parent or parent-substitute of the same sex.

Recent investigations have shown that, at least in laboratory animals, testosterone influence on the foetal hypothalamus plays a decisive role in development of behavioural sex.[19] This observation does not, however, challenge the psychological importance of identification.

With considerable simplification, one may say that to be a mother equals to be like mother, to reject motherhood is a rejection of mother. Between these two extremes one may postulate various attempts at compromise. At one end of the spectrum are those women who remain virgins throughout their lives, next those who live in an infertile marriage, then spontaneous aborters, those wanting induced abortions and those with a number of obstetric complications. In other words, if the unconscious rejection of motherhood is overcome sufficiently to permit a pregnancy, it might nevertheless operate strongly enough to result in various complications, including para-partum neurotic reactions.

We wish to emphasize that we believe the key conflict to be the ambivalence between the instinct of procreation and the rejection of the feminine role. The former is of course reinforced by social convention, the family's, including the husband's expectations, and perhaps a neurotic wish for someone to possess and be dependent on oneself. In modern Western society the rejection of motherhood is in turn reinforced by a demand on the woman to be economically productive, not only reproductive. There is no doubt that the emancipation of woman has increased her difficulties in solving her conflict.

It is extremely difficult to test these hypotheses in a scientific way. Few attempts have been made and the evidence is scarce. In one study of identical twins discordant for motherhood, i.e. pairs where one twin was a mother the other not, it was found that in 8 pairs the twins admitted different contact with their mother. In 7 of these pairs the twin closer to the mother was a mother herself. When the health of the twins with children was considered in relation to the cause of childlessness in the co-twins, some interesting observations were made. (1) In pairs where the co-twin was unmarried, or had married after menopause, the index twin showed mainly psychiatric over-morbidity compared with her co-twin. (2) When the co-twin was married but voluntarily childless, the index twin was more somatically ill; and finally (3) in pairs where the co-twin was sterile for organic causes, the index twin was also more prone to gynaecological diseases. In the majority of the pairs the twins probably share a common basic attitude towards motherhood due to their identical genetic set-up and common early environment. This is illustrated by the fact that the mean age at first pregnancy of the probands was significantly higher than that of primiparae in the general population. Therefore it seems justified to suppose that the childlessness of the co-twins and the over-morbidity of the index twins are, at least partly, expressions of the same phenomenon. As the twins of this sample were all over forty years old, the study was designed to cover the long-term course, and the findings must be judged with caution.[16, 21] They seem, however, to lend some support to the main theory.

In our retrospective study we found a strong correlation between the number of post-partum neurotic symptoms and a history of earlier spontaneous abortions. When aborters were compared with matched controls from the same sample, it was found that there were significantly more aborters who had a high number of symptoms, but also more who were symptom-free the year after the subsequent, successful pregnancy. By closer study, it was found that there were among the aborters more women who admitted a closer contact with their father during childhood and who were also free from neurotic symptoms during that time. There were also more aborters who had lost their father and were more neurotic during childhood. In contrast, women with a closer contact with their mothers and satisfactory mental health during childhood were commoner in the control group. These seem to be the only controlled studies supporting the assumption of an association between early attachment, complication of pregnancy and para-partum neurotic reactions.[15, 20]

In our prospective study, some patterns are emerging which seem to lend further support to these views. For several reasons we chose the conscious attitude towards the present pregnancy at first examination (i.e. whether the pregnancy was planned or unplanned, wanted or unwanted) as a starting-point. A negative and, still more an ambivalent attitude implied a high risk of neurotic symptoms post-partum. Women with such attitudes had had more often than others unsatisfactory relations with their mothers during childhood and adolescence, and they had been insufficiently informed about sexual matters, particularly about menarche. They had had sexual experiences earlier than other women, and more frequently had had more than one sexual partner. In their marriages they were the dominant partner, their sexual adaptation was poorer, they had more frequently an unsatisfactory relationship with their husbands, who often wanted more children than they themselves did. They also admitted a stronger inclination for a professional life than for motherhood. In contrast, women who had grown up with sisters only, or were only children, had significantly more often a positive attitude to their pregnancies. This seems to indicate that a feminine dominance in the family makes it easier to accept motherhood, at least as far as the conscious attitude is concerned.

In summary, women with bad or unsatisfactory relations with their mothers during infancy and adolescence, and women with early object-losses had, largely, poorer sexual adaptation before marriage, a negative attitude to the pregnancy and more post-partum neurosis. These observations also support the main hypothesis.

So far we have only been able to identify women with a conscious rejection of the pregnancy. As already mentioned, we believe that a number of women suppress their rejection, but it still remains a forceful factor in them.

These theories still await confirmation from greater and different samples. The study of further groups of women with para-partum neurosis and other psychological (as well as physiological) patterns is still at its very beginning.

4

Conclusion

The data already available clearly show, however, that para-partum neurotic reactions should be of prime importance to those responsible for preventive medicine. The enormous profits in terms of better health achieved by the ante-natal clinics ought to show the way. To us it seems quite natural to think of psychological ante-natal clinics, staffed by gynae-cologists and general practitioners trained in psychological medicine and collaborating with psychiatrists. Such clinics would be wise investment not only in the service of the present, but above all, for future generations.

REFERENCES

1. ARENTSEN, K. 1966 *Om psykoser opstået efter fødsler med saerligt henblick på prognosen*. (On psychoses beginning after childbirth with special consideration of the prognosis.) Odense: Andelsbogtrykkeriet.
2. BAKER, A. A. 1967. *Psychiatric disorders in obstetrics*. Oxford: Blackwell.
3. BISKIND, L. 1958. Emotional aspects of pre-natal care. *Postgrad. Med.*, 633.
4. DEUTSCH, H. 1944. *The psychology of women*. New York: Grune & Stratton.
5. DEUTSCH, H. 1948. *Problems of early infancy*. New York: Grune & Stratton.
6. EBERHARD, G., JOHNSON, G., NILSSON, L. and SMITH, G. J. W. 1965. Clinical experimental approaches to the description of depression and anti-depressive therapy. *Acta psychiat. scand.*, **41**, suppl. 186.
7. ENGSTRÖM, L., AF GEIJERSTAM, G., HOLMBERG, N. G. and UHRUS, K. 1964. A prospective study of the relationship between psycho-social factors and course of pregnancy and delivery. *J. psychosom. Res.*, **8**, 151.
8. GORDON, R. E., KAPOSTINS, E. E. and GORDON, K. K. 1965. Factors in post-partum emotional adjustment. *Obstet and Gynec.*, **25**: 2, 158.
9. GORDON, R. E. and GORDON, K. K. Factors in post-partum emotional adjustment. Presented at the American Orthopsychiatric Association Annual Meeting. Washington.
10. HAMILTON, J. A. 1962. *Post-partum psychiatric problems*. Saint Louis: C. V. Mosby Company.
11. JACOBSON, L., KAIJ, L. and NILSSON, Å. 1965. Post-partum mental disorders in an unselected sample: frequency of symptoms and predisposing factors. *Brit. med. J.*, **1**, 1640.
12. JACOBSON, L., KAIJ, L. and NILSSON, Å. 1967. The course and outcome of the post-partum period from a gynaecological and general somatic standpoint. *Acta obstet. gynec. scand.*, **46**, 183.
13. JANSSON, B. 1964. Psychic insufficiencies associated with childbearing. *Acta psychiat. scand.*, **39**, suppl. 172.
14. KAIJ, L., JACOBSON, L. and NILSSON, Å. 1967. Post-partum mental disorder in an unselected sample. The Influence of parity. *J. psychosom. Res.*, **10**, 317.
15. KAIJ, L., MALMQUIST, A. and NILSSON, Å. 1969. Psychiatric aspects of spontaneous abortion. II. The importance of bereavement, attachment and neurosis in early life. *J. psychosom. Res.*, **13**, 53.
16. KAIJ, L. and MALMQUIST, A. 1971. Motherhood and childlessness in monozygous twins. I. Early relationship. *Brit. J. Psychiat.*, **118**, 11.
17. KANE, F. J., HARMAN, W. J., Keeler, M. H. and EWING, J. A. 1968. Emotional and cognitive disturbance in the early puerperium. *Brit. J. Psychiat*, **114**, 99.
18. KRÜGER, H. 1965. Zur Psychodynamik der Gestationspsychosen. *Z. Psychother, med. Psychol.*, **15**, 230.
19. MACCOBY, E. E. 1967. The development of sex differences. London: Tavistock.
20. MALMQUIST, A., KAIJ, L. and NILSSON. Å. 1969. Psychiatric aspects of spontaneous abortion. I. A matched control study of women with living children. *J. psychosom. Res.*, **13**, 45.
21. MALMQUIST, A. and KAIJ, L. 1971. Motherhood and childlessness in monozygous twins. II. The influence of motherhood on health. *Brit. J. Psychiat.*, **118**, 22.
22. MARCÉ, L. V. 1858. *Traité de la folie des femmes enceintes, des nouvelles accouchées et des nourrices*. Paris: Baillière et Fils.

23. McDONALD, R. L. 1965. Personality characteristics in patients with three obstetric complications. *Psychosom. Med.*, **27**, 383.
24. NILSSON, Å., KAIJ, L. and JACOBSON, L. 1967. Post-partum mental disorder in an unselected sample. The psychiatric history. *J. psychosom. Res.*, **10**, 327.
25. NILSSON, Å., KAIJ, L. and JACOBSON, L. 1967. Post-partum mental disorder in an unselected sample. The importance of the unplanned pregnancy. *J. psychosom. Res.*, **10**, 341.
26. NILSSON, Å. 1970. Para-natal emotional adjustment. *Acta psychiat. scand.*, Suppl. **220.**
27. PAFFENBARGER, R. S. 1964. Epidemiological aspects of parapartum mental illness. *Brit. J. prev. soc. Med.*, **18**, 189.
28. PAFFENBARGER, R. S. and McCABE, L. J. 1966. The effect of obstetric and perinatal events on risk of mental illness in women of childbearing age. *Amer. J. publ. Hlth.*, **56**, 400.
29. PITT, B. 1968. "Atypical" depression following childbirth. *Brit. J. Psychiat.*, **114**, 1325.
30. PROTHEROE, C. 1969. Puerperal psychoses: a long-term study 1927–1961. *Brit. J. Psychiat.*, **115**, 9.
31. PUGH, T. F., JERATH, B. K., SCHMIDT, W. M. and REED, R. B. 1963. Rates of mental disease related to childbearing. *The New Engl. J. Med.*, **268**, 1224.
32. RHEINGOLD, J. C. 1964. *The fear of being a woman.* New York: Grune & Stratton.
33. ROBIN, A. A. 1962. The psychological changes of normal parturition. *Psychiat. Quart.*, **36**, 129.
34. TETLOW, C. 1953. Psychoses of childbearing. Read at the Quarterly Meeting of the Royal Medico-Psychological Association held at Warwick.
35. THOMAS, C. L. and GORDON, J. E. 1959. Psychosis after childbirth: ecological aspects of a single impact stress. *Amer. J. med. Sci.*, **238**, 363.
36. TOD, E. D. M. 1964. Puerperal depression: a prospective epidemiological study. *Lancet*, ii, 1264.
37. WINOKUR, G. and WERBOFF, J. 1956. The relationship of conscious maternal attitudes to certain aspects of pregnancy. *The psychiat. Quart.*, Suppl.
38. YALOM, I. D., LUNDE, D. T., MOOS, R. H. and HAMBURG, D. A. 1968. "Postpartum Blues' syndrome": a description and related variables. *Arch. gen Psychiat.*, **18**, 16.

XXI

LACTATION—ITS PSYCHOLOGIC COMPONENTS

NILES NEWTON
M.A., PH.D. (Columbia)
Associate Professor, Division of Psychology
Department of Psychiatry, Northwestern
University Medical School, Chicago
U.S.A.

MICHAEL NEWTON
M.A. (Cambridge), M.B.B.CH. (Cambridge)
M.D. (Pennsylvania), F.A.C.O.G., F.A.C.S.
Clinical Professor
Department of
Obstetrics and Gynaecology
Pritzker School of Medicine
Division of Biological Sciences
University of Chicago
Chicago, U.S.A.

1

Introduction

The rapidity with which lactation failure spreads through human groups suggests that it is triggered by psychologic factors. For instance, national surveys have indicated that the percentage of babies who were completely bottle fed on discharge from hospitals in the United States increased from 35% to 63% in just ten years (1946–1956).[43] A further 10% increase in complete bottle feeding was found in 1966.[44] In the course of twenty years in Bristol, England, the number of three-month-old breast-fed infants dropped from 77 to 36%.[66] In an obstetric clinic in France the proportion of babies getting *no* breast milk increased from 31 to 51% in just five years.[67] This decrease is so rapid that hereditary factors could not be operative and major physiologic changes in function would be unlikely in the absence of radical stresses, such as starvation or epidemic disease. Human emotions and behavior, however, may change rapidly in keeping with the rapid changes observed in rates of breast-feeding.

Human lactation is sensitive to a wide variety of interrelated factors which will be discussed in the following order:

1. Individual psychological factors in the mother and in the baby which appear to be related both to the initiation and the continuation of breast-feeding.

2. Group psychological factors, including group attitudes, and sociological and historical trends which appear to be related to the initiation and continuation of breast-feeding.

3. Psycho-physical mediating mechanisms, through which individual and group psychological factors actually influence the production of milk in women attempting to breast-feed.

4. The practical management of lactation based on the factors discussed in 1, 2, and 3.

2

Individual Psychological Factors

Verbalized Attitude of Mother

Breast-feeding performance is closely related to what the mother says about her attitudes toward breast-feeding. Newton and Newton[56] interviewed 91 patients in the immediate post-partum period. Replies to questions were written down verbatim as nearly as possible and judged by two independent referees who did not know the patients or their breast-feeding history. Feeding procedures were the same for all mothers. Babies were brought out to the mothers six times a day, staying with the mother for forty-five minutes to an hour each time. This allowed the mother with favorable attitudes toward breast-feeding to relax with her baby, cuddling it and suckling it, up to four or five hours a day. The mothers judged to have positive attitudes toward breast-feeding gave more milk (p less than 0·01) and were more successful (p less than 0·01) than those judged to express negative feelings toward breast-feeding, as shown in Table I.

TABLE I

Relation of Attitudes toward Breast-feeding to
Breast-feeding Performance

Verbalized attitude toward breast-feeding	Mean amount of Milk obtained by baby at 4th-Day Feedings	Successful nursing by mothers*
	gm	%
Positive	59	74
Ambivalent	42	35
Negative	35	26

* as judged by no need for bottle supplement after 4th hospital day.

Four subsequent studies have confirmed the finding that breast-feeding performance is related to verbalized attitudes toward breast feeding.[28, 53, 71, 84]

Physical Response of Mother

The survival of the human race, long before the concept of "duty" evolved, depended upon the satisfactions gained from the two voluntary acts of reproduction—coitus and breast-feeding. These had to be sufficiently pleasurable to ensure their frequent occurrence.

The physiologic responses in coitus and lactation are closely allied. Uterine contractions occur both during suckling[45] and during sexual excitement.[34] Nipple erection occurs during both.[37, 55] Milk ejection has been observed to occur during sexual excitement in women.[9] Moreover, the degree of ejection appears to be related to the degree of sexual response.

Extensive breast stimulation occurs during breast-feeding. Breast stimulation alone can induce orgasm in some women.[34] Emotions aroused by sexual contact and breast-feeding contact both involve skin changes. Sexual excitement causes marked vascular changes in the skin.[37] The breast-feeding act raises body temperature as measured in submammary and mammary skin area.[1] Masters and Johnson[38] found that nursing women had a higher level of sexual interest than non-nursing post-partum women. Nursing mothers not only reported sexual stimulation from suckling but also, as a group, were interested in as rapid a return to active intercourse with their husbands as possible.

Feelings of aversion for the breast-feeding act appear to be related to dislike of nudity and sexuality. The Newsons,[47] after interviewing more than 700 English mothers, commented "For many mothers, modesty and feeling of distaste form a major factor in their preference for the artificial methods.' Salber and her associates,[72] working with American mothers who had never attempted to nurse, stated "The idea of nursing repelled them. They were excessively embarrassed at the idea or too 'modest' to nurse." Adams[2] found that primiparas who stated a desire to bottle-feed showed significantly more "psycho-sexual disturbances" in various measures collected in interviews and by tests (p values ranging from 0·05 to 0·001). Sears et al.[73] found that mothers who breast-fed were also significantly (p less than 0·02) more tolerant in sexual matters such as masturbation and social sex play. Nor are these feelings limited to those of Anglo-Saxon culture. Upper-middle-class Ladinos of Guatemala are reported to "express notions of modesty, distaste and boredom in regard to breast-feeding."[75]

Both psychologic feelings of frigidity toward the breast-feeding act and physiologic measures of response have been related to breast-feeding failure. Both Bloomfield[3] and Newson and Newson[47] found indications of a positive relation between enjoyment of breast-feeding and duration of breast-feeding. Newson and Newson,[47] using questions that probed beyond the conventional answers, found that 66% of the mothers who breast-fed for two weeks or more "actively enjoyed the experience", often describing the tenderness and closeness engendered by the breast-feeding act. Hytten *et al.,*[28] however, report that none of the primigravidas who breast-fed for three months "found it physically or emotionally pleasurable".

On the physiologic level the thermal skin response and the nipple-erection reflex appear to be related to milk production. Abolins[1] reported a "strong positive correlation" between milk supply and rise in temperature of mammary skin due to nursing. Gunther,[17] in a study of nipple protractility in breast-feeding mothers, found that those whose total nipple protractility was 2·5 cm usually experienced successful breast-feeding, whereas those with just 0·25 to 0·50 cm less protractility were notably less successful in establishing breast-feeding. Masters,[37] studying nipple erection as part of sexual excitement, observed an increase of 1 to 1·5 cm in nipple length that was due to stimulation. This suggests that the nipple-erection reflex may lead to more efficient nursing.

Other Maternal Behavior and Attitudes

In many mammals motherly interest and care are almost synonymous with the course of lactation. There is also evidence that maternal behavior and maternal attitude may be related to breast-feeding behavior in women.

Potter and Klein[60] did a detailed study of 25 nursing couples in a Brooklyn, New York, hospital. A rating of the mother's "nursing behavior" was obtained by observation of the way she handled the baby at breast-feeding time. Each mother was also rated on "maternal interest" through a lengthy interview centering on such questions as doll play in childhood, interest in other people's babies and number of children desired. As calculated from the tabular data presented by Potter and Klein, the high correlation of $+0·648$ (p less than 0·001) is found to exist between the nursing-behavior index and the maternal-interest index. Home visits[60] to 16 mothers indicated that all those who rated low on the maternal-interest scale had discontinued nursing immediately upon discharge from the hospital. Of those who had ranked high on the maternal-interest scale, all but 1 had continued to nurse.

Other studies indicate a relation between breast-feeding and motherly interest. Both Brown *et al.*[7] and Adams[2] questioned nulliparas concerning feeding choice during pregnancy. Both found that bottle-feeding choice was significantly correlated with mother-centred reasons for feeding choice, whereas those planning to breast-feed tended to give reasons concerned with the welfare of the baby. We[58] observed a significant relation (p less than 0.05) between ratings of reactions of mothers to the first sight of their babies and ratings of attitudes toward breast-feeding as expressed during a later interview to a different observer who did not know the first rating. Mothers judged to react to their babies with joy and delight more frequently expressed the desire to breast-feed them.

Three studies have concentrated on the behaviour of mothers of older children with past attempts to breast-feed. Two studies[22, 73] dealing with populations in which breast-feeding was on the average so brief that it might be considered "problem lactation" found no statistically significant relations between maternal behaviour and duration of breast-feeding except that Sears et al.[73] did report differences in the area of sexuality as previously mentioned. Freeman[15] worked with children from the Institute of Child Guidance, New York City, who constituted a population in which some well established lactation existed. She studied 100 cases randomly selected from those breast-fed for one year or more and 100 cases randomly selected from those breast-fed for one month or less. The former were more than twice as likely to have been rated as suffering from maternal "overprotection" than those receiving little or no breast-feeding, who were more than twice as likely to be rated as "rejected".

A recent investigation of the relation of lactation to maternal behavior by Newton, Peeler and Rawlins[59] controlled some of the variables that have made previous research studies suggestive but not conclusive. Nursing and non-nursing post-parturient mice were paired and given adoptive litters. Nursing and non-nursing post-parturient human beings were matched for parity and educational status. No significant differences in maternal behavior between pair members were found on some items of maternal behavior. However, nursing and non-nursing mothers differed significantly in their willingness to have the baby in bed with them. Seventy-four per cent of the nursing and 29% of the non-nursing mothers did so. The nursing members of mouse pairs manifested a similar significantly heightened drive to be in close contact with the young.

Life Experiences of the Mother

Some life experiences of the mother appear to be related to breast-feeding success, especially labor and breast-feeding of previous children, although more remote experiences associated with the breast-feeding mother's own infancy may also play a part.

The importance of obstetric experience is suggested by N. Newton's[53] finding that primiparas who had slow labors were significantly (p less than 0·05) more likely to have negative attitudes toward breast-feeding. Jackson and her co-workers[30] studied the relation of breast-feeding to labor difficulty with the use of a scale that gave points for the amount of anesthesia required, length of labor and use of forceps. The more difficult the labor, as rated by this scale, the lower the rate of breast-feeding.

Previous attempts to breast-feed may also determine attitudes. Bloomfield,[3] working with a sample in which only 16% breast-fed for three months, found that 66% of the mothers who had been this successful once repeated the performance. Robinson[65] in a study of 3,266 infants, gained the clinical impression that multiparas who failed in previous lactations were likely to take the infants off the breast when they returned to household duties. They failed and "were quite sure they would fail again".

Recent research with other mammals suggests the possibility that mother-baby contact in the mother's own infancy is also related to the ability to breast-feed in adulthood. For instance, four female macaque monkeys raised in partial isolation in individual wire cages were finally impregnated in spite of the "inadequacy of their sexual behavior".[19] The maternal behavior of all four mothers was completely abnormal, ranging from indifference to abuse. Whereas the usual macaque mother requires the efforts of more than one human attendant to separate her from her baby, these mothers paid no attention when their infants were removed for feeding by hand, necessitated by the mother's refusal to nurse. Eventually, two of the mothers did permit fairly frequent nursing, but at the same time became more violently abusive toward their offspring.[19] Similar abnormal maternal behavior has been observed in rat and goat mothers that had been subjected to partial mother separation in their own infancy.[18, 36]

Personality

Of three recent studies specifically concerned with the relation of personality to breast-feeding, only Call's[8] inadequately controlled exploratory report deals with the most pertinent problem—the relation of personality to success in breast-feeding among those who try. He found indications that women who continued to breast-feed after starting were likely to be more maternal and less conventional. Women who decided to bottle-feed appeared to be the least anxious; yet of those who actually put the baby to the breast, it seemed to be the calmer mother who was most likely to continue.

Plans to bottle-feed or breast-feed appear to be related to certain other personality characteristics measured in pregnancy, in women expecting their first babies. Adams[2] found that bottle-choice women responded to pregnancy with significantly (p less than 0.01) more dependency as measured during interview. They also showed significantly more disturbed behaviour on eight items of the Blackey test, as compared with one item for the breast-choice group. Brown et al.,[6] working with women of higher and lower social class, found a personality difference that crossed class lines. Both clinic and private patients showed significant (p less than 0.01) differences in the Fc response on the Rorschach test. This may be interpreted to mean that the breast-choice mothers placed more importance on the exchange of affection with other people than bottle-choice mothers.

Infant's Behavior and Emotions

Breast-feeding is a co-operative process between two people; smooth function depends on the behavior of the baby as much as on the behavior of the the mother. Behavior problems in the baby can occur at the level of inefficient sucking, dislike of the nursing situation, and lack of responsiveness.

Inefficient sucking by the baby is sometimes related to medical management techniques. Brazelton[5] found a high relation between the ability to nurse effectively and the amount of barbiturate medication given to the mother during labor. On the first day only 30% of the feedings of babies from heavily medicated mothers were rated as effective as compared with 65% of those of babies from the lightly medicated (p equal to 0·03). The differences for the second day were 25% vs. 65% (p equal to 0·002), for the third day 35% vs. 75% (p equal to 0·001) and for the fourth day 55% vs. 87% (p equal to 0·001). Not until the fifth and sixth days were the babies of heavily medicated mothers as alert and effective in nursing situations as those of less heavily medicated mothers. This finding has now been confirmed and extended. The study of Kron et al.[35] indicates that newborn infants whose mothers had received a single dose of obstetric sedation during labor sucked at significantly lower rates and pressures and consumed less nutrient than those born to mothers who had received no obstetric sedation. Drug effects persisted at a significant level throughout the four-day period that the infants remained in the newborn nursery.

Another frequent way in which the baby comes to reject breast-feeding is by being taught other techniques of sucking that are not appropriate to the breast. Davis et al.[11] studied neonates fed by bottle, cup and breast for ten days. Interest in sucking continued to rise in those fed by breast. They showed a significantly (p less than 0·01) longer sucking response on a standard sucking test from the fourth to the tenth day as compared with those fed by bottle. This finding is in keeping with the observation that supplementary bottle feeding interferes with the milk supply.[16, 57] Gunther[17] has suggested that the rubber nipple acts as a supersign stimulus to the infant in the same way that an oyster catcher, presented with her own eggs and wooden ones of twice the size, will sit on the larger, artificial ones.

The pleasantness of the feeding situation may also influence the baby's attitude towards breast-feeding. Robinson[65] observed that "many infants whose mothers fed them strictly by the clock refused point-blank to take the breast after the age of three months and had to be bottle fed or starve. The breast was not refused if the mother was easy-going and fed her infant by instinct rather than by the clock." Scheduling of a few large feedings causes the breast to be overfull, so that when ejection occurs, the milk may spurt out, choking the infant. Cutting out the air supply, even temporarily, may be a quick way to instill fear or ambivalence. Ejection-reflex failures can also teach the baby to dislike the breast; it may be frustrating to have little milk available at some times and an abundance at others. Newton and Newton[50] found that breast-feeding was significantly (p less than 0·01) more successful when there was less fluctuation in the amount of milk obtained from one feeding to the next.

Responsiveness may also influence the baby's enjoyment and co-operation with breast-feeding. Middlemore, as quoted by Gunther,[17] accurately described responsive and frigid breast-feeding on the part of the baby. She stated: "The active satisfied babies established the sucking reflex and rhythm quickly ... and showed their pleasure by seeking the nipple when it was withdrawn." These are contrasted to the inert ones: "they did not move much or cry at the breast.'

The reaction of older babies to breast-feeding is even more clearly observable. The total body shows signs of eagerness—rhythmic motions of hands, feet, fingers and toes may occur along with the rhythm of sucking. Erection of the penis is common in male babies. After feeding, there is often a relaxation that is characteristic of the conclusion of satisfactory sexual response. The sensuous enjoyment of breast-feeding is likely to increase the baby's desire to suckle his mother frequently and fully, thus stimulating the secretion of milk.

3

Group Psychological Factors

Feelings Related to Female Status

The impact of an industrial money economy—with the breaking up of the wider family unit as the main economic unit of society—has had far-reaching effects on the role of women and the value placed on woman's unique biologic contributions.[53] When the wider family group stops co-operating in home manufacture and home production of food and material, women and children in the family become economic liabilities unless they go out to work and earn money. Children are no longer associated with rise in social status; large families may pull down the social standing of a family in industrial culture. If economic matters are related to man's emotions, children are no longer as desirable and beloved, and the status of women as bearers of children has fallen. Furthermore, women who stay at home, while more and more of the economic activity leaves the home, are no longer contributing so much to society economically. Feelings of security may depend in part on the feeling of being needed and essential.

N. Newton[53] has emphasized the point that women's joy and acceptance of the female biologic role in life may be an important factor in their psychosexual behavior, which includes lactation. She found through interviewing women under controlled conditions in the post-partum period that women who desired to bottle-feed also were significantly (p less than 0·05) more likely to say that men have a more satisfying time in life. Adams[2] similarly found that nulliparas who planned to breast-feed significantly (p less than 0·05) more frequently stated their satisfaction with woman's role in life.

This line of thinking and evidence tends to fit in with historical attitudes toward breast-feeding. Periods of great wealth and luxury in the Western world—the age of Imperial Rome, Athens in the time of Pericles, the era of Louis XIV in Paris,[69] early eighteenth-century England and Colonial America,[4, 69]—were characterized by the rejection of breast-feeding by large numbers of women who used wet-nursing or artificial feeding in the form of pap to sustain infants. In these eras upper-class women may have tended to be objects of amusement rather than real contributors to the work of the societies. Thus, they may have tended to feel somewhat worthless and in-secure. However, in what Toynbee calls "times of trouble" breast-feeding has been popular.[81]

Feelings Related to Region, Education, Social Class and Work

Woman's role in life, as determined by her cultural locale, education, social class and work, has been repeatedly shown to be related to her breast-feeding behavior. Breast-feeding rates differ with even slight variations in region or culture. Thus, Meyer's[43] 1956 survey indicated that more than half the babies discharged from hospitals in Arizona, Colorado, Georgia, Idaho, New Mexico, Oklahoma and Utah were still getting some breast milk, whereas only 20% or less of those discharged from hospitals in Connecticut, Maine and Massachusetts were still wholly or partially breast-fed. The effect of size of community was shown in an extensive California study, in which the duration of breast-feeding was found to increase with increase in size of community where the mother lived most of her life.[23] The effect of sub-cultural groups can be seen in a study of women in Victoria, Australia, where Greek-speaking and Italian-speaking mothers had a lower artificial feeding rate than English-speaking mothers.[48] Marked national differences in breast-feeding were found in a cross-cultural study involving London, Paris, Stockholm, Brussels, and Zürich. Not only was the overall incidence different, but significant differences in the type of weaning curves were observed.[26]

Breast-feeding rates are very sensitive to differences in education and social class in some cultures. American mothers with high-school education have a lower breast-feeding rate than those with college education.[47, 64, 71] Higher education may also favor breast-feeding in the developing country of Uganda.[83] A cross-cultural study found higher breast-feeding rates associated with high social status in Zürich and Stockholm, but not in Brussels and Paris where no sign of class differences in breast-feeding was noted.[26] British and American studies found that the highest social status definitely favored breast-feeding.[47, 64, 70, 71, 87]

However, the relation between social class and breast-feeding appears sometimes to be bimodal. Those of the very lowest social groups, like those of the highest, are sometimes reported with higher breast-feeding rates than the middle group,[23, 64, 71] but this is not always true.[47, 87]

These discrepancies may be partly a matter of spreading fashions, influencing different social groups at different times. Differences in how breast-feeding is measured may also cause confusion. For instance, in Cork, Ireland a 1954 study[10] found that in comparison with social Groups 4 and 5, the financially well-off Groups 1 and 2 were less likely to start breast-feeding (50% *vs.* 67%), but those who started were more likely to continue. Thus, by six months the statistics were reversed: 14·6% of social Groups 1 and 2 babies were breast-fed beyond six months, as compared with 8·4% of Groups 4 and 5 babies. However, in contrast to this, a 1965 study in California found just the opposite. The highly educated mothers with four or more years of college started breast-feeding more frequently than others, but were less inclined to continue breast-feeding once started.[23]

Another confusing factor in assessment of breast-feeding rates may be the fact that some mothers reported as breast-feeding, actually did so only partially. Salber and Feinleib[70] found that among Boston mothers reported as nursing their babies for three months or more, 70% also gave the bottle, and 71% introduced solid food before the baby was three months old.[70]

Woman's work-load certainly influences breast-feeding but here again, the situation is complex and depends not on the work alone but on how the work is carried out. Work itself interferes little with breast-feeding in cultures that are accepting enough of the baby so that they permit the baby to accompany the woman as she works. Many non-Western cultures of both the simple and the complex types depend heavily on women's work contributions; yet breast-feeding flourishes for two or more years with each baby because the work does not involve mother-baby separation.[42]

On the other hand, even very simple cultures can manifest emotional indifference to breast-feeding when the mother is the chief source of economic support and when her work requires her to be away from the baby for long periods. This is true of the women of Alor in the Lesser Sundas.[42] Jelliffe[32] emphasizes that the need for tropical women to go out to work all day is a cause of increasingly early weaning in urban groups and more sophisticated rural groups as well.

Effect of Feelings of Others

Many people working with mothers acquire a strong suspicion that the attitude of husband, family, and friends may have a real bearing on breast-feeding behavior. However, this is difficult to document. There does not appear to have been any statistical effort made to correlate fathers' attitudes toward nursing and its success. Grandmothers' ardor for breast-feeding does not appear to be related to breast-feeding rates.[84] Bloomfield[3] noted that mothers acted more like their friends, 80% of whom preferred bottle-feeding, than like their own mothers, 75% of whom approved of breast-feeding.

The effect of medical personnel is more clearly delineated. The enthusiastic physician can develop a practice in which the breast-feeding rates of his patients are far above that usual in the rest of the society.[33, 79, 82] A recent example is the breast-feeding program started by an American obstetrician in 1959. In two years the hospital breast-feeding rate of her practice jumped from 33 to 65%, and 52% of those who started breast-feeding continued to five months as compared with 15% previously.[62]

Enthusiasm about lactation in cultures with declining lactation rates, however, is frequently considered improper: the physician may lose status because of it. Two recent studies in the United States[7] and England[27] have analyzed the feelings of medical personnel toward breast-feeding, finding a general lack of strong enthusiasm of the type that appears to be associated with successful medical breast-feeding programs.

Lack of interest or rejective feelings in any area may tend to hinder the dissemination of knowledge in that area. This makes it hard for those who are interested to obtain facts. This is true of breast-feeding. As early as 1920 Sedgwick and Fleischner[74] were dismayed because so much more time was being spent in American medical schools teaching about artificial feeding than about breast-feeding. Rejective feelings have also made it necessary to hide the fact of breast-feeding, thus impeding the flow of knowledge by observation. Just twenty years ago in rural Mississippi, breast-feeding in church was acceptable; seventy-five years ago in Indiana, upper-class women naturally took their babies to afternoon parties to nurse them as needed. Now in the United States there is a strong taboo on nursing in public or even showing photographs of nursing babies, whereas bottle-feeding in public and pictures of bottle-feeding babies are totally acceptable. Thus, a young girl often starts breast-feeding without ever once having had a chance to observe another woman breast-feeding. She is ignorant, even if she is interested.

4

Psycho-physical Mediating Mechanisms

The Milk-ejection Reflex

This is a neurohormonal mechanism, regulated in part by central-nervous-system factors. The primary stimulus is suckling applied to the nipple, which triggers the discharge of oxytocin from the posterior pituitary gland that is carried to the breast in the blood. The oxytocin acts on the myoepithelial cells around the alveoli, causing them to contract, and thus pushing out the milk into the larger ducts, where it is more easily available to the baby.[51]

The psychologic importance of the milk-ejection reflex in human beings was first emphasized by Waller[80] in his book, *Clinical studies in lactation.* He used case histories to illustrate the fact that milk ejection can be inhibited by embarrassment, and can be conditioned so that it is set off by the mere thought of the baby far away.

Newton and Newton[49] inhibited the milk-ejection reflex experimentally in a mother through distractive techniques that did not appear to disturb the baby. These consisted of placing the feet in ice water, painfully pulling the toes, and asking the solution of mathematical problems, punishing mistakes with electric shocks.

Table II shows how the amount of milk obtained by the baby varied. On control days, when there was no disturbance, the baby obtained significantly (p less than 0·01) more milk than when the mother was subjected to disturbance. The amount of milk rose to near normal, however, when oxytocin was injected to set off the milk-ejection reflex artificially.

TABLE II

*Effect of Maternal Disturbance and Oxytocin on
the Amount of Milk Obtained by the Baby*

Maternal disturbance	Mean amount of milk obtained by infant during standardized feeding
No distractions-no injection	168
Distraction-saline injection	99
Distraction-oxytocin injection	153

The relation of the reflex as set off by natural stimuli to the overall success of breast-feeding was studied experimentally.[50] The baby was first allowed to nurse fully to set off the milk-ejection reflex. Then the breasts were each pumped for five minutes. Finally, 3 units of oxytocin (Pitocin) was injected, and each breast was pumped again for five minutes. The unsuccessful breast-feeding mothers showed some failure in natural ejection, since 47% of the total milk obtained was available only after artificial ejection. The percentage for successful breast-feeding mothers was 27. The difference is statistically significant (p less than 0·01).

Another way of demonstrating the relation of the milk-ejection reflex to the success of breast-feeding was to study the clinical signs that accompany milk ejection. The following signs, which can be easily recognized and reported by the mother, were studied: milk dripping from the breast opposite the one being nursed; uterine cramps during nursing due to the action of oxytocin on the uterus; and cessation of nipple discomfort during a feeding as the baby begins to obtain milk, thus easing the negative pressure. Newton and Newton[50] compared 53 successful breast-feeders (no supplementation after the fourth day) with 50 unsuccessful breast-feeders (supplementation required after the fourth day). The total average milk-ejection symptoms were significantly (p less than 0·01) higher in the successful group.

The milk-ejection reflex appears to be very sensitive to small differences in oxytocin level, suggesting that minor psychosomatic changes may influence the degree to which the milk is available to the baby. Wiederman *et al.*[85] found that the intravenous threshold dose of oxytocin needed for response was 0·25 to 10mU.

Sucking Stimulation

Possibly even more important than the ejection reflex to the success of breast-feeding is the amount of sucking stimulation permitted. Far less sucking seems to be permitted in cultures where negative attitudes towards breast-feeding are common than in those where breast-feeding is almost universal. It may be a frequent human reaction to try to cut down and regulate the disliked stimulus, which in this case is sucking at the breast. Cultures that seem to emphasize breast-feeding tend to encourage it for at least two years.

Ford,[14] in his survey of 64 pre-literate cultures, found records of weaning age in 46: none of these cultures normally weaned any baby before six months; one culture weaned between six months and a year; 14 weaned some or all babies between one and two years. In 31 cultures the earliest recorded age of weaning any infant from the breast was two or three years.

Regulated, restricted, short breast-feeding, in the extreme form that is now occurring in some Western industrial countries, has developed only comparatively recently. Thus, Waller,[81] in England in 1943, wrote about feeding schedules as follows: "Not long ago the regulation spacing in this country was two hours; some twenty-five years ago it gave place to three hours, and later still to four." In 1906 Southworth,[76] an American physician, writing in a standard pediatric textbook, advised four nursings on the first day, six on the second, ten a day for the rest of the first month, eight feedings a day for the second and third months, seven feedings a day for the fourth and fifth months and six a day for the sixth to the eleventh months. He approved of night feedings through the fifth month.

There is considerable evidence in human beings that the restriction of sucking actually inhibits lactation. Salber[68] assigned 1057 neonates to one of three feeding groups during their hospital stay. Those on true self-demand, after initial weight loss, showed the most rapid weight gain and were nearest their birth weight at one week as compared with the schedule-fed infants. Neonates on three-hour schedules gained faster and were nearer their birth weight at one week than infants on four-hour schedules. Moreover, artificial sucking stimulation in the form of "emptying" the breast by hand or machine in cultures where the baby is not allowed to suck more than six times a day has been repeatedly recommended as a method of increasing yields.[63, 82] Egli et al.[12] experimentally cut down on sucking by substituting a bottle for all but three feedings daily. This caused a significant (p less than 0·05) decrease in breast milk obtained by the baby; furthermore, two days after ample sucking was re-instituted, the milk yield increased significantly (p less than 0·05), reaching its previous high level. Reducing feedings from six to five caused the "not-enough milk" syndrome to occur in about a third of primiparas studied and some few multiparas.[21] Illingworth and Stone[29] experimentally assigned one group of two-day-old babies to demand feeding, and another group to continued rigid schedules of six feedings a day. The demand babies ate more frequently, gained significantly more weight by the ninth day, caused only half as much nipple soreness in the mothers, and were significantly more likely to be breast-feeding at one month. Other studies on the effect of sucking on lactation are reviewed elsewhere.[51, 59]

Other Sensory Contact

The milk-ejection reflex and sucking stimulation depend primarily on sensory stimulation of the nipple, but other sensory stimulations, particularly auditory, visual, olfactory and tactile, may be important. Hartemann et al.,[20] in a study of mothers of premature babies, gained the clinical impression that the desire to nurse fades if the mothers do not have contact with their babies. They recommend letting mothers of premature babies have their babies as soon as possible to see and feel, to keep up their interest in nursing. McBryde[40] found that when Duke Hospital changed from routine separation of mother and baby to routine rooming-in of baby with mother, the breast-feeding rate jumped from 35·0 to 58·5%.

Research on other mammals suggests that tactile stimulation may be important. In goats, licking and nuzzling as well as soft vocalization is described[25] as a prelude to getting the neonate in a favorable position for nursing. If the mother is separated from the neonate and put back in the herd, even for a few minutes, this instinctive process is stopped. If she can be persuaded to nurse her young at all thereafter, she continues to be indifferent and gives the teat only when in "the mood".[46] This weaker maternal receptiveness causes her to accept other kids as well as her own. Hersher et al.[24] studied the nursing behavior of goat mothers that had been separated from their young within five to ten minutes after birth and then returned to them within an hour. Tests of nursing behavior two months and three months later indicated that mothers that had experienced brief sensory separation from their kids nursed other kids as long as their own. Control-group mothers nursed their own kids about six times as long as they nursed other kids.

In human cultures where breast-feeding is enjoyable enough to continue its full course, mother-baby separation is not easily tolerated by the mother or baby. Matthews[39] describes the mother-baby sensory contact among the Yorubas of Nigeria observed in 1948 to 1950, when the usual breast-feeding period was eighteen to twenty-two months as follows:

> A strict breast-feeding routine would be difficult to attain because mothers, determined and obstinate, are not easily separated from their babies for long. Cots and cradles are not welcomed. The baby will remain from birth until about the second year of life almost constantly in close physical contact with the mother, who will feed it at regular intervals, usually determined by the onset of crying.

Similar descriptions come from anthropologic accounts from Asia, North America, South America, Africa and the Middle East.[42] Mother and baby very frequently stay in continuous close sensory contact with each other (even when not in the act of nursing) in cultures characterized by late weaning and few lactation difficulties.

In contrast to this, Western cultures raise many barriers against sensory contact between mother and baby. Modern Western styles of female dress make breast-baby contact difficult. Families no longer sleep all together in one room. Narrow beds built for one person only are fashionable, and the baby, especially, is expected to sleep alone. Many hospitals in the Western world now practise separation of mothers and babies at birth, except for brief feeding times, and when the baby and mother return home the ideal is a separate room where the baby spends much of his time. These customs are relatively new. For instance, housing the baby away from the mother started in American hospitals only about sixty years ago.[4]

Here, again, the trigger mechanisms may lie in attitude changes within family life that accompany full industrialization and the money economy. A common way in which human beings express mixed feelings or ambivalence is to put distance between themselves and the object in question.

5

Management

General

Several important principles underly the management of lactation:

1. Management extends throughout the obstetric cycle from the onset of pregnancy until the baby is weaned.

2. The psychologic and physical aspects of management cannot be separated.

3. Physicians and others who attend obstetric patients should be constantly aware of their own attitudes toward lactation. A casual hostile word or a thoughtless action of neglect may be very damaging to a woman who is uncertain or ambivalent about her role in lactation.

Ante-partal Care

A preventive concept of obstetrics requires that physicians (and midwives) take responsibility for the education of all their pregnant patients in the hygiene, physiology and psychology of normal pregnancy. Information about breast-feeding is an especially important part of such a program, since such information is not easily available elsewhere. The aim should always be to give confidence to those whose personality makes it likely they will enjoy the experience and have an abundance of milk, rather than pushing the negatively inclined mother into placing a baby on the nipple for two or three weeks, which might be an unsatisfactory experience for both.

The initial ante-partal history should cover relevant details of the patient's previous breast-feeding experiences. The breasts should be carefully examined: an appropriate comment is that the breasts are adequate for successful lactation (which is almost invariably true). Data on breast-feeding and the breast should be included in the standard ante-partal record form.

The waiting room in clinics and physicians' offices can have readily available books and pamphlets that can help to relieve fears and dispel misinformation. Particularly to be recommended are *Nursing your baby*[61] and *The womanly art of breast-feeding*,[86] which will soon be available in Britain and affiliated areas from the Souvenir Press Ltd, 95 Mortimer Street,

London. Booklets on breast-feeding produced by companies profiting from the sale of cow's milk formulas should be carefully evaluated before distribution. They frequently recommend such limitation of sucking that lactation failure may be produced. Films such as "Breast feeding is a family experience" which is available from Childbirth Education Association of Seattle, 7337 27th Avenue, N.W., Seattle, Washington 98107, can be shown in ante-partal classes and in schools as part of biology and family life education classes. Even more effective than a film is a breast-feeding demonstration by a relaxed mother of an older baby who can show a group of expectant mothers how easily and modestly nursing can take place. She can also answer questions about breast-feeding.

At some point in pregnancy, preferably after exposure to factual information about breast-feeding, it is necessary for the physician (or midwife) to ascertain the patient's feelings about breast-feeding her baby. It is best if this can be done without requiring the patient to commit herself irrevocably, since the arrival of the baby may help her reach a decision that she was unwilling to make earlier.

By whatever means the physician gains an impression of his patients' wishes, his role is to support those who wish to breast-feed, and further advise those who are doubtful. *For those who appear definitely adverse to breast-feeding an attempt to overpersuade is likely to do more harm than good.* It may, in fact, damage the rapport between the patient and her attendant that is so necessary for good obstetric care.

If the patient is interested in breast-feeding, then it is desirable during her later pregnancy to introduce her to women who have successfully breast-fed their children and are interested in helping to give emotional support to others who wish to do so. An organization of mothers who have nursed successfully and stand ready to help other mothers who seek to learn the "womanly art" is the La Leche League International, 9616 Minneapolis Avenue, Franklin Park, Illinois 60131. The League now has branches in over 700 different communities mainly in the United States and Canada, but it is also represented in England, Ireland, New Zealand, Australia and some non-English-speaking countries. Other scattered nursing groups besides those affiliated with the La Leche League also exist. In Great Britain the National Childbirth Trust, 9 Queensborough Terrace, Bayswater, London W2, has shown interest in giving emotional support and information concerning breast-feeding as well as labor.

For physicians interested in keeping lactation support more closely under their own supervision, the method devised by an American obstetrician, Dr. Carolyn Rawlins, merits consideration. She chose mature kindly women from her own practice, who had nursed their own babies, to serve as breast-feeding counselors. Patients expressing desire to nurse were invited to the doctor's home in the ninth month of pregnancy for a meeting which included a discussion of breast-feeding and a personal introduction to a breast-feeding counselor.

Early Post-partum Care

The establishment of a successful lactation is in large part determined by the patient's care during the first few post-partum days. Under adverse circumstances such as are all too frequently present in modern hospitals, even the mother who is most enthusiastic about nursing her baby may be discouraged. In a favorable environment, however, the ambivalent mother is helped to breast-feed successfully.

To give maximal assistance to the mother, the environment must take into account the two most important factors in the establishment of lactation—provision of adequate sucking stimulation and promotion of the ejection reflex. This involves both the physical surroundings and the emotional climate. Although the physician obviously cannot control every factor, it is his responsibility to see that his patient has the best opportunity available to learn to nurse her baby successfully.

One of the problems besetting the management of breast-feeding in the modern specialized hospital is the fact that obstetricians take care of the mother and pediatricians take care of the baby, and frequently neither will accept full responsibility for the management of a function such as lactation, which involves both mother and baby intimately. When possible, close co-operation between obstetrician and pediatrician is essential. Specifically, each should understand the other's attitude toward breast-feeding and be familiar with the measures the other usually takes in regard to it. The same co-operation is necessary between different groups of nursing personnel.

Environment

Since sucking stimulation hastens the appearance of milk and promotes adequate secretion, arrangements which permit this are essential. Babies permitted to nurse within eight hours after delivery were found to have lost significantly less weight on the third day post-partum than those permitted no access to the breast for twenty-four hours or more.

When the mother has not received heavy sedation or deep anesthesia for labor and delivery, the normal healthy baby should be encouraged to suck immediately after delivery and as desired thereafter. Such babies suck readily and well when placed in their mothers' beds after removal from the delivery table. This response may be affected by the management of the mother during labor and delivery. A recent study indicates that when the mother receives heavy premedication, the baby may be unable to take hold and suck well until the fifth day of life.[5]

In the first few hours following delivery, observation of both mother and baby is important. Intensive-care units, in which both mother and baby receive skilled constant care together, are best for the establishment of lactation and the mother-baby relationship.[77] Following the immediate recovery period, the best arrangement is for the mother and baby to be placed in close proximity to each other (rooming-in). If this is not possible, it is expedient to have the baby brought to the mother eight times a day starting three hours after birth, provided both are in good health. The baby should stay with the mother for one hour for each of the daytime feedings, but for less time at night, when the mother is normally asleep. The mother should be encouraged to nurse and cuddle her baby as much as she desires when he is in the room with her.

Emotional Support

Friendly, sympathetic help assists the mother with a positive or ambivalent attitude to achieve lactation success, and particularly encourages early and adequate function of the ejection reflex. By far the most important part of the medical team in this respect is the nursing staff and their aides. A thoughtless word by anyone can undo much good. The nurse should always be ready to praise and encourage the nursing mother. She should help her find comfortable positions for nursing.[54] She should insure privacy as far as possible during nursing and promote a comfortable, unhurried atmosphere. The physician himself should always be aware of his responsibility for the action of these other members of his team in regard to breast-feeding and can show his interest by asking about feeding at each visit to the patient. A husband and mother who have positive attitudes toward breast-feeding can also be a source of emotional support to the patient.

Additional Measures

Lactation may be aided in several other ways that are primarily physical in nature. But accepting attitudes on the part of the mother's attendants and emotional support in administration are necessary for their full effectiveness.

1. The use of all bottles, supplementary, complementary, or prelacteal, reduces the amount of sucking stimulation received by the breast.[57] This in turn causes less milk to be secreted. Furthermore, the baby who sucks bottles develops a measurably weaker sucking reflex by four days of age, so that he gives less vigorous sucking to the breast when he is applied. In one study involving 884 patients, the simple expedient of giving supplementary food by spoon instead of bottle doubled the length of breast-feeding.[78]

2. A good uplift brassiere should be worn. It should not be too tight since this can restrict blood flow through the breast. The mother should put on a clean brassiere daily, or even oftener when there has been dripping of milk.

3. There is no necessity for special cleaning of the nipples before nursing. The breast-feeding mother should be encouraged to splash water over her breasts at bath or shower-time daily, but she should not use soap on her nipples. Soap removes the protective skin oils and leaves the nipple more prone to damage. Alcohol has also been demonstrated to be destructive to the nipple during lactation.[52] There is some evidence that substances containing petrolatum impede healing. However, plain unmedicated hydrous

lanolin applied after feedings is indicated when the mother's nipples are sensitive.

Later Post-partal Care

The first few days after the patient arrives home from the hospital are crucial in the establishment of successful lactation. The main problems which the young mother has are still related to sucking stimulation and the ejection reflex. With regard to the former, the advice given by Southworth in Carr's *Practice of pediatrics*, published in 1906, is still worth remembering since at that time successful breast-feeding was the rule rather than the exception.[76] He advised ten nursings a day for most of the first month, eight the second and third months, seven the fourth and fifth months, and six a day for the sixth through eleven months. He also approved of night feedings up through the fifth month. The problem of insufficient sucking may arise several weeks after delivery, when social and domestic responsibilities begin to demand more of the mother's attention. Rest and increased sucking for 48–72 hours often improve the milk supply.[12]

There are many things which can inhibit the injection reflex after the patient gets home. Lack of privacy, the demands of husband or other children or the disapproval of a mother or mother-in-law can quickly reduce the flow of milk to a dribble. The physician should be aware that these untoward events may occur and should try to help his patients to avoid them in advance. A woman usually needs help at home. This should come from a motherly woman who understands breast-feeding, not from a mother or mother-in-law who has never breast-fed and disapproves of the whole idea. In these days of early discharge from hospitals, adequate follow-up at home by a competent nurse interested in and understanding of breast-feeding is of great value.

Apart from the emotional climate surrounding the nursing mother at home, drugs which assist the function of the ejection reflex may be of value. A mild tranquilizer, such as one of the phenothiazine derivatives or alcohol in the form of sherry or beer, may be used. Artificial production of ejection by the intranasal use of synthetic oxytocin (Syntocinon) may be helpful.

Cessation of Lactation

When no artificial limits are set on the duration of lactation, and adequate food is available for the baby in addition to human milk, breast-feeding gradually decreases as the baby learns to eat and drink by himself. Under such circumstances nursing becomes a source of comfort to both mother and baby rather than a means of providing nourishment. Evaluation of lactation practices of preliterate and traditional human cultures suggest that the great majority of human beings throughout history have been nursed for two or three years or longer. This method of handling lactation has therefore been well tested. In contrast to this long-term effect of the human mammal, by-passing lactation or limiting it to several weeks are not yet known.

If weaning occurs suddenly because of illness of mother or baby or by reason of some externally imposed regimen, both mother and baby may experience some emotional disturbance. The mother, in addition, may have painfully swollen breasts.

When cultural pressures, social demands and personal feelings indicate that weaning is desirable, it should be accomplished so slowly that the breasts do not become overfull and the baby shows no increased irritability or failure of appetite. A good rule to follow is to drop no more than one feeding every two weeks, and never to refuse a breast to a baby who cries for it. As other food is plentifully available, and as the lack of sucking stimulation reduces the mother's milk supply, the day does eventually come that the baby can peacefully and happily accept a bottle or a biscuit instead of his last remaining scheduled nursing.

6

Summary and Conclusions

The rapid decline in breast-feeding as it is occurring in many parts of the world today[41] almost certainly is closely related to psychologic changes triggered by changes in group interaction and influenced by economic and historical trends. Breast-feeding behavior appears to be associated with the following variables in the mother: verbalized attitudes toward breast-feeding; physical responsiveness; other types of maternal behavior; life experiences, particularly in connection with labor and previous lactation; and possibly certain other personality characteristics. However, breast-feeding depends not only on the individual response of the individual mother but also on the reaction of the infant to the breast-feeding situation and on certain social variables such as definition of the female role in society, social class and educational status and attitudes fostered by interaction with others in modern industrial culture. These factors in turn may influence actual production of milk through the psycho-physiologic mediating mechanisms of the milk-ejection reflex, sucking stimulation and possibly also more generalized central nervous system effects resulting from auditory, visual, olfactory and tactile contact between mother and infant.

A woman who is interested in nursing her baby requires assistance and support throughout her reproductive cycle from pregnancy until the baby is weaned:

Ante-partum care should include:

1. an adequate lactation history and sustained interest in the patient's feelings on this subject;
2. opportunity for the patient to meet and talk with mothers who have breast-fed successfully;

3. provision of information about breast-feeding as part of a general program of ante-partum education or by personal discussion, as well as by the use of appropriate films or books.

Post-partum management both in hospital and at home should include:

1. provision of sufficient sucking stimulation to produce adequate secretion of milk by:
   (a) initiation of breast-feeding within an hour after birth if mother and baby are both in good condition and delivery has not been complicated, and as soon as possible in other mothers and babies;
   (b) encouragement of demand feeding without limitation of sucking time at each feeding.
   (c) avoidance of prelacteal, supplementary, or complementary bottles while lactation is being established, since these reduce sucking stimulation, and use of a spoon or dropper if liquids must be given.
2. Prevention of inhibition of the milk ejection reflex by:
   (a) privacy and freedom from embarrassment during nursing;
   (b) peaceful surroundings, limitation of visitors in hospital and at home, and home help provided by a woman who has herself breast-fed successfully.
   (c) use of mild analgesics or tranquilizers as needed;
   (d) use of intranasal oxytocin before nursing to produce artificial ejection of milk when indicated;
   (e) continued emotional support from physician, nursing personnel, and from a woman who has breast-fed successfully.

Care during later lactation pertains primarily to the mother, particularly when minor breast-feeding difficulties arise. It should include:

1. sufficient rest and sleep, a noncompetitive life, and a diet superior in proteins, minerals and vitamins;
2. provision of solid or semisolid food for the baby only when he is ready to take it (at least by 6 months of age);
3. slow weaning at a time mutually acceptable to mother and baby;
4. management of specific complications as they arise.

REFERENCES

1. ABOLINS, J. A. 1954. Das Stillen und die Temperatur der Brust. *Acta obstet. gynec. scand.*, **33**, 60.
2. ADAMS, A. B. 1959. Choice of infant feeding technique as function of maternal personality. *J. cons. Psychol.*, **23**, 143.
3. BLOOMFIELD, A. E. 1962. How many mothers breast feed? Survey in general practice. *Practitioner*, **188**, 343.
4. BRACKEN, F. J. 1953. Infant feeding in American colonies. *J. Amer. diet. Ass.*, **29**, 349.
5. BRAZELTON, T. B. 1961. Psychophysiologic reactions in neonate. II. Effect of maternal medication on neonate and his behavior. *J. Pediat.*, **58**, 513.

6. BROWN, F., CHASE, J. and WINSON, J. 1961. Studies in infant feeding choice of primiparae. II. Comparison of Rorschach determinants of accepters and rejecters of breast feeding. *J. project. Techn.* **25**, 412.

7. BROWN, F., LIEBERMAN, J., WINSON, J. and PLESHETTE, N. 1960. Studies in choice of infant feeding by primiparas. I. Attitudinal factors and extraneous influences. *Psychosom. Med.*, **22**, 421.

8. CALL, J. D. 1959. Emotional factors favoring successful breast feeding of infants. *J. Pediat.*, **55**, 485

9. CAMPBELL, B. and PETERSEN, W. E. 1953. Milk let-down and orgasm in human female. *Hum. Biol.*, **25**, 165.

10. CURTIN, M. 1954. Failure to breast feed: review of feeding history of 1007 infants. *Irish J. med. Sci.*, **6**, 447.

11. DAVIS, H. V., SEARS, R. R., MILLER, H. C. and BRODBECK, A. J. 1948. Effects of cup, bottle and breast feeding on oral activities of newborn infants. *Pediatrics*, **2**, 549.

12. EGLI, G. E., EGLI, N. S. and NEWTON, M. 1961. Influence of number of breast feedings on milk production. *Pediatrics*, **27**, 314.

13. EPPINK, H. 1968. An experiment to determine a basis for nursing decisions in regard to time of initiation of breast feeding. Unpublished dissertation. Health Sciences, Wayne State University. University Microfilms, Inc.: Ann Arbor. No. 69–14, 668.

14. FORD, C. S. 1945. *A comprehensive study of human reproduction*. New Haven: Yale Univ. Press (Publications in Anthropology No. 32).

15. FREEMAN, M. 1932. Factors associated with length of breast feeding. *Smith College Studies in Social Work*, **2**, 274.

16. GRULEE, C. G. 1943. Breast feeding. Papers presented at International Assembly of Inter-State Post Graduate Medical Association of North America, p. 135.

17. GUNTHER, M. 1955. Instinct and nursing couple. *Lancet*, i, 575.

18. GUZE, H. 1958. Effects of pre-weaning nursing deprivation on later maternal, hoarding and sexual behavior in rat. *Dissertation Abstr.* **18**, (6), 2227.

19. HARLOW, H. F. and HARLOW, M. K. 1962. Social deprivation in monkeys. *Scient. Am.*, **207**, 136.

20. HARTEMANN, J., REBON, M. and DELLESTABLE, P. 1962. Effects of attraction of mother and child on maintenance of nursing. *Bull. Féd. Soc. Gynéc. Obstét. franç.*, **14**, 770.

21. HARTEMANN, J. and RICHON, J. 1962. Maternal nursing and reduction of number of infant feeding times. *Bull. Féd. Soc. Gynéc. Obstét. franç.*, **14**, 773.

22. HEINSTEIN, M. Behavioral correlates of breast-bottle regimes under varying parent-infant relationships. *Monogr. Soc. Research Child Develop.* **28**, (4), 1.

23. HEINSTEIN, M. 1965. *Child rearing in California*. Berkeley: Bureau of Maternal and Child Health, Department of Health.

24. HERSHER, L., MOORE, A. U. and RICHMOND, J. B. 1958. Effect of post-partum separation of mother and kid on maternal care of domestic goat. *Science*, **128**, 1342.

25. HERSHER, L., RICHMOND, J. B. and MOORE, A. U. 1963. Maternal behavior in sheep and goats. In *Maternal behavior in mammals* (H. L. Rheingold, ed.), pp. 203–232. New York: Wiley.

26. HINDLEY, C. B., FILLIOZAT, A. M., KLACKENBERG, G., NICHOLET-MEISTER, D. and SAND, E. A. 1965. Some differences in infant feeding and eliminating training in five European longitudinal samples. *J. Child Psychol. Psychiat.*, **6**, 179.

27. HUNTINGFORD, P. J. 1962. Attitude of doctors and midwives to breast feeding. *Develop. Med. Child Neurol*, **4**, 588.

28. HYTTEN, F. E., YORSTON, J. E. and THOMSON, A. M. 1958. Difficulties associated with breast feeding. *Brit. med. J.*, i, 310.

29. ILLINGWORTH, R. S. and STONE, D. G. H. 1952. Self-demand feeding in maternity unit. *Lancet*, i, 683.
30. JACKSON, E. B., WILKIN, L. C. and AUERBACH, H. 1956. Statistical report on incidence and duration of breast feeding in relation to personal-social and hospital maternity factors. *Pediatrics*, **17**, 700.
31. JELLIFFE, D. B. 1956. Breast feeding in technically developing regions. *Courrier (Paris)* **6**, 191.
32. JELLIFFE, D. B. 1962. Culture, social change and infant feeding, current trends in tropical regions. *Amer. J. Clin. Nutr.*, **10**, 19.
33. KIMBALL, E. R. 1951. Breast feeding in private practice. *Quart. Bull. Northw. Univ. med., Sch.*, **25**, 257.
34. KINSEY, A. C., POMEROY, W. B., MARTIN, C. E. and GEBHARD, P. H. 1953. *Sexual behaviour in the human female: by staff of Institute for Sex Research, Indiana University.* Philadelphia: Saunders.
35. KRON, R. E., STEIN, M. and GODDARD, K. E. 1966. Newborn sucking behavior affected by obstetric sedation. *Pediatrics*, **37**, 1012.
36. LIDDELL, H. S. 1961. Contributions of conditioning in sheep and goat to understanding of stress, anxiety and illness. In Conference on Experimental Psychiatry. Western Psychiatric Institute and Clinic, 1959. *Lectures on Experimental Psychiatry: Pittsburgh Bicentennial Conference Mar. 5–7, 1959* (H. W. Brosin, ed.), pp. 227–255. Pittsburgh: University of Pittsburgh Press.
37. MASTERS, W. H. 1960. Sexual response cycle of human female. *West. J. Surg.*, **68**, 57.
38. MASTERS, W. H. and JOHNSON, V. E. 1966. *Human sexual response.* Boston: Little, Brown.
39. MATTHEWS, D. S. 1955. Ethnological and medical significance of breast feeding; with special reference to Yorubas of Nigeria. *J. trop. Pediat.*, **1**, 9.
40. MCBRYDE, A. 1951. Compulsory rooming-in in ward and private newborn service at Duke Hospital. *J. Amer. med. Ass.*, **145**, 625,
41. MCGEORGE, M. 1960. Current trends in breast feeding. *N.Z. med. J.*, **59**, 31.
42. MEAD, M. and NEWTON, N. 1967. Cultural patterning in perinatal behavior. In *Childbearing: its social and psychological aspects* (S. A. Richardson and A. F. Guttmacher, eds.), pp. 142–244. Baltimore: Williams and Wilkins.
43. MEYER, H. F. 1958. Breast feeding in United States: extent and possible trend. *Pediatrics*, **22**, 116.
44. MEYER, H. F. 1968. Breast feeding in the United States: report of a 1966 national survey with comparable 1946 and 1956 data. *Clin. Pediat.*, **7**, 708.
45. MOIR, C. 1934. Recording the contractions of human pregnant and non-pregnant uterus. *Trans. Edinb. obstet. Soc.*, **54**, 93.
46. MOORE, A. U. 1960. Maternal neonate bond in sheep and goat: its formation and significance for later life in herd. Paper presented at 1960 APA meeting Chicago, Ill., September 1–7 (mimeographed from author).
47. NEWSON, L. J. and NEWSON, E. 1962. Breast feeding in decline, *Brit. med. J.*, **2**, 1744.
48. NEWTON, D. B. 1966. Breast feeding in Victoria. *Med. J. Aust.*, **2**, 801.
49. NEWTON, M. and NEWTON, N. 1948. Let-down reflex in human lactation. *J. Pediat.*, **33**, 698.
50. NEWTON, M. and NEWTON, N. 1950. Relation of let-down reflex to ability to breast feed. *Pediatrics*, **5**, 726.
51. NEWTON, M. and NEWTON, N. 1962. Normal course and management of lactation. *Clin. Obstet. Gynec.*, **5**, 44.
52. NEWTON, N. 1952. Nipple pain and nipple damage. *J. Pediat.*, **41**, 411
53. NEWTON, N. 1955. *Maternal emotions: a study of women's feelings toward*

menstruation, pregnancy, childbirth, breast feeding, infant care, and other aspects of their femininity. New York: Hoeber.

54. NEWTON, N. 1955. *The family book of child care.* New York: Harper.
55. NEWTON, N. 1958. Influence of let-down reflex in breast feeding on mother-child relationship. *Marriage & Family Living,* **20,** 18.
56. NEWTON, N. and NEWTON, M. 1950. Relationship of ability to breast feed and maternal attitudes toward breast feeding. *Pediatrics,* **5,** 869.
57. NEWTON, N. and NEWTON, M. 1951. Recent trends in breast feeding: review. *Amer. J. med. Sci.,* **221,** 691.
58. NEWTON, N. and NEWTON, M. 1962. Mothers' reactions to their newborn babies. *J. Amer. med. Ass.,* **181,** 206.
59. NEWTON, N., PEELER, D. and RAWLINS, C. 1968. Effect of lactation on maternal behavior in mice with comparative data on humans. *Lying-in: J. Reprod. Med.,* **1,** 257.
60. POTTER, H. W. and KLEIN, H. R. 1957. On nursing behavior. *Psychiatry,* **20,** 39.
61. PRYOR, K. 1963. *Nursing your baby.* New York: Harper.
62. RAWLINS, C. 1963. Tested program for breast feeding success. Unpublished speech given at University Medical Center, Jackson, Mississippi.
63. RICHARDSON., F. H. 1925. Universalizing breast feeding in community. *J. Amer. med. Ass.,* **85,** 668.
64. ROBERTSON, W. O. 1961. Breast feeding practices: some implications of regional variations. *Amer. J. publ. Hlth.,* **51,** 1035.
65. ROBINSON, M. 1951. Infant morbidity and mortality: study of 3266 infants. *Lancet,* i, 788.
66. ROSS, A. I. and HERDAN, G. 1951. Breast-feeding in Bristol. *Lancet,* i, 630.
67. ROUCHY, R., TAUREAU, M. and VALMYRE, M. J. 1961. Current trends in maternal breast feeding. *Bull. Féd. Soc. Gynéc. Obstét. franç.,* **13,** 471.
68. SALBER, E. J. 1956. Effect of different feeding schedules on growth of Bantu babies in first week of life. *J. trop. Pediat.,* **2,** 97.
69. SALBER, E. J. 1960. Rejection of breast feeding. *Med. Tms.,* **88,** 430.
70. SALBER, E. J. and FEINLEIB, M. 1966. Breast feeding in Boston. *Pediatrics,* **37,** 299.
71. SALBER, E. J., STITT, P. G. and BABBOTT, J. G. 1958. Patterns of breast feeding. I. Factors affecting frequency of breast feeding in newborn period. *New Eng. J. Med.,* **259,** 707.
72. SALBER, E. J., STITT, P. G. and BABBOTT, J. G. 1959. Patterns of breast feeding in family health clinic II. Duration of feeding and reasons for weaning. *New Eng. J. Med.,* **260,** 310.
73. SEARS, R. R., MACCOBY, E. E. and LEVIN, H. 1957. *Patterns of child rearing.* Evanston: Row, Peterson.
74. SEDGWICK, J. P. and FLEISCHNER, E. C. 1921. Breast feeding in reduction of infant mortality. *Amer. J. publ. Hlth.,* **11,** 153.
75. SOLIEN DE GONZALES, N. L. 1963. Breast feeding, weaning and acculturation. *J. Pediat.,* **62,** 577.
76. SOUTHWORTH, T. S. 1906. Maternal feeding. In *Practice of pediatrics* (W. L. Carr, ed.), pp. 89–107. Philadelphia: Lea.
77. STELLA, SR. M. 1960. Family-centered maternity care. *Hosp. Progr.,* **41,** 92.
78. UNGAR, R. 1949. Kinderärztl. *Praxis,* **17,** 285.
79. VERMELIN, H. and RIBON, M. 1961. Management and results of maternal breast feeding at maternity hospital of Nancy. *Rev. franç. Gynéc.,* **56,** 119.
80. WALLER, H. K. 1938. *Clinical studies in lactation.* London: Heinemann.
81. WALLER, H. K. 1943. Reflex governing the outflow of milk from breast. *Lancet,* **214,** 69.
82. WALLER, H. K. 1950. Early yield of human milk and its relation to security of lactation. *Lancet,* i, 53.

83. WELBOURN, H. F. 1958. Bottle feeding: problem of modern civilization. *J. trop. Pediat.*, **3,** 157.

84. WICKES, I. G. and CURWEN, M. P. 1957. Lactation and heredity. *Brit. med. J.*, **2,** 381.

85. WIEDERMAN, J., FREUND, M. and STONE, M. L. 1963. Human breast and uterus: comparison of sensitivity to oxytocin during gestation. *Obstet. and Gynec.*, **21,** 272.

86. *Womanly Art of Breast Feeding.* 1963. La Leche League International: Franklin Park, Illinois.

87. YANKAUER, A., BOEK, W. E., LAWSON, E. D. and IANNI, F. A. J. 1958. Social stratification and health practices in child bearing and child rearing. *Amer. J. publ. Hlth.*, **48,** 732.

XXII

INFANTICIDE

PHILLIP J. RESNICK

M.D.

Instructor in Psychiatry
Case Western Reserve University
Cleveland, Ohio
U.S.A.

A simple child,
That lightly draws its breath,
And feels its life in every limb,
What should it know of death?

W. Wordsworth[77]

1

Introduction

For the lay person, no crime is more difficult to comprehend than the killing of a child by his own parent. However, upon closer examination most cases of infanticide have quite understandable motives. There were 10,920 murders in the United States in 1966. One out of 22 was a child murdered by his parent.[36] In England and Wales, the percentage of murders which are infanticides is substantially higher.[73] Obstetrics has made great strides in reducing infant and maternal mortality. It is hoped that foreknowledge of certain behavior patterns will prove helpful to the obstetrician in the prevention of these family tragedies.

2

Historical Background

The killing of children goes back as far as recorded history. Reasons have included population control, illegitimacy, inability of the mother to care for the child, greed for power or money, superstition, congenital defects, and ritual sacrifice.[56] The practice of stabilizing buildings by enclosing children in their foundations is still symbolically represented by our foundation stones.[67] There was an ancient concept that those who create may destroy that which they have created. Roman law formalized this concept under *patria potestas*, which recognized a father's right to murder his children. Among Mohave Indians, half-breeds were killed at birth.[18] A merciless environment forced Eskimos to kill infants with congenital anomalies as well as one of most sets of twins.[23] The killing of female infants was common in many cultures. In China, this practice was widespread as late as the 1880s. Daughters were sacrificed because they were unable to transmit the family name and imposed the burden of paying their marriage portion. [43, 58] It is claimed that the widespread murder of children in ancient times was first stemmed by the influence of the Christian religion.[63]

3

Definition of Terms

In the medical literature, all child-murders are usually lumped together under the term "infanticide". "Filicide" refers to cases in which the murderer is a parent of the victim. In the author's opinion, two distinct types of filicide are evident. One is the killing of an unwanted neonate within the first few hours of life. The other is the murder of a child after its role in the family has been more firmly established. In this chapter filicide will be operationally defined as the killing of a son or daughter older than 24 hours. A new word, *neonaticide* has been proposed for the killing of a newborn before this age.[59, 60] Neonaticide is a separate entity, differing from filicide in the diagnoses, motives, and disposition of the murderer.

4

Description of the Murderers and Victims

Review articles on both filicide and neonaticide were recently published by the author.* A total of 168 cases of child murder were collected from the world literature dating back as far as 1751. There were 88 maternal filicides, 43 paternal filicides, 35 maternal neonaticides, and 2 paternal neonaticides. It may be seen from Table I that the mothers in the neonaticide group are significantly younger than those in the filicide group. While most (88%) of the maternal filicide group are married, only 19% of the maternal neonaticide group enjoyed that status. All but one of the fathers were married. The ages of the filicide victims ranged from a few days to as old as 20 years (Table II). The most dangerous period for the victims is the first six months of life. This, of course, is the time of maternal post-partum psychoses and depressions. The younger the child, the more likely is the suicidal mother to think of him as a personal possession and feel inseparable from him. The

* See Editor's Foreword.

TABLE I

Age of Murderers

Age (years)	Maternal neonaticide No.(%)	Maternal filicide No.(%)	Paternal filicide No.(%)
15–19	11(42)	0	0
20–24	9(35)	11(18)	0
25–29	1(4)	16(26)	8(50)
30–34	2(8)	15(25)	5(31)
35–39	3(11)	9(15)	1(6)
40–44	0	6(10)	2(13)
45–50	0	4(6)	0
Subtotal	26(100)	61(100)	16(100)
Unknown	9	27	27
Total	35	88	43

TABLE II

Age of Victims

Age	Maternal filicide No.(%)	Paternal filicide No.(%)
24 hours to 6 months	26(30)	9(24)
6 months to 2 years	20(23)	6(16)
2–3 years	15(17)	8(21)
4–7 years	15(17)	7(19)
8–11 years	7(8)	4(10)
12–20 years	5(5)	4(10)
Subtotal	88(100)	38(100)
Unknown	11	17
Total	99*	55*

* The totals exceed the number of cases because there were multiple victims in 15 instances.

older children were more likely to be defective. Slightly more than half of the victims were girls, but this was not statistically significant. The sex and age patterns of the victims offer no support to theories that Oedipal or adolescent issues precipitated the fatal attacks.

The diagnoses as given in the case reports are compiled in Table III. Only a few of the women in the neonaticide group were psychotic, but psychosis was evident in two-thirds of the maternal filicide group. The unreliability of diagnostic labels from country to country and from decade to decade must be kept in mind; nonetheless, these figures do suggest that neonaticide and filicide are committed by two different psychiatric populations. A serious element of depression was found in only 3 of the maternal neonaticide cases compared with 71% of the maternal filicide group. Finally, suicide attempts accompanied more than one-third of the filicides, but none occurred among the neonaticide cases.

TABLE III

Diagnoses

Diagnosis	Maternal neonaticide No.(%)	Maternal filicide No.(%)	Paternal filicide No.(%)
Schizophrenia	1(3)	25(29)	4(9)
Psychosis, other	0	22(25)	9(21)
Nonpsychotic	8(23)	10(11)	10(23)
Character disorder	9(25)	11(13)	5(12)
Melancholia	0	8(9)	6(14)
No psychiatric diagnosis	9(25)	4(5)	6(14)
Manic-depressive	0	3(3)	0
Retarded	2(6)	1(1)	2(5)
Neurosis	1(3)	2(2)	0
Delirium	2(6)	1(1)	1(2)
Epilepsy	3(9)	1(1)	0
Total	35(100)	88(100)	43(100)

TABLE IV

Methods of Filicide

Method	Maternal filicide No.(%)	Paternal filicide No.(%)
Head trauma	12(13)	12(28)
Strangulation	13(14)	7(17)
Drowning	15(17)	2(5)
Cutting or stabbing	8(9)	6(14)
Shooting	8(9)	3(7)
Suffocation	9(10)	2(5)
Thrown from height	9(10)	1(2)
Gas	8(9)	2(5)
Poison	5(6)	2(5)
Manual assault	0	3(7)
Starvation	3(3)	0
Burning	0	2(5)
Subtotal	90(100)	42(100)
Unknown	4	5
Total	94*	47*

* The totals exceed the number of cases because of multiple methods in some instances.

5

Methods of Infanticide

Head trauma, strangulation, and drowning are the most common methods of both filicide and neonaticide. It may be seen from Table IV that fathers tended to use more active methods such as striking, squeezing, or stabbing, whereas mothers more often drowned, suffocated, or gassed their victims. Unusual methods of filicide included putting sulphuric acid in a nursing bottle[39] and biting to death.[62] One father put his son on a drill press and drilled a hole through his heart.[62] Methods of neonaticide rarely used in filicides are exposure, neglect, and confinement in a closed space. Less common methods of neonaticide include dismemberment, decapitation, acid, lye, throwing to pigs, and burying alive. The need to stifle the baby's first cry makes suffocation the method of choice for mothers attempting to avoid detection.[54] The drownings are most often accomplished in toilets. Case reports of up to 48 stab wounds or decapitation may reflect the bitterness of the abandoned girl, who sees the child in her lover's image.[51, 64] Some mothers use extreme cleverness to avoid discovery of their deed. In India, these methods have included drowning in milk and poisoning by rubbing opium on the mother's nipples.[46] Some midwives killed newborns by thrusting a needle under the eyelid or into the anterior fontanel.[27, 34] A needle from one such unsuccessful attempt was found at autopsy in the brain of a 70-year-old man.[34] Asch[5] has recently suggested that a "large proportion" of previously unexplained crib deaths may in reality be covert infanticides.

6

Motives for Infanticide

In order to provide a framework for viewing child murder, the infanticides will be divided into five categories. The comparative frequency of each is shown in Table V. This classification is based on the explanation given by the murderer and is independent of diagnosis. When overlapping occurred in the proposed groups, each case was classified by the single most important motive.

It is apparent from Table V that the motives which cause a mother to kill her newborn are considerably different from those which drive a mother to murder an older offspring. Whereas the majority of filicides are undertaken for an "altruistic" motive, the great bulk of neonaticides are committed simply because the child is not wanted.

TABLE V

Classification of Infanticides by Apparent Motive

Motive	Maternal neonaticide No.(%)	Maternal filicide No.(%)	Paternal filicide No.(%)
'Altruistic'			
Associated with suicide	0	37(42)	13(30)
To relieve suffering	1(3)	12(14)	2(5)
'Acutely psychotic'	4(11)	21(24)	7(16)
'Unwanted child'	29(83)	10(11)	8(19)
'Accidental'	1(3)	6(7)	10(23)
'Spouse revenge'	0	2(2)	3(7)
Total	35(100)	88(100)	43(100)

Classification of Filicide by Apparent Motive

1. "Altruistic" filicide. The fact that almost half the filicides involved an explicit altruistic motive is the most important factor that distinguishes filicide from other homicides. Two subgroups are evident among these murders committed "out of love":

(a) Filicide associated with suicide. When they killed themselves these parents claimed that they could not abandon their children. One mother left a suicide note saying, "Bury us in one box. We belong together, you know."[69] There are scattered reports of cases where both husband and wife planned the murder of the entire family, usually because they could see no way out of their poverty.[6, 11, 40, 42] Some mothers extended their suicides even further by burning down their homes.[20]

(b) Filicide to relieve suffering. These parents killed to relieve the victim's suffering, which may have been real or imagined. Euthanasia was the ostensible reason why one couple decided to gas themselves along with their 20-year-old encephalitic son. Carp[11] postulated that their deed was due to an inability to accept the narcissistic injury and their need for revenge. The suffering was delusional in the case of a 29-year-old married woman who choked her three-year-old son to death after becoming convinced that a spell was causing the child to grow smaller.[9] Also classified within this group are those parents who killed their children in a misguided effort to prevent them from suffering at the hands of paranoid persecutors. In one case, a 50-year-old widow murdered her 11-year-old daughter rather than allow her to be taken into an imagined white slavery ring.[47]

2. "Acutely Psychotic" Filicide. This designation includes parents who killed under the influence of hallucinations, epilepsy, or delirium. It does not include all of the psychotic child murders. This is the weakest category, because it contains those cases in which no comprehensible motive could be ascertained. Various descriptive explanations have been offered for these crimes, including Kretschmer's "short circuit" reaction[41] and Wertham's "catathymic crisis".[71] Both occur when an affective impulse is translated directly into a violent action. Reichard and Tillman[57] take issue with the need for a new diagnostic entity; their hypothesis is that these murders may represent an attempted defense against the outbreak of a schizophrenic psychosis. The following example is abbreviated from Bender:[9]

> The patient, a 43-year-old Scottish woman, had always been an even-tempered, devoted mother and wife. Her husband was aware of no change in her until two days before the crime. She began to act in a wild manner and kept saying, "There is nothing wrong with me." The neighbors observed her leaning out of the window of her fifth-floor apartment when she suddenly thrust her struggling nine-year-old daughter out to her death. She told the ambulance driver she had only done what the Lord advised. After hospital admission she became increasingly bewildered, disturbed, resistive, and, at times, mute and catatonic. She rapidly exhausted herself and died three weeks later.

Hopwood[37] reports that in crimes resulting from epileptic automatism it is not uncommon for individuals to have total amnesia for the event and to go on as though nothing happened. He tells of one epileptic mother who placed her baby on the fire and the kettle in her cradle. Alcohol was rarely found to be a direct cause of filicide. However, there is one case report in which a 38-year-old married woman cut the throat of her four-month-old infant in a hallucinated, delirious paroxysm after a four-day drunken orgy.[37]

3. "Unwanted child" filicide. These murders were committed because the victim was not desired or was no longer wanted by the parent. Illegitimacy caused one girl to kill her 16-day-old infant after giving birth incognito in an out-of-town hospital.[43] Two married women killed their youngsters because the youngsters had not been fathered by their husbands.[66, 75] Wertham[72] tells of a dull 25-year-old widow who was offered marriage only if she parted with her two children. After being refused placement by social agencies, she decided to dispose of them by use of a hatchet, knife, and gasoline for burning.

4. "Accidental" filicide. These murders are usually the result of a fatal "battered child syndrome".[38] They are called "accidental" because homicidal intent is lacking. More fathers than mothers killed in violent outbursts, often in the overzealous application of discipline. The following example is taken from Adelson.[2]

> A mother reported that her three-year-old daughter kept taking the nursing bottle away from her 13-month-old sibling. Following an instance of this activity, the mother poured the contents of a pepper shaker into the child's mouth. The child "swallowed" the material, started to gasp, and was rushed to a nearby hospital. The pepper had occluded her air passages, and she was dead on arrival. The mother had been involved in two previous child batterings.

Filicide by accident may also occur as an epiphenomenon. Delay[16] quotes an example of a man who could gain sexual pleasure only from sadistic acts. On the pretence of disciplining his 14-year-old daughter, he tied an apron over her face with a tight strap. After beating her with an electric cord, he planned to masturbate, but instead found his daughter dead.

5. *"Spouse revenge" filicide.* This final category consists of parents who killed their offspring in a deliberate attempt to make their spouses suffer. The prototype is found in the story of Medea. After killing their two sons, Medea told her unfaithful husband, Jason, "Thy sons are dead and gone. That will stab thy heart."[49]

Rheingold[62] tells of a recently separated 29-year-old woman who beat her three-year-old daughter to death with a claw-hammer. Her husband had wanted to take the girl, but she preferred to "offer the baby to God" rather than let him have her. She believed her husband had left her for another woman. Rheingold felt that the patient regarded her daughter as a rival and projected the daughter-rival onto the female rival. In this author's opinion, it seems equally likely that aggressive feelings toward the rival were acted out upon her daughter.

Special Motives in Neonaticide

The most common reason for neonaticide among married women is extramarital paternity. One example[48] is a woman who became impregnated by her brother-in-law while her husband was in prison. After cool deliberation and careful planning, she murdered her infant at birth to avoid suspicion of her affair. It is commonplace for fathers to show some jealousy of their newborn children. The one case[42] in which both the husband and wife consciously planned the murder of their expected infant is an extreme example of this. The 28-year-old father and 17-year-old mother made no preparations for the birth of their baby except to dig a grave in the cellar. Both parents had physical deformities and feelings of inferiority. They were deeply in love and could not bear the thought of a third party interfering in their relationship. The husband initially proposed the crime against the "annoying animal that deformed his beloved wife's virginal figure". He assisted in the delivery at home, strangled the infant, and buried it.

The stigma of having an illegitimate child is the primary reason for neonaticide in unmarried women today, as it has been through the centuries. In 1826 Scott wrote the following: "A delicate female, knowing the value of a chaste reputation, and the infamy and disgrace attendant upon the loss of that indispensable character and aware of the proverbial uncharitableness of her own sex, resolves in her distraction, rather than encounter the indifference of the world and banishment from society, to sacrifice what on more fortunate occasions, it would have been her pride to cherish."[65]

The very livelihood of these women was often at stake, particularly among domestic servants. A typical example is this case taken from Harder.[33]

A 19-year-old single girl, who lost both her parents by age 12, became a domestic servant in the country. She was impregnated by a man she knew only slightly, and he disappeared upon learning of her condition. Although the thought of killing the expected child filled her with horror, she saw no other way out. When the baby came a month earlier than expected, she strangled it upon hearing the first cry. When the body was found, she confessed at once. She did not regret what she had done, because she felt that the child had no chance in life anyway because of its illegitimacy. As is common in this type of neonaticide, she confided in no one, concealed her pregnancy, and delivered clandestinely.

Hirschmann and Schmitz[35] divided women who killed their illegitimate infants into two major groups. The women in the first group are said to have "a primary weakness of the characterological superstructure". In the second group are women with strong instinctual drives and little ethical restraint. All but a small minority of our 35 cases would fall into the former group. These women are usually young, immature primiparas. They submit to sexual relations rather than initiate them. They have no previous criminal record and rarely attempt abortion. Gummersbach[30] points out that passivity is the single personality factor which most clearly separates women who commit neonaticide from those who obtain abortions. Women who seek abortions are activists who recognize reality early and promptly attack the danger. In contrast, women who commit neonaticide often deny that they are pregnant or assume that the child will be stillborn. No advance preparations are made either for the care or the killing of the infant. When reality is thrust upon them by the infant's first cry, they respond by permanently silencing the intruder.

The women in the second group—those with strong instinctual drives and little ethical restraint—are more callous, egoistic and intelligent. They tend to be older, strong-willed, and are often promiscuous. Their crime is usually premeditated and not out of keeping with their previous life style. For example,[35] one 38-year-old divorced woman killed her newborn infant which was the result of a liaison with a married father of four children. This woman had a police record for both prostitution and procuring. She had a previous stillborn outside of marriage, but neonaticide could not be proven.

7

Psychodynamics

The Medea complex was first named by Wittels[76] as the unconscious hatred of a mother for her maturing daughter as a potential rival. Stern[67] correctly pointed out that Medea had no daughters, and therefore called Wittels' definition a misnomer. Stern redefined the Medea complex as the mother's death-wishes toward her offspring, usually as revenge against the father.

Rheingold goes further by stating that the filicidal impulse exists to some degree in every mother.[61] It is not uncommon for mothers to seek psychiatric help because of obsessional filicidal thoughts. Little concern has been expressed in the literature about these mothers acting upon their impulses.[4, 12, 22] However, McDermaid and Winkler[44] point out in their syndrome of "child-centred obsessional depression" that filicide may be an exception to the general belief that obsessional ideas are not carried out.

To illustrate how infanticide may be unconsciously multi-determined, three cases treated by the author will be presented. The first two cases are altruistic filicides associated with suicide.

Case 1. Mrs. A., a 31-year-old wife of a military pilot and mother of four (Betty, aged five; Carol, four; and sons aged two and seven), drove off a cliff with her five-year-old daughter. She spent six months in the orthopaedic ward of another hospital and then was transferred to my psychiatric service.

Her present illness could be dated from the birth of her last child when she began to feel tense and inadequate as a mother. She obtained some relief by spending increased time outside her home; this led to two sequential extramarital affairs. Three months before the filicide she and the children accompanied her husband to Alaska. As her sleep pattern became disturbed by the long daylight hours, she became irritable and depressed. She was hospitalized after taking an entire bottle of tranquilizers, but felt she could not establish rapport with her psychiatrist. Covering up her illness with superficial smiles, she was discharged in one week. At home she became agitated, slept poorly, and was unable to complete her housework.

Mrs. A. reported that two days before the killing, her psychiatrist had told her that if she could not talk to him she might commit suicide. The patient misconstrued this to mean that she should commit suicide. One day before the murder she told her husband that she was sick and needed help. He told her, "The children don't want you, and I don't want you. Why don't you get out?" She felt she was mentally ill but had no place to turn for help. She believed her girls were being raised too materialistically. While there still might be a chance for her younger daughter, Carol, she felt that Betty was a "completely ruined *monster*".

On the fatal day she deliberately took Betty along for a drive. She felt that Betty just could not get along without her. She did not want Betty to have to go through life as she did, with no mother in the home. The patient drove off the cliff and sustained a compound fracture of her mandible and a fracture of her left radius. She reported that her daughter shook her and said, "Mommy, Mommy, we have to get out of here." The formerly beautiful daughter had her forehead pushed in and "tissue like scrambled eggs coming out of her head." The patient said, "Oh, my God, what have I done? I've made a *monster* out of her."

She then felt she had to kill her daughter and herself. She could not bear to think of her daughter going through life with those scars. She recalled feeling that she had had internal scars as a child. After trying unsuccessfully to choke Betty, she picked up a rock and kept striking her on the head until she was dead. She then avulsed a third of her own scalp by hitting herself with the same rock. Failing thus to kill herself, she tried throwing herself down the mountain and cutting her wrist. Deciding that Betty should at least have a funeral, she attempted to climb up the mountain, where she was found thirty-six hours later.

Mrs. A. described her mother as a materialistic, pretentious woman who worked and was rarely in the home. The patient had never been able to express anger to her mother. She described her father as kind and gentle but weak and childish. In later life he was diagnosed as a paranoid schizophrenic. There was one brother two years older than the patient. The patient had childhood memories of wanting to die if her mother died during an illness. She did well in school and went on to get a college degree.

From the time of her marriage at age 22, sexual relations were unsatisfactory. She felt her frigidity ruined her husband's masculinity. She described her daughter, Betty, as a brilliant, beautiful child with blond hair and olive skin. The patient showed her the most affection and loved her "more than anything else in the world". Betty reminded her of her own mother, but even more of herself when she was a child. When she punished Betty it was like punishing herself. She came to feel that Betty belonged more to her and that Carol belonged more to her husband.

The final diagnosis was schizophrenic reaction, schizo-affective type. After four months of psychiatric hospitalization, the patient was discharged and returned to live with her family and a housekeeper.

Case 2. Mrs. B. a 28-year-old wife of an enlisted man and mother of two (Allan, aged six and Billy 14 months), shot herself and killed her 14-month-old son in March 1966.

The patient dated her present illness from 1963, when she developed prickling sensations which she described "as if ants were crawling over my body". The following year she received six months of outpatient psychiatric care before she and her sons accompanied her husband to Germany. In October 1965 when she learned she was pregnant with a third child, she became anxious and depressed, requiring hospitalization for one month. A tubal ligation after delivery was recommended, but the necessary concurrence by a second psychiatrist could not be obtained. The patient was quite disappointed.

For two months before the murder she became increasingly depressed, felt as if she were in a fog, and just wanted to stay in bed. One week before the shooting her psychiatrist wrote in her chart that, in view of the nonconcurrence regarding a tubal ligation, he could foresee nothing but tragedy for this woman and her two children. Upon arriving home on the fatal day, her husband found Billy shot to death and the patient suffering from two bullet wounds. Mrs. B. had amnesia for the shooting. Two months later the patient had a sodium amobarbital (Amytal) interview and gave the following account of the tragic day:

"That morning I felt I was going into labor because of a severe backache. I was depressed thinking how hard it was to raise even the two children. I heard the previous day at the psychiatrist's office that the tubal ligation could only be done for suicidal tendencies. I got up from the kitchen where I was drinking coffee and got my husband's gun. I shot myself through the left breast and sat down again. I walked into Billy's room. When I heard him call 'Mama', that was it. I thought: 'Who is going to take care of my Billy?' I said 'Billy', and pulled the trigger. I did it on impulse. I didn't meant to hurt him; I never meant to hurt him. After I saw the blood on him, I panicked. How could I do such a thing to a boy I loved? I thought I couldn't be Billy's mother and do what I did to him. Poor Billy. I loved him. He'll never be dead in my heart. I called my husband to come right home. When I went back upstairs and found that Billy was dying, I shot myself again in the chest."

Mrs. B was the eighth of nine children. Her mother was described as kind, understanding, and hardworking. Billy was born on the seventh anniversary of her mother's death. Her father was quick-tempered; he left the running of the household to his wife. The patient felt very close to an older sister who had pretty blond hair, "just like Billy." Her first memory was the death of this sister when the patient was three years old. Her younger sister was born about the same time. The patient became sexually involved with older men at age six. She performed various sexual acts for money until age 15, when she was sentenced to a residential school for delinquent girls. From the time of her marriage at age 18, she had little communication with her husband. Her husband reports that she initially despised the idea of having children and became unbearable during each of her pregnancies.

The final diagnosis was schizophrenic reaction, chronic undifferentiated type. Two weeks after the shooting she delivered a healthy male infant. A tubal ligation was performed during her psychiatric hospitalization. She did not respond to psychotropic drugs or ECT and was eventually transferred for long-term psychiatric care.

Psychiatric mechanisms that occur in filicide associated with suicide will be illustrated by material from case 1. The suicidal mother often thinks of her child as an extension of herself. This is demonstrated by Mrs. A's feeling that punishing Betty was like punishing herself. At first glance it may be difficult to see how the term "altruistic" could be applied to a mother beating her daughter to death. However, the depressive murderer usually picks an "overloved" individual for his victim.[8] The suicidal mother may identify her child with herself and project her own unacceptable symptoms onto the victim.[9] By this mechanism Mrs. A. viewed Betty as a "ruined monster" that had to be destroyed. At the same time, she wanted to prevent her daughter from suffering the same "motherlessness" that she had endured. This motive of sparing the victim from the same fate as the parent was quite common. All of these factors contribute in converting suicides to filicides.

Ideally, in each case of filicide what occurred in the early object relationships of the murderer to cause him to express his aggression in this manner should be known. In many cases there is evidence that the aggression acted out on the child was displaced from the murderer's mother, father, spouse, or sibling. Some filicides were carried out after the murderer had been criticized by his mother.[66] Meyerson[45] observed a reversal of role in fantasy, in which the child becomes the parent and the parent becomes the child; it was at the point where the parent felt the child was rejecting him that the homicidal rage was expressed.

In both cases 1 and 2 the patients had felt abandoned by their mothers when they were children. These feelings were revived in Mrs. A. when her husband told her to "get out". She identified Betty with her own materialistic mother. By murdering her daughter, Mrs. A. was able to vent the anger that her mother had never tolerated. In case 2 Mrs. B. had had from childhood association of death with birth. When her feelings of abandonment were reawakened by the onset of labor, she turned her rage on Billy. The filicidal drive of both patients may also be seen as an attempt at "reunion with mother" through death.

The following case, abstracted from DeVallet and Scherrer,[17] is an example of aggression displaced from a spouse. A 32-year-old woman drowned two of her three children and attempted to drown herself. Her two victims had ichthyosis, the same incurable skin disease as her husband. She claimed she had killed them to relieve their suffering from the disease. Although she never reproached her ichthyotic husband, it was found that she had nothing but disgust for him, especially his conjugal demands. The special care and bathing she gave the victims was a thinly veiled defense against the anger she had transferred from her husband to the children.

Zilboorg[78] reports a case where a mother's filicidal impulse stemmed from seeing her child as a living testimony to her incestuous attitude toward her father. Olive[50] found a 40% incidence of actual incest among a group of 15 filicidal women. He felt they had eroticized relationships with their murdered children; destructive wishes aimed at the initial incest-object were reactivated and vented on the current incest-object—the child. One feature which stood out in several of the neonaticides was the inability of the unwed girl to reveal her pregnancy to her mother. This may be due to the girl's shame or to fear that her mother's response would be anger, punishment, or rejection. In addition, unresolved Oedipal feelings may cause some of these girls to have the unconscious fantasy that their pregnancy is proof of incest. The following case is an example of this speculation:

Case 3. Mrs. C., a 36-year-old, married, childless secretary, committed neonaticide at age 17. She did not have her first psychiatric contact until she made a suicide attempt almost two decades later.

Four months before her suicide attempt she found a letter which indicated that her husband had been unfaithful. As with each previous adversity she encountered, she felt that this was retribution for her killing. She became anorectic and lost 22 pounds over a four-month period. She developed insomnia, indecisiveness and inability to concentrate at her work. She began to feel that others could read her mind and influence her through voodoo. She had frightening dreams and fantasies in which she and her husband were beaten, murdered and crucified. When she looked in the mirror she saw herself as a devil. She became totally preoccupied with how "evil" she was, especially because of her neonaticide. Feeling that she deserved to die, she drank a glass of corrosive liquid which caused esophageal stricture, eventually necessitating a colon-esophageal transplant.

The patient was the third of four sisters. Mrs. C. described her father as a jolly, outgoing, talkative laborer who brought home his paycheck weekly, but was more like a roomer than a husband. He "ran around", and the patient often heard her mother speak of the "other woman". Her mother was described as a strong-willed, decisive, brusque woman, who often hurt the patient's feelings. Even the tone of her voice could make the patient feel as though she was being hit. Mrs. C. was constantly seeking her mother's approval, but never felt that she received it. Her first memory occurred at age three. Her father had taken her out in a new dress and showed her off to some men. They kidded him by saying that she was too cute to be his. From age eight to eleven the patient had a recurent dream in which a terrifying monster came at her from behind but never quite reached her. As far back as Mrs. C. could remember, her parents slept in separate bedrooms. When she was fifteen, her parents separated permanently. However, her father would come back and have the patient launder his shirts.

Only a few times, mainly for her high school graduation affairs, did the patient date the boy who impregnated her. She passively submitted to sexual relations to avoid his disapproval. She did not know what to do about her pregnancy, but she was quite certain she could never let her mother know. She corsetted herself and successfully concealed the pregnancy from her family. She declined to go on to college even though a scholarship awaited her. Fortuitously alone at home when she began labor, she gave birth in the bathroom to a male child. She strangled the infant with her hands and then hung it on a towel rack with a hanger until she had cleaned up. She wrapped the body in old clothes and put it in a dresser drawer overnight. The next day she put it in the rubbish and her crime was never discovered. She was amazed at her own coolness. She claims she had no feeling of guilt at the time—"It was just something that had to be done." However, since the killing she has tried to do good "to even things up". She regarded non-specific throat symptoms at age twenty and an ovarian cyst at age twenty-three as justified punishment. She felt it would be appropriate for her to die in childbirth as a final balancing of the scales. After the neonaticide, the patient got a job as a secretary. She had an extended affair with a narcotics addict that ended after he had served a prison sentence. She felt it was her "lot in life" to put up with this man even though he treated her badly. The man, who subsequently became her husband, was married when she met him at a ten-year high school class reunion. During their affair, she was very conscious of being the "other woman" of whom she had so often heard her mother speak.

The final diagnosis was psychotic depression. The patient's psychotic thinking cleared early in her three-month hospital stay. After her discharge, she was seen weekly for one year as an outpatient.

Whereas some infant murders result from psychosis, this case may be looked upon as a psychosis resulting, in part, from a neonaticide. When Mrs. C. learned of her husband's infidelity, she developed murderous impulses toward him. In view of her past murder in reality, it was difficult for her to experience these wishes at a conscious level. Instead they took the form of fears in her psychosis that both she and her husband would be murdered. It is noteworthy that, as Mrs. C.'s neonaticide injured her infant's throat, so the method of suicide she selected damaged her own throat.

Various elements in the patient's history suggest that unresolved Oedipal feelings may have been instrumental in this neonaticide. Her first memory questions her blood relationship to her father. Throughout her childhood, the patient was unable to feel close to her mother. During psychological testing, her response to Rorschach Card IV was of particular interest. She appeared terrified, threw down the card, and cried for a long time. She said it was dreadful, like the monster in her repetitive dream. Several months later she admitted that her first thought upon seeing the card was that of her mother in a fur coat. After her parents' separation, Mrs. C. took over the rather intimate chore of doing her father's laundry. In spite of protesting, she proceeded to become the "other woman" in relation to her husband. The sum of these factors suggests that Mrs. C. may have failed to reveal her pregnancy to her mother because of the unconscious idea that it would be viewed as proof of incest.

8

Paternal Infanticide

It may be seen from Table V that fathers were over-represented in the "unwanted child" and "accidental" categories. Fathers are more likely to kill when there is doubt about paternity and when the progeny is viewed as a financial burden or an impediment to their career.

Although it is not uncommon for fathers to murder older children, it is quite rare for a father to kill a newborn infant. Fathers have neither the motive nor the opportunity of mothers. Only two case reports of neonaticide were found in which the father was the sole killer. One mentally deficient 32-year-old man poisoned his newborn child because he felt that his own poor health might result in his death, leaving no one to provide for his wife and child.[31] The other father was a bright 26-year-old man who was forced into marriage by his wife's pregnancy.[52] He saw the coming child as a bar to his ambition. On one occasion he put poison into his wife's soup in an attempt to cause the infant to be stillborn. He strangled the infant while delivering his wife himself, and told her it was stillborn. When questioned, he admitted the deed with no remorse. Although free of overt psychosis at the time, he developed a full-blown picture of schizophrenia three years later.

9

Reaction to the Deed

After the "altruistic" and "acutely psychotic" killings there is often immediate relief of tension. This explains the failure of some parents to complete their suicide. However, upon realization of the gravity of their act, they may attempt suicide even if it was not planned. The murderer may appear dazed and confess in a mechanical way, or he may deny his own identity and the deed. Following the initial reaction there may be an increase of symptoms, but more often there is a tendency to recover.[9] These parents usually run to seek help, making no attempt to conceal their crime. By contrast, the "unwanted" and "accidental" infanticide murderer often goes to great lengths to dispose of incriminating evidence.

The reaction of the spouses is rarely mentioned in the literature. Upon discovering Medea's deed, Jason exclaimed, "Accursed woman! by Gods, by me and all mankind abhorred as never woman was, who hadst the heart to stab thy babes, thou their mother, leaving me undone and childless."[49] The husbands in cases 1 and 2 said their first impulse was to get a divorce. Both felt that they could never trust their wives alone with the remaining children. The husband in case 1 seemed to have more difficulty in forgiving his wife's infidelity than her filicide. After considerable soul-searching and some rocky trial visits home, they resumed their marriage.

Although the husband in case 2 initially regretted that his wife didn't "finish the job on herself", he later decided he still loved her. When his six-year-old son asked if his mother would shoot him also, he replied, "I don't think so." He continued to keep a gun collection in the home. It might be speculated that this patient's actions were influenced by her husband's unconscious impulses.

The reaction of the hospital staff to the prospect of caring for the child-murderers was one of anxiety and hostility. After the patients arrived in the ward there was some abatement of these feelings. Considerable resistance was also encountered among hospitals and psychiatrists in arranging subsequent care for these patients. In the same fashion, the relative infrequency with which infanticide is mentioned in either the medical or popular literature may be due to the repugnance of the theme.

10

Disposition

It may be seen from Table VI that, among the filicide cases, fathers were more likely to be executed or sent to prison, whereas mothers were more often hospitalized. This pattern was constant even after correction for the higher proportion of fathers in the "unwanted child", "accidental", and "spouse revenge" filicide categories. All the patients in these three groups were sentenced to prison, probation, or execution. Mothers who commit

TABLE VI

Disposition

Disposition	Maternal neonaticide No.(%)	Maternal filicide No.(%)	Paternal filicide No.%
Prison or Probation	16(57)	20(27)	22(63)
Hospital	5(18)	50(68)	5(14)
Acquitted or no action taken	7(25)	0	0
Execution	0	0	3(9)
Suicide	0	4(5)	5(14)
Subtotal	28(100)	74(100)	35(100)
Unknown	7	14	8
Total	35	88	43

neonaticide are less likely to be hospitalized than mothers who commit filicide. This difference is in keeping with the lesser number of psychoses in the neonaticide group. Victoroff[70] notes that there is some appreciation that a mother who destroys her own child constructs enough guilt in this act to punish her sufficiently for her crime. Juries often find that the woman accused of neonaticide does not correspond to their imagination of a murderess. For no other crime is there such a lack of convictions.[30] Even those who are convicted often receive only probation or minimal prison sentences.

11

Legal Considerations

To understand the current legal status of infant murder, it is instructive to review the English laws regarding this crime. In the reign of James I, the law presumed an illegitimate newborn found dead to have been murdered by its mother unless she could prove by at least one witness that the child was born dead.[70] In 1803, the same rules of evidence and presumption became required as in other murders.[26] Death sentences for this crime were almost invariably commuted.[43] Juries hesitated to find a verdict of guilty and send the accused to the gallows. Abse states, "those juries knew that at or about the time of birth, dogs, cats, and sows ... sometimes killed their own young. They were not prepared to extend less compassion and concern to a mentally sick woman than they would to an excitable bitch."[1]

A desire to make the punishment more appropriate to the crime led to the Infanticide Act of 1922. This act reduced the penalties to those of manslaughter for a woman who killed her newly born child while the "balance of her mind was disturbed from the effect of giving birth."[43] Critics of this law suggest that if a woman were insane at the time of the crime, she should be held not responsible, rather than be convicted of a lesser crime.[7]

Several countries in Europe provide lesser penalties for infanticide than for adult murder. These universally apply only to the mother; if a father kills a newborn child, he is charged with murder.[33, 54] In the United States, there is no legal distinction between the murder of adults and the murder of infants. Although it is a common occurrence to find dead newborn infants in sewers, alleys, and incinerators in any metropolitan community, convictions are rare because of the difficulty in proving the guilt of those responsible.[3] Several states have passed laws against the more easily prosecuted offense of concealment of birth.

In order to convict an individual of infanticide, it must be proven that he killed the infant by a specific act of commision or omission.[15] It must also be proven that the infant breathed and had a viable separate existence from the mother after being fully extruded from the birth canal. Proving live birth was made easier by Swammerdam's discovery in 1667 that fetal lungs would float on water if respiration had occurred.[56] However, this test was found to be not infallible, and even careful microscopic examination of neonatal lungs today does not always reveal a definitive answer.[3] The other vexing forensic problem is to prove that the child was completely born. It is theoretically possible for a woman to cut the throat of her half-born infant, report the incident to the authorities, and therefore escape prosecution for either murder or concealment. Such cases have been reported.[13, 14]

12

Prevention

There are conflicting opinions in the literature about the likelihood of a parent's killing a second child. At one extreme, Elsasser[21] suggests that the death sentence for these parents can be an "act of grace". On the other hand, Batt[8] does not even advise against future pregnancies for the mother who kills during a post-partum depression. However, only one study[68] reports a follow-up on filicides. Recurrent depressions often requiring re-hospitalization were common. Occasionally, there is an attempt to repeat the act. Due to the gravity of the prognosis, careful consideration must be given to each case before hospital discharge. The likelihood of a woman killing a second newborn child after standing trial for neonaticide is very slim. There are a few reports in which a mother did kill two[19, 74] or three[10, 25] successive newborns. However, in all but one case, the previous neonaticides were undiscovered and unpunished. There is a greater chance of recidivism if the crime was consistent with the life style of the mother.

Three-quarters of the parents who committed filicide showed psychiatric symptoms prior to their deed. Some mothers talked openly of suicide and even expressed concern about the future of their children. It is discouraging that a full 40% of these parents were seen by a physician shortly before their crimes. Obstetricians should be alert to the filicidal potential of all depressed parents, particularly mothers considering suicide. The danger is increased if there is a strong parental identification with an "overloved" child. A direct question about the fate of the children may be helpful in assessing the inseparability of the parent-child bond. Absolute indications for hospitalizing these parents are their fears about harming their children and overconcern about their children's health. Evidence of hostility toward the favorite child of a loathed spouse is another cause for concern.

On the other hand, direct medical intervention to prevent neonaticide is much more difficult. It is common for these mothers not to seek any pre-natal care at all. It is not possible to get accurate figures on the incidence of neonaticide because so many cases are never discovered. Published figures do suggest a decline of neonaticide in the last century. [13, 14, 24, 28, 29, 53, 55] Several factors may contribute to this decline. Effective birth control measures are now widely available. Since the advent of antibiotics, abortions are rarely life-threatening. Homes for unwed mothers have become available as a shelter from the "scoff and scorn of a taunting world", and placement of unwanted children can often be arranged. Finally, welfare payments today have reduced the prospect of being destitute. Yet, in spite of these advances, thousands of neonaticides still occur in the United States alone each year. One way to further reduce the incidence of neonaticide would be a liberalization of abortion laws. Although this approach is far from ideal, it would offer a woman a less cruel alternative than killing her newborn infant. Each infanticide is tragic, not only for the infant, but also for the ongoing effect which the crime has on the life of the parent. To convey the ongoing anguish of these parents, I will conclude with Medea's thoughts upon her double filicide:

> To die by other hands more merciless than mine—
> No; I who gave them life will give them death.
> Oh, now no cowardice, no thought how young they are,
> How dear they are, how when they first were born—
> Not that—I will forget they are my sons.
> One moment, one short moment; then forever sorrow.[32]

REFERENCES

1. ABSE, L. 1967. Infanticide and British Law. *Clin. pediat. (Bologna)*, **6**, 316.
2. ADELSON, L. 1964. Homicide by pepper. *J. forens. Sci.*, **9**, 391.
3. ADELSON, L. 1959. Some medicolegal observations on infanticide. *J. forens. Sci.*, **4**, 60.
4. ANTHONY, E. J. 1969. A group of murderous mothers. *Acta psychother. (Basel)*, **7**, (Supp.) pt. 2:1.
5. ASCH, S. S. 1968. Crib deaths: their possible relationship to post-partum depression and infanticide. *J. Mt. Sinai Hosp.*, **35**, 214.
6. BAKER, J. 1902. Female criminal lunatics: a sketch. *J. ment. Sci.*, **48**, 13.
7. BARTHOLOMEW, A. A. and BONNICI, A. 1965. Infanticide: a statutory offence. *Med. J. Aust.*, **2**, 1018.
8. BATT, J. C. 1948. Homicidal incidence in depressive psychoses. *J. ment. Sci.*, **94**, 782.
9. BENDER, L. 1934. Psychiatric mechanisms in child murderers. *J. nerv. ment. Dis.*, **80**, 32.
10. BUHTZ, G. 1942. Totung von Drei neugeborenen Kindern durch die eigene eheliche Mutter. *Arch. Kriminol.*, **110**, 14.
11. CARP, E. A. D. E. 1947. Psychologic study of murder of own child; Case. *Ned. T. Geneesk.*, **91**, 1766.
12. CHAPMAN, A. H. 1959. Obessions of infanticide. *Arch. gen Psychiat.*, **1**, 12.
13. CURGENAVEN, J. B. 1888–9. Infanticide, baby-farming and the Infant Life Protection Act, 1872. *Sanit. Rec., London*, **10**, 409, 461.
14. CURGENAVEN, J. B. 1889–90. Infanticide, baby-farming and the Infant Life Protection Act, 1872. *Sanit. Rec., London*, **11**, 4, 415.
15. DEADMAN, W. J. 1964. Infanticide. *Canad. med. Ass. J.*, **91**, 558.
16. DELAY, J., LEMPERIERE, T., ESCOUROLLE, R. and DEREAX, J. F. 1957. Contribution a l'étude de l'infanticide-pathologique. *Sem. Hop. Paris*, **33**, 4068.
17. DeVALLET, J. and SCHERRER, P. 1939. Un cas de psychose de dégoût conjugal avec réaction infanticide. *Ann. med. psychol.* (pt. 2), **97**, 80.
18. DEVEREUX, G. 1948. Mohave Indian infanticide. *Psychoanal. Rev.*, **35**, 126.
19. DOERR, F. 1916. Doppel-Kindsmord. *Arch. Kriminol.*, **65**, 148.
20. DONALIES, G. 1949. Selbstmord und Brandstiftung. *Nervenarzt*, 20, 133.
21. ELSASSER, G. 1939. Zur Frage des "Familien- und Selbstmordes," *Allgemeine Zeitschrift für Psychiatrie und ihre Grenzgebiete mit Beilage Zeitschrift für psychische Hygiene*, **110**, 207.
22. FEINSTEIN, H. M., PAUL, N. and PATTISON, E. 1964. Group therapy for mothers with infanticidal impulses. *Amer. J. Psychiat.*, **120**, 882.
23. GARBER, C. M. 1947. Eskimo infanticide. *Sci. Monthly*, **64**, 98.
24. GILLI, R. 1952. L'infanticidio nella Provincia di Firenze nel Cinquantennio. *Minerva med.-leg.*, **72**, 135.
25. GLOS. 1905. Eine rückfallige Kindsmorderin. *Arch. Kriminol.*, **20**, 49.
26. GREAVES, G. 1862–3. Observations on some of the causes of infanticide. *Tr. Manch. statist. Soc.*, **1**.
27. GRIFFITHS, W. H. 1873. Infanticide. *Lancet*, ii, 519.
28. GRZYWO-DABROWSKI, W. 1928. L'avortement et l'infanticide à Varsovie après la Guerre. *Ann. Med. lég.*, **8**, 545.
29. GUARESCHI, G. 1940. L'infanticidio commesso su gemelli. *Arch. Antrop. crim.*, **60**, 870.
30. GUMMERSBACH, K. 1938. Die kriminalpsychologische Persönlichkeit der Kindesmödernnen und ihre Wertung im gerichtsmedizinischen Gutachten. *Wien. med. Sschr.*, **88**, 1151.

31. HACKFIELD, A. W. 1934. Crimes of unintelligible motivation as representing an initial symptom of an insidiously developing schizophrenia; study of comparative effects of penitentiary vs. hospital regime on such cases. Amer. J. Psychiat., 91, 639.

32. HAMILTON, E. 1942. Mythology. Boston: Little, Brown and Co.

33. HARDER, T. 1967. The psychopathology of infanticide. Acta. psychiat. scand., 43, 196.

34. HAUN, K. July 1927. Beitrag zur Lehre vom Kindesmord. Dtsch. Z. ges. gerichtl. Med., 10, 58.

35. HIRSCHMANN, V. J. and SCHMITZ, E. 1958. Structural analysis of female infanticide. Z. Psychother. med. Psychol., 8, 1.

36. HOOVER, J. E. 1966. Uniform Crime Reports—1966. Washington, D.C.: U.S. Government Printing Office.

37. HOPWOOD, J. S. 1927. Child murder and insanity. J. ment. Sci., 73, 98.

38. KEMPE, C. H, SILVERMAN, F. M., STEELE, B. F., DROEGEMUELLER, W., and SILVER, H. K. 1962. The battered-child syndrome. J.A.M.A., 181, 17.

39. KOCKEL. 1930. Mord durch Schwefelsaure. Dtsch. Z ges. gerichtl, Med., 15, 253.

40. KOMINE, S. 1938. Parent suicide and child murder in Japan (abstract). Amer. J. Psychiat., 95, 487.

41. KRETSCHMER, E. 1934. A textbook of medical psychology, trans. by E. B. Strauss. London: Oxford University Press.

42. LEY, A. 1940. Infanticide et jealousie. Rev. Droit pen., 40, 30.

43. MATHESON, J. C. M. 1941. Infanticide. Med.-leg. Rev., 9, 135.

44. MCDERMAID, G. and WINKLER, E. G. 1955. Psychopathology of infanticide. J. clin. expl. Psychopath., 16, 22.

45. MEYERSON, A. T. 1966. Amnesia for homicide ("pedicide"): its treatment with hypnosis. Arch. gen. Psychiat., 14, 509.

46. MODY, C. R. 1849. An essay on female infanticide; to which the prize offered by the Bombay Government for the second-best essay against female infanticide among the Jodajas and other Rajpoot tribes of Guzerat was awarded, Bombay.

47. MORTON, J. H. 1934. Female homicides. J. ment. Sci., 80, 64.

48. NIEDENTHAL, R. 1938. Eine Verbrechersippe. Öff. Gesundh. Dienst. III, 24, 966.

49. OATES, W. and O'NEILL, E. JR. (eds.). 1938. "Medea", by Euripides. In The complete Greek drama, 1. New York: Random House.

50. OLIVE, R. O. 1967. Filicide (abstract). Roche Report: Frontiers of Hospital Psychiatry, 4, (no. 22), 3.

51. PAUL, C. 1942. Infanticide sadique. Ann. med.-leg., 22, 173.

52. PFISTER-AMMENDE, M. 1937. Zwei Fälle von Kindstotung in Psychiatrischev. Beurteilung. Schweiz. Arch. Neurol. Psychiat., 39, 373.

53. PINKHAM, J. G. 1883. Some remarks upon infanticide, with report of a case of infanticide by drowning. Boston med. surg. J., 109, 411.

54. POLLACK, O. 1950. The criminality of women. Philadelphia: University of Pennsylvania Press.

55. PUPPE, G. 1917. Zur Psychologie und Prophylaxe des Kindesmordes. Dtsch. med. Wschr., 43, 609.

56. RADBILL, X. 1968. History of child abuse and infanticide. In The battered child (R. E. Helfer and C. H. Kempe, eds.). Chicago: University of Chicago Press.

57. REICHARD, S. and TILLMAN, C. 1950. Murder and suicide as defenses against schizophrenic psychosis. J. clin. Psychopath., 11, 149.

58. Relative prevalence of infanticide in Japan and China. 1885. Tokyo, Trans. (Discussion) 47, Supple. 12, 137.

59. RESNICK, P. J. 1969. Child murder by parents: a psychiatric review of filicide. Amer. J. Psychiat., 126, 325.

60. RESNICK, P. J. 1970. Murder of the newborn: A psychiatric review of neonaticide. *Amer. J. Psychiat.*, **126**, 1414.

61. RHEINGOLD, J. C. 1967. *The mother, anxiety, and death; the catastrophic death complex.* Boston: Little, Brown and Co.

62. RHEINGOLD, J. C. 1964. *The fear of being a woman; a theory of maternal destructiveness.* New York: Grune and Stratton.

63. RYAN, W. B. 1857. Child-murder in its sanitary and social bearings. *Sanit. Rec., London*, **4**, 165.

64. SARRAT, J. 1911–12. De l'infanticide dans ses rapports avec les psychoses transitoires des femmes en couches. *Faculté de Médecine et de Pharmacie de Lyon*, **40**.

65. SCOTT, D. 1826. Case of infanticide. *Edinb. med. J.*, **26**, 62.

66. SLATER, A. L. 1961. Infanticide—report of two cases. *Med. J. Aust.*, **48**, 819.

67. STERN, E. S. 1948. The Medea complex: mother's homicidal wishes to her child. *J. Ment. Sci.*, **94**, 321.

68. TUTEUR, W. and GLOTZER, J. 1966. Further observations on murdering mothers *J. forens. Sci.*, **11**, 373.

69. TUTEUR, W. and GLOTZER, J. 1959. Murdering mothers. *Amer. J. Psychiat.*, **116**, 447.

70. VICTOROFF, V. M. 1955. A case of infanticide related to psychomotor automatism; psychodynamic, physiological, forensic and sociological considerations. *J. clin. exp. Psychopath.*, **16**, 191.

71. WERTHAM, F. 1937. The catathymic crisis: clinical entity. *Arch. Neurol. Psychiat.*, **37**, 974.

72. WERTHAM, F. 1949. "Medea in modern dress", in *The show of violence* by F. Wertham. Garden City, New York: Doubleday.

73. WEST, D. J. 1966. Murder followed by suicide. Cambridge, Mass: Harvard Univ. Press.

74. WINNIK, H. Z. 1963. Psychopathology of infanticide, a case study. *Israel Ann. Psychiat. Related Disciplines*, **1**, 293.

75. WISEMAN, R. 1855. Medico-legal investigation: child murder. *Edinb. med. J.*, **1**, 492.

76. WITTELS, F. 1944. Psychoanalysis and literature, in *Psychoanalysis today* (S. Lorand, ed.). Albany, N.Y.: Boyd Printing Co.

77. WORDSWORTH, W. "We Are Seven", in *The home book of verse.* Vol. I, 316. 1965. (B. E. Stevenson, ed.). New York: Holt, Rinehart, and Winston.

78. ZILBOORG, G. 1931. Depressive reactions related to parenthood. *Amer. J. Psychiat.*, **87**, 927.

XXIII

ILLEGITIMACY

ALFRED WHITE FRANKLIN

M.B., B.CH., F.R.C.P.

Physician in Charge, Department of Child Health,
Saint Bartholomew's Hospital, E.C.I
Paediatrician, Queen Charlotte's Maternity Hospital
London
England

1

Introduction

Illegitimacy is defined as the state of a person born out of wedlock. A growing tenderness towards all who are deemed unfortunate in the modern world has produced attempts to soften the semantic asperity of the old English word "bastard", once used to describe the person in that state. The name of illegitimate child, less severe, is deplored by many because it implies some fault in the child. Modern usage has "child or baby of an unmarried mother". This describes exactly as the essential difference between legitimate and illegitimate, the fact that the mother is not recognized in law as enjoying the civil state of marriage. The distinction, known to Roman law, has been drawn in all stable ordered societies that are based on the family as the social unit and that are prepared to protect by law the ownership and the inheritance of land and property. The child has usually taken the social status of the mother, and not the father, and has no rights of inheritance. Most of the other legal disabilities have been removed in Britain. Nevertheless, if society allows its male citizens no more than one legal wife at any one time, some law is needed to deal with a human being who results from an extra-marital sexual relationship.

The pejorative implication of bastardy has long been diminished in the case of royalty, and consequently of the upper strata of any aristocracy into which Royal mistresses of sufficient fertility have been advanced. Descendants can well regard the heraldic bar sinister with pride. The exasperation remains for the possessor of an hereditary title whose legitimate wife furnishes only girls, while a mistress gives him sons. Many notable bastards have left their mark upon the world—Moses, Julius Caesar and Ernest Bevin, a notable British Foreign Secretary, among them.

Royalty, aristocrats and plutocrats are able to protect their illegitimate offspring, and their example is now being followed by persons who enjoy the status of personalities in the public eye. For all the others, whatever the law ordains and whatever society thinks about illegitimacy in general, the particular unmarried mother and her child face an ordeal through the social labelling process. Neighbours gossip, friends take sides, parents are blamed— "what can you expect", "look at the way she was spoilt as a child", "how badly she was brought up", "I always knew she'd come to a bad end". Many expectant unmarried girls, even in these lax days, are ashamed of what pregnancy reveals, while some show a brazenness that could be explained as the product of inverted shame. The girl often conceals her pregnancy from work or flat mates, parents and relations, and sometimes goes so far as to exclude its existence from her own consciousness. She becomes hypersensitive to the reactions of others, or to what she imagines those reactions to be.

Illegitimacy, because of the emotional reaction to it, which no application of reason can disperse, forces special attitudes and deviant relationships between the unmarried mother and the professional workers she must consult. Professional people, social or moral welfare workers, health visitors, doctors of all kinds, act and react not only as ordinary folk but also as professionals, as members of the society which makes the rules as well as advisers and aids to those who break them. If illegitimacy is still a problem situation, it is worth examining the reasons. It is worth examining too how it comes about that illegitimate babies are born at all in an age which publicises contraception, promotes the sale of contraceptives, and permits of easily obtainable abortion. In this Chapter I propose to discuss the incidence, the causation (aetiology), the disabilities (symptoms), the management and the prevention. Some reference must be made to adoption and to the care of the unsupported mother.

2

Incidence

The incidence of illegitimacy in England and Wales in 1968 is given as 85 per thousand total live births. In the quinquennia 1881-5 and 1921-5 the figures were 48 and 43, a steady rate over nearly half a century. The circumstances of war appear to raise the figure, which reached 60 in the first and 94 in the second World Wars, with a peak just short of one in ten in 1945. Peacetime brought a reduction back to 45 in 1949. The rising incidence from 1949 to 1959 of 45 to 50 suggested that some new factors might be operating, and the further steady rise during the last few years, to 66 in 1962 (55,376) and, as stated above, to 85 in 1968 (66,806) needs to be explained, although there is a "clinical impression" that the incidence is once more declining.

Variations within any country, and between different countries, can be great, even between neighbours such as Scotland and England and Wales. The rate has always been higher in Scotland, an observation which seems not to support the popular notion that volatile personalities and tropical nights are important in causation. In the latter half of the nineteenth century Banff and Wigtown attracted statistical attention (Seton[19]) with a figure often as high as 25% (250 per thousand). In one parish, in the ten years from 1866, 59 mothers between them had 147 illegitimate babies, 2 having 5 each, 6 having 4 each, 11 having 3 each and 40 having 2 each. Local worthies varied their explanation: between night courtship, the incontinence of youth and want of moral training on the one hand, and on the other "non-resident concubinage", a prudent avoidance of marriage when incomes are very low, and the absence of that urban convenience, the prostitute.

Figures have always tended to be higher in the Scandinavian countries and this may have promoted the recent legislation in favour of the unsupported mother and her illegitimate child. In Sweden and in Denmark figures per thousand live births were 102 and 100 in the quinquennium 1881–5, 145 and 106 in the quinquennium 1921–25 and in 1963–4 131 and 89. Corresponding 1963–4 figures in Norway, the Netherlands and France are 39, 17 and 59. Experience of the great depression in the United States revealed a rise of illegitimate births by 12% between 1929 and 1934 while the legitimate birthrate fell. Economic depression and living on the dole seemed to depress marriage rates but to increase fertility. Discriminatory taxation against marriage and a high cost of marrying in relation to average income level could in theory produce the same results. No writer has yet suggested that the illegitimacy rate is an index of either morality or continence.

Difficulties of Assessment

Human behaviour can be interpreted in a way that is acceptable to the modern statistical analytical method only when it is compartmentalized. The enterprise is difficult, and data are hard to define or identify. Because the observers are themselves part of the scene that is being observed, bias from preconceived ideas, beliefs, assumptions, attitudes to life, to our fellows, to ourselves, is absolutely unavoidable. In the absence of exact data, progress in understanding fully the causes for illegitimate birth is slow, and efforts at prevention and at helpful management are often ineffective, clumsy at best, and at worst harmful.

Clearly too, the distribution of the compartmental fault or failure will vary between different cultures and, as is shown in times of war, in the same culture when living conditions alter dramatically. A list can be constructed from the literature and from experience of the recognized, or more properly the recognizable, causes of illegitimacy. Such classification reflects what appears to be the most probable explanation in each case—"appears to be" rather than "is", because there are often reasons within reasons and the central truth may escape detection even with the most refined analysis.

3

Aetiology

Personal Inadequacies

The birth of an illegitimate baby is the visible evidence of a failure by mother and father, both together, of a fault in one or more compartments of their lives. A life is a whole but 'no man is an island'. Nor is any woman. All who form part of society have legal, moral and social obligations, although it is fashionable in England at present not to accept them all but rather to select those which are found agreeable and to reject the rest. Collisions, head on, between those whose selections clash, are as uncomfortable as they are unavoidable. So, alas! are failures. But as well as legal, moral and social compartments which have no greater importance than society agrees at any time to give them, there are biological compartments which cannot be controlled by human reason. Emotional stability, intellectual potential and a tendency towards abnormal psychological reactions labelled psychotic and psychoneurotic, vary between person and person. Inadequacies, both in mastering inner drives and in adjusting to external stresses, can also determine failure.

Premarital Intercourse

Premarital intercourse is common enough not to be accounted a fault, a crime, or even a sin. Indeed to establish that everything works well in this important piece of married life before rather than after the legal knot is tied would seem to mark a prudent couple, and is the custom in some societies. Comparisons of marriage dates and estimated dates of conception have been interpreted as showing that in England and Wales the latter precede the former one time in four. The Registrar-General now estimates from confidential questions the annual number of live births taking place before the completion of the seventh month after the marriage date. The 1968 total was 74,531. When illegitimate are substracted from total live births and without allowing for the truly premature, at least one legitimate birth in every ten shows conception to have occurred before marriage. Sometimes the accidental death of the husband-to-be, or the discovery that he is already married, prevents timely marriage and hence birth in wedlock of children conceived out of it.

Common Law Marriages

Regular co-habiting of a man and a woman in a union blessed by neither church nor state contributes another large section. Easier divorce is claimed as the cure for this situation. But it is only an assumption that every man whose legal marriage fails wishes to make another legal contract; he might prefer the idea of freedom protected by the law relating to bigamy. In these two categories the presumption is that two people fall in love, that some circumstance, or simple prudence, stands in the way of immediate marriage, and that as far as illegitimate children are concerned, they can count on a settled and full family life. Such a situation has been called by Bowlby[3] "socially acceptable" to distinguish it from one which results in a social problem of greater or less complexity.

Adolescent Sexuality

Sexual experiment among young adolescents has often led to pregnancy in past years. How far society is wise to encourage this natural curiosity as a proper expression of the adventurousness of youth, is difficult to judge. It needs balancing by the use of contraceptives, of which the "pill" is the most popular, or of ready and free abortion. No one can yet assess the short, let alone the long, term results of these tamperings with biological processes.

Notions of Morality

It is impossible to prophesy what the effect will be on morals and behaviour of the acceptance of the dogma that chastity has no value. Fears of venereal disease and of illegitimate pregnancy no longer deter, since the former is easily cured and the latter easily aborted. "Whosoever looketh on a woman to lust after her hath committed adultery with her already in his heart" must have remained a counsel of perfection for the majority of Christians in the last two thousand years. Yet as a guide to conduct, even if lacking now the force of a moral law, it has probably helped to prevent many illegitimate births; the veto ordained by religion still operates. The ability to subdue or sublimate strong sexual passion must, too, have played some part by strengthening character and improving behaviour in other directions.

To prove these arguments needs solid evidence, and it may be that sexual frankness and free expression in the kind of sexual intercourse that carries with it no family responsibility will even be beneficial to human behaviour. What to an older generation looks like the rule of sex may look to the young like the deposing of chastity and the enthronement of charity. Chastity's attendants were often hypocrisy and repression. Charity's handmaidens are compassion and service. While never displayed towards the Establishment or to those known in earlier times as "elders and betters", who tend to be scorned rather than respected and noisily flouted rather than obeyed, yet charity with compassion and practical service marks one of the most notable attitudes of youth throughout the world today. Youth is involved in an attempt to realise a true brotherhood of man.

4

Investigations

A society that agrees to the abolition of brakes on human machines has a duty to take strong action to make the roads on which they travel safe, as well as to provide a complete breakdown service for the inevitable accidents of which illegitimate birth is undoubtedly one. The assumption in all this, that any adolescent or young adult given the opportunity, will sooner or later find the sexual urge too strong to resist, may or may not be true.

Studies of the *dramatis personae* could bring enlightenment. Cross sections of "normal" populations are not easy to examine in depth, although samples can be dredged up for questioning about their sex lives. It is easier to look at captive groups such as the university students who patronised a student health service and who were observed by Giel and Kidd.[9] Their records on entry could be examined after the pregnancy was diagnosed. For a university student a pregnancy is a major educational disaster, and presumably this leads to caution—an idea strengthened by the higher proportion in the Faculty of Arts than in that of Science, where educational aims would be stronger. Yet in a group of 1,422 women students in Edinburgh the incidence of pregnancy was 7·74 per 1,000. Giel and Kidd[9] compared the content and frequency of the medical consultations of 57 of these girls, before the pregnancy and excluding any pregnancy consultations, with the records of 57 randomly selected controls. The unmarried mothers showed more consultations, and more of them had evidence of psychiatric disability. For example, half the control group had no consultation, as compared with just over one quarter of the mothers; one in ten of the controls had five or more consultations, as compared with nearly one-third of the mothers. The mothers had a significantly greater incidence of neurotic symptoms, and more of them came from unstable homes. The effect was to drive the girls to sexual intercourse in a search for emotional security. Sexual relations help to give emotional security when they do form part of what binds together a man and a woman living a family life in a family setting, and they can lead a boy and girl towards a secure relationship which in the end need not depend absolutely on continued sexual activity. But there is no actual promise of emotional security in sexual relations, especially when the main object is the pleasure that the act provides. That emotional security can be found through sexual intimacy is a damaging delusion when either partner uses the other, the sexual act being the end in itself.

Other aims than sensual pleasure and emotional security are recognizable by all who deal with unmarried mothers and who have eyes to see. Pregnancy and/or a baby provide the most convincing technique for flouting parental authority or, although less effectively, for bringing a reluctant lover to the point of matrimony. More subtle explanations or statements of the sequence of events are available. Swainson[21] saw a conflict due to the ambivalent role in university girls of training for a graduate course and preparation for marriage, a conflict between head and heart, with a pregnancy forcing the issue between the two.

Leontine Young[24] diagnosed many of her girls as mentally sick people who prescribed a pregnancy for themselves or inflicted this self-punishment as a symbol of hatred felt for, but not to be expressed against, mother. Such subtleties do not appeal to the general public, either lay or professional, and obstetricians and paediatricians can be included among the professional general public. They much prefer the concept of the wronged or raped girl, sometimes sober and overpowered or, better still, doped with drugs or alcohol and then "taken advantage of". Such human wickedness of course occurs, especially in times of war or revolution or wherever the normal landmarks for behaviour are obscured. To suggest this as the usual cause for illegitimacy in the United Kingdom in the twentieth century would not be credible. A serious attempt to "know the reason why" would need the establishment of a psychiatric service in maternity hospitals and units to study many of the relationships between pregnant women, their children, their own parents, their husbands, the nursing staff, the doctors, the fact of pregnancy itself, and the prospect of motherhood in action. Observations of the normal and of such abnormality as illegitimacy would shed light on both.

In the absence of observations of this kind on a normal "maternity population" including a proportion of the unwed, some attempts have been made to discover explanations by questioning the unmarried mothers themselves in mother-and-baby homes. Experience of this kind of enquiry in a transit camp used as a "mother-and-baby" home during the Second World War showed among 460 unmarried mothers whose babies survived the first month of life how a pattern of reputed explanations could seize the girls' imaginations (Franklin[7]). "One girl after another gave the same story of rape in a railway carriage, or of mixed drinks on a lonely gun-site". By contrast, a note on fathers reads: "Married men having serious affairs outnumbered the rakes and rogues", an observation to be balanced by the statement that "the man in the case is missing from these records, as, so often, he is in life." Of the 460, 69 came from institutions or foster homes or were themselves either illegitimate or orphaned. This group contributed about half the girls judged to be difficult, a judgement strengthened by the later finding that they were the most likely to change their minds about adoption and, marginally, the least likely to marry. Of the 62 difficult girls only 14 came from apparently good homes.

The explanations given by girls then and now include ignorance or absence of contraceptives, inadequate sex instruction, alcohol and late-night parties, and ill-placed reliance on the man's promise to avoid the pregnancy. Are these reasons, or excuses? In Manchester University Anderson, Kenna and Hamilton[1] from the Psychiatric Department conducted a study of extramarital conception in adolescence in the Department of Obstetrics between 1953 and 1955. Their 62 adolescent primigravidae provided "an unselected sample of twentieth-century adolescents using the ordinary maternity facilities of their society". Aware of the earlier observations of Hans Binder in Basel[2] on 350 unmarried mothers, they sought especially, but failed to find, the psycho-social factors that he stressed. But of Binder's group only about one-third were minors, and the groups were hardly comparable. Binder's adverse factors included lower social classes, economic stringency during childhood, parental disputes and the disruption of the primary home. In fact about two-thirds of the Manchester group had suffered disruption of family relationships at some time; but these workers, like Binder, had no control figures comparison with which they could establish statistically whether the psycho-social factors really were causative.

In view of Leontine Young's[24] conclusions, described below, it is of interest that five of the Manchester girls expected to become pregnant and not one had considered abortion. Parkes[18] described three reactions of girls who conceived extra-maritally: personal rejection leading to panic and attempted abortion, denial, and acceptance. Of the Manchester girls 59 accepted, 3 denied, none panicked. The conclusions reached are not surprising, since 37 out of the 62 married the putative fathers, and with many, about two-thirds of the total, the diagnosis was really of accident complicating premarital intercourse and "formal marriage seemed merely to set a public seal on a contract already struck". Although about one-quarter resulted from casual or experimental intercourse, none of the girls was promiscuous. The amount of sex education in this group was small, so that ignorance could have been one factor. Only one of the babies was adopted, the others remaining with the unmarried mothers in their parents' homes so that these were, virtually, all in Bowlby's "socially acceptable" group.

Whether or not it is helpful to try to establish the exact cause among the "socially acceptable" group, the "socially unacceptable" require study, partly because the girl may need treatment to avoid a recurrence, partly because the babies need to be cared for, and partly because rational means of prevention, which can only follow accurate diagnosis, could reduce the number of family social problems. Most studies have shown a relatively high contribution of illegitimate births from mothers who were themselves illegimate.

The most exciting report is that of Leontine Young in her book *Out of Wedlock*, first published in 1954 and based on experience of 350 unmarried mothers. Certain patterns of behaviour during and after pregnancy emerge, and appear linked in a cause-and-effect manner with patterns of upbringing and parental outlook, and the inter-relationship between members of the family. Her most valuable insight is into the girl described as mother- or father-ridden. She has also interesting things to report about the adolescent unmarried mother, accounting for 40% of her clients, the unmarried father, and about casework. Her most dramatic conclusion is that one group of unmarried mothers, a "socially unacceptable" one, is of especial importance. because the girls need and should benefit from psychiatric treatment, or from understanding and facing the real underlying causes of their disturbed behaviour. The girl has a compulsion to act out an infantile fantasy before being able to achieve adult maturity. It is the pregnancy that is the evidence of being an adult and it is the pregnancy that is the compulsive necessity. The baby is unimportant, the child into which the baby will grow is excluded from thought. The father of the child is no more than the necessary instrument by which pregnancy is accomplished. There is no need for an emotional or even a social relationship, so that the girl hardly seems to know who he is. He appears and he disappears. The "urge for a baby has been separated from its normal matrix, love for a mate".

Leontine Young analyses the factors and circumstances in the past life, home and childhood that have produced the girl's psychological problem which finds expression in an out-of-wedlock child. Sometimes, having acted out her fantasy, the girl is cured. Sometimes she fails completely to comprehend the nature of her problem and the compulsive process is repeated. The picture that emerges is of a girl who achieves pregnancy easily, carries it well and does nothing to disturb it—in short of a girl who seems to want to be contentedly and successfully pregnant. The critical background is not so much a broken home as an unbalanced home, dominated ruthlessly by mother or father in such a way as to prevent the development of the daughter to maturity and emotional independence. The dominant parent attacks and destroys the personality of the mate, emotionally castrates a son, and gets in the way of a daughter's outside emotional relationships. Whether seduced and loved to excess by her mother or rejected and punished, the girl turns the hatred that she feels subconsciously for her mother against herself, and the pregnancy is a self-inflicted punishment. The dominance of the father ends in the daughter's pregnancy, the ultimate expression of her rebellion. These girls chose as lovers selfish, irresponsible cads, memory of whom was later clothed in romance or made the target of vindictive fury.

In 1960 two medical social workers at Queen Charlotte's Maternity Hospital in London decided to see whether such extraordinary phenomena could be discovered at their hospital. They matched 50 white ante-natal patients, primigravidae holding British passports and unmarried at the birth of the baby, with 50 women similarly qualified but married, and they were able to confirm Leontine Young's findings (Franklin[8]). However, it must be stressed that most of the premarital intercourse accidents would have been excluded by marriage in the ante-natal period and that Queen Charlotte's, by being a hospital not confined to serving a locality, does not attract a representative group of pregnant women.

Among those unmarried mothers whose attitudes and behaviour place them outside the normal are a group who inhabit a world of fantasy. Their complicated tales are full of drama and tragedy. Because their fabrications sustain them, satisfy any moral scruples that they may have and beckon them towards a blissful, extravagant future, they compel belief not only to their inventor but, by the contagion of enthusiasm, to the whole audience of doctors, midwives and friends. It is with real grief that we learn in the end that the framed bedside picture of the handsome father was bought in a junk shop, that the daily tribute of flowers has been ordered and paid for by the girl herself, and that she has manufactured in her own brain the promises that he will be coming from Paris or Buenos Aires at once to marry her, having somehow disposed of the obstacle of his impossible wife. These Münchausen maidens dwell in the unreal world of dreams, their lies being for them protective truth; but their babies are all too real and their problems defy solution. Statisticians, in an effort to find explanations for the sexual irregularities evidenced by their cold figures, think of poverty, custom, climate, religion, illiteracy and environment. But neither the behaviour of Leontine Young's mother-, or father-ridden daughters, nor that of Münchausen maidens could be explained by these terms.

Virginia Wimperis, in her classic book *The unmarried mother and her child*, steers a middle course. Her wish is to keep both mother and child securely among the normal citizens, while recognizing that there is something to be learned from psychiatric studies. Her aim is to inform social planners and to improve social policies. Central to her argument is the Midboro Survey conducted by Valerie Hughes. In this town of a quarter of a million inhabitants in 1949 the illegitimacy rate was 5·6%, and records and questionnaires were provided for 278 girls, many under sixteen years old with a peak incidence of twenty to twenty-four years. First-born babies came earlier to the unmarried than to the married. The majority (164) of the fathers were described as "fiancé" or "friend", known for anything from one to ten years. Acquaintance was claimed by 20 to be casual, by 53 to be short (up to three months), and about 40 there was no information. Social level ("the phrase has no precise modern meaning"), educational level, and mental level were not relevant. No information about the girls' own family background was collected through which a comparison could be made with Leontine Young's or Hans Binder's figures. Nevertheless, in the book by Virginia Wimperis,[23] one of the two mothers who tell their stories, herself the illegitimate daughter of a father-ridden girl, comes straight from the pages of *Out of wedlock*.[24]

Professor Crew,[5] among others, has suggested that illegitimacy is an index of ignorance, and that education in contraceptive techniques, supported by easier divorce, would largely solve the problem. In Midboro in just over half of the sample, mother or father or both were barred from marriage, but between 26 and 40% were free; and Virginia Wimperis finds it "not clear why they did not marry", especially as in many it seemed to be a deliberate decision. Stable cohabitation in "unofficial families" (Spence), all looking straightforward and being socially acceptable to neighbours, was the situation in 40%. In about 10% there was unstable cohabitation, the pattern being of an ordinary mother, a deserted wife with children to support, setting up house with a manual worker. About half of the remainder were illegitimate babies born to single women not cohabiting.

Wimperis, filled with compassion for the girls and even more for the tribulations of their children, stands at the opposite pole from Hans Binder[2], the Swiss psychiatrist. Involved in decisions about abortion, he wished to study the psychological problems which follow unmarried motherhood. He selected 350 cases at random from the official guardianship files of Basel. He found a preponderance of the unskilled, the uprooted and the underpaid. He found that many had grown up in disturbed, shaken, chaotic relationships. He noted of one group that, although not "light minded", the girls' first sexual experience was a matter of chance, without passion or love. Such girls were not disturbed. The largest group had frequent love affairs, hungering for the affection of which they felt themselves to have been starved, making demands upon the man which he was unwilling to satisfy, and ending even more disturbed emotionally and morally. He noted, too, a small promiscuous group, superficial in character, with originally a good capacity for love, but so damaged that only sexuality remained, readily indulged, perhaps satisfying vanity, but giving no pleasure.

What is important is the understanding of the problem which has led the girl to the point of an unmarried pregnancy. The compulsion to classify can be turned to advantage if the classification is based not on preconceived ideas and prejudices, but on observed data. The data must include the emotional life history of the parents. Some groups will be common to all cultures, others will be rarer in one than another. All should arouse sympathy and be met with compassionate understanding and without sentimentality.

5

Disabilities

The hazards for the unmarried mother, according to Christine Cooper[4], are emotional, physical, mental and legal. Greenland[10] omits mental and substitutes social and moral. Legal hazards are certainly common to all whose existence is by definition outside the law; but the socially acceptable, the premarital accidents and those regularly cohabiting, who form such a high proportion of the illegitimate population, ought not to suffer severely from any of the other disabilities.

The unmarried mother who keeps her child and returns to her own family is cushioned to some extent from strains; the one who has her child adopted may grieve, may be cured of her infantile fantasy or, without treatment, may repeat a pregnancy. The unmarried unsupported mother who tries to keep her child is the one who needs the goodwill and the active help of the community. In my own war-time study (Franklin[7]), where an element of selection entered since the women could not, for one reason or another, have the support of their own parents, 298 were followed up out of 460. Those whose babies were adopted were less easy to follow, only 82 of 179 having kept in touch with matron. Exactly half were married. More of those who kept their babies kept in touch but a smaller precentage had married, 70 out of 216. It was unusual in this wartime population for the child's father to marry its mother, the reverse of what happens when mother and father both belong to the same community.

Dorothy Levy[13] in the United States followed the fate of 54 of 72 unmarried mothers, and found that having the baby adopted doubled the chances of marriage. She observed that many of the single women who had kept their babies had made a success of it. Macdonald too[16] was surprised that the children's condition was "better than might have been expected". Information about 240 of the original 265 living in a Midland town, was collated with a five-year follow-up study. Half were living with the putative father at the time of conception and of those followed 30% were married within five years and another 40% cohabiting. Of the 15% of single women who kept the baby, 5% had had other babies. Morris,[17] after examining Birmingham records from 1950 to 1954, reported that of each 20 illegitimate babies, 17 were at home with mother or a near relative, 2 had been adopted by non-relatives, and 1 was in a residential or foster home. In this series the great majority were in the socially acceptable group. Of the children admitted to care, two-thirds owed this to their illegitimate status and the rest to the mother's mental inadequacy, illness or neglect. He makes no comment on marital status. For the purposes of this discussion it is assumed that the hazard for the unmarried mother is *not* thereafter to be married.

The hazard of a drift into prostitution is diminished now that younger women have become less strict about the preservation of virginity. The need for professional prostitution, too, might be expected to be smaller because of "the pill", legal abortion, and easy divorce. But allowing always that some women are natural harlots and that sexual intercourse with harlots has its own attraction for the perverse male, the proportion of promiscuous women is small in all reports on illegitimacy.

The hazard of a second pregnancy is also small. The exception is the unmarried mother in stable co-habitation, the growth of whose family is legitimate in all but name. The absence of a legal bond between mother and father is liable to cause the mother anxiety lest in one of those emotional crises which form an integral part of most marriages, the father walks out. On the other hand, as time passes, the parents may completely forget that they are not married legally. Leontine Young's mother- or father-ridden daughters run the risk of repeating their self-inflicted punishment, unless they are helped to an insight into the true nature of their compulsive act.

The hazard to the young mother's personality is a loss of self-esteem and confidence. Crumidy and Jacobziner[6] studied 100 unmarried primigravidae under the age of twenty-one in East Harlem. That they were mainly negro and Puerto Rican does not necessarily vitiate results. "They seemed", the author wrote, "to be a challenge to themselves, the neighbourhood and the community." This caused an initial hostility towards assistance, so that unorthodox techniques in social work were called for.

Hardest to prevent is the socio-economic disadvantage of the unsupported unmarried mother who keeps her child. A baby-minder during infancy enables such a mother to continue earning, but as the years pass, the difficulties increase. Whether encouragement should be given to this group so as to increase its size at the expense of adoption can only be decided when long-term comparative studies of adopted children are made and examined. What form encouragement could take is discussed under "management".

6

Management

A married woman, learning of her first pregnancy usually rejoices. For an unmarried woman, who is within the range of "normal", the news may give little cause for gladness, and it is usually kept from the man. Experience shows how difficult it is for most girls to tell their own parents, the prospect of confessing to them producing more anxiety than the prospect of the birth itself (Crumidy and Jacobziner[6]). It is natural for the pregnant wife, in contemplation of the baby to be, to wish to have it, to see it, to hold it, to feed it and to love it; it is as natural for the unwed mother to question every single one of these wishes.

Ante-natal advice and post-natal management, must take account of these differences. The unwed expectant mother needs a friend, one who will be on her side, without censure and without envy. The world outside seems hostile because, perhaps, it reflects the verdict of her own conscience. She feels unloved and rejected. Compassion and acceptance must therefore move her helper, but these feelings must not lead the helper into too close an identification, lest emotional involvement warp judgement. Both parts are difficult to play successfully, since both need either rare gifts for spontaneous, intuitive empathy or a depth, as rare, of self-analysis of motive and conduct.

Possible lines of action should certainly be discussed. Socially acceptable babies usually go to the cohabiting home or to grandparents, where the feeding and management are not affected by the label of illegitimacy. For the socially unacceptable the options must remain open. The mother must allow time for careful thought after the baby's birth. Now that girls come of age at eighteen, fifteen-year-olds, and certainly all older mothers should see and handle the babies of whose foetal presence and movements they have been aware during the preceding months. The mother is legally responsible until the baby is adopted. Hilda Lewis,[14, 15] whose work for unmarried mothers and their babies has been justly acclaimed, has stressed this point and the folly of encouraging the mother not to see her baby. She makes a plea for the better training of the staffs of maternity hospitals in the emotional and social problems of illegitimacy. A promise that a woman need never see her baby introduces extra tensions into a situation already tense enough. Sometimes there is anxiety lest inadvertently mother and baby might meet. Experience shows that they ought to meet as a matter of course.

Breast feeding, which is not popular today, should not be pressed; but neither should it be forbidden. The mother gains from feeling that, at least for the period when her baby depended on her, she was able to give it all that it needed. It is natural that she should love it at this time and that she should grieve at parting, if her decision is adoption. Grief is a stage in emotional healing; the excision of grief always leaves a troublesome scar. Forced marriage, in the interests of respectability but in the absence of the true foundations on which durable marriage rests, seems to be in the interests neither of mother nor baby—nor of father.

The temptation for the too sympathetic adviser is to lighten the load to the level at which it is a load no longer. The expectant mother is moved out of her circle before her shape proclaims her state. She is delivered where she is unknown, an anaesthetic is promised, so that she feels nothing of her labour, and she is told that she need not see the baby, certainly not feed it at the breast, and that it will be adopted without delay. So this biological adventure is reduced to a minor operation, removed from the spheres both of feeling and of experience. Such a denial of reality cannot be commended as wise. Parallel follow-up studies on two groups of unmarried mothers— those who have been deprived of experience and the rest—would teach what is the best advice. However, until such a study has been made, the unmarried mother must be helped to face the consequences of her actions and to gain maturity through the experience of reality.

Should the mother be encouraged to decide during her pregnancy what she will do with her baby? Bowlby[3] is in favour of this on the grounds that all the factors are known at this stage, the potential of the mother and the socio-economic environment. But what is not known is the effect on the woman of having successfully borne a child. Nor can the condition of the baby be predicted, whether it will be normal or a mongol, have a congenital defect, e.g. spina bifida, or suffer from the effect of a damaging birth.

The Scandinavian countries Sweden and Denmark, whose high illegitimacy rates were noted in the discussion on incidence, have adopted extremely liberal policies for management. In Denmark early in this century Mothers' Aid Centres were set up to help single women in difficulties. The rise in popular demand for abortion drew attention to the troubles of women who, far from being unmarried, could be described as over-married, burdened as they were with the care of large families in poor housing under tight economic circumstances and in an unhappy marital atmosphere. A Pregnancy Measures Act was passed in 1937 (amended in 1960) for the help of any or all mothers, whether married or single. The Act was not operative until October 1939, the interval being occupied with preparing eleven

Mothers' Aid Centres for their enlarged responsibilities. These include family planning, sex education, contraceptive advice, marriage guidance counselling and adoption arrangements, as well as preparing the information upon which rested the decision to terminate the pregnancy. Dr. Hoffmeyer[11] describes how the materialistic approach has over the years given place to the emotional aspects of the problems of maternity.

Scandinavian populations are small and, compared with those in the United Kingdom, are scattered. Making allowance for this and for cultural and religious differences, any factual information about abortion is worthy of study by our community which is only now bringing abortion out of the back streets and into the open. Abortion in Denmark is by no means "on demand". There are four classes of indication: medico-social, ethical, eugenic and defective. The first includes dangers to life and health from physical, mental or psychic disabilities. The second—ethical—group allows abortion when conception results from a criminal act, incest, rape or sexual intercourse with a girl under the age of fifteen. The third depends on advice from the Institute of Human Genetics and from doctors conversant with teratogenic factors. The last is for those mothers who are considered unfit to care for children through mental or severe physical handicap. Acute panic, suicide threats and depressive states, induced by the first knowledge of pregnancy, are regarded as transient and not usually as indications for abortion. Under these laws, abortion is not regarded as the remedy for illegitimacy. Unmarried mothers could have abortions under any of the four groups of indications, but more often counselling with both moral and material support helps the unmarried mother to continue her pregnancy and to contain the problem. The 1937 Act gave a new status to the illegitimate child, attempting to remove many of the disabilities the prospect of which previously weighted the decision in favour of killing him in early foetal life. The Act with its 1960 amendment gives the illegitimate child the same right to his father's name and to inherit, as a child born in wedlock. The father, who must be identified by the mother or selected by a judge from those who might be the father, is bound to support the child. Where there is delay in payment, Mothers' Aid advances the money and it is the duty of the municipal authority, not the mother, to recover the cost of maintenance, which may be stopped out of the father's wages.

Support for the unmarried mother and her child goes farther (Mothers' Aid in Denmark 1965[20]). Special Collective Houses are available for some mothers. Here a mother can live with her baby while taking a training course in some career compatible with her continuing care of her child. After two years, her rehabilitation is considered complete and she moves out into the world with her child.

The supporters of these policies could easily be accused, both by cynics and by prudes, of encouraging immorality and of subsidizing sin. Mothers' Aid figures (Hoffmeyer et al.[12]) indicate, on the contrary, a decline in illegitimacy from 100 per 1,000 in the 1930s to 66 per 1,000 in 1955. A subsequent rise to 89 per 1,000 in 1963 is explained by the presence in the population of a large cohort of girls born between 1944 and 1949, since girls of fifteen to nineteen produce 40% of the illegitimate children in Denmark.

Despite these compassionate plans, the problem of precocious sex in teenagers remains, and is accepted as evidence of emotional isolation and of frustration in parental relationships. It may be recalled that Leontine Young concludes that, when the girl's pregnancy is the result of a compulsion, she cannot use contraceptives nor can she seek abortion, since both of these would involve her in a responsibility for the pregnancy which she is unwilling to face. Fostering or adoption by grandparents or a non-relative with understanding moral support and careful attempts at explanation remains the only practical steps for this difficult group.

The unmarried mother is no longer an outcast, but she is still not wholly accepted by society. Clark E. Vincent,[22] examining unmarried mothers with a sociologist's eye, puts their problems and our compassionate solutions into the perspective of society. They remain, he observes, a threat to the legitimate family. He suggests that support for illegitimacy weakens the group regard for legitimacy. As the status of the former rises, so the status of the latter declines. Less shame and less dishonour for the unmarried mother mean less pride and less honour for the married one.

7

Prevention

Can illegitimacy be prevented? If it can, by what techniques? Armed with pencil and paper and using his powers of reason, the social reformer can write down the list of available methods—sex education, contraceptive provision (with instructions), abortion and infanticide. The simplest preventive measure would be for every boy and girl to be given sex education before puberty and then to avoid sexual intercourse until marriage. If this is too difficult for wayward human flesh, contraception might be made obligatory for all extra-marital intercourse, although the rule would need strengthening by dire penalties for its breach. And as no contraceptive method when put into practice by human beings is one hundred per cent effective, the accidental pregnancy would have, by law, to be aborted or, were it diagnosed too late, would need to be made harmless by a legalised infanticide.

What will *not* prevent illegitimacy is to fill the world with erotic stimuli, to neglect religion, to remove by precept and example all control of human desires, to provide some sex education too late and to expect the young to use contraceptives when their adventurous nature leads them to look on contraception as a cowardly practice. Abortion at present may or may not be available and may or may not be requested, while abhorrence places a veto on infanticide. As with so much in modern life, the techniques are fashioned, waiting for use, but the human spirit, uncontrollable by the human intellect and the human will, tormented by desires and deaf to the voice of conscience, demands the right to choose.

Unfortunately, the complexities of human relationships, compulsive actions and the confusions of family life still remain. Only when self-discipline is seen to be a worthy aim, despite its seeming to be no more than its own reward, will the problem of illegitimacy be truly solved. Yet the social reformer should not despair. Let him turn his attention to the illegitimate child, to study how best to help him to become a mature, adjusted adult, strengthened rather than demoralised by the knowledge of the circumstances of his birth.

REFERENCES

1. ANDERSON, E. W., KENNA, J. C. and HAMILTON, M. W. 1960. A study of extramarital conception in adolescence. *Psychiat. Neurol. (Basel)*, **139**, 313.
2. BINDER, H. 1941. *Die unehelihe Mutterschaft.* Bern: Huber.
3. BOWLBY, J. 1952. *Maternal care and mental health.* Geneva: W.H.O., H.M.S.O.
4. COOPER, C. 1955. The illegitimate child. *Practitioner*, **174**, 488.
5. CREW, F. A. E. 1948. *Measurements of the Public Health.* Edinburgh: Oliver and Boyd.
6. CRUMIDY, P. M. and JACOBZINER, H. 1966. A study of young unmarried mothers who kept their babies. *Amer. J. publ. Hlth.*, **56**, 1242.
7. FRANKLIN, A. W. 1954. Discussion on adoption. *Proc. roy. Soc. Med.*, **47**, 1044.
8. FRANKLIN, A. W. 1966. Leontine Young and Tess of the d'Urbevilles. *Brit. med. J.*, **1**, 789.
9. GIEL, R. and KIDD, C. 1965. Some psychiatric observations on pregnancy in the unmarried student. *Brit. J. Psychiat.*, **3**, 591.
10. GREENLAND, C. 1957. Unmarried parenthood, ecological aspects. *Lancet*, i, 148.
11. HOFFMEYER, H. 1965. Medical aspects of the Danish legislation on abortions. *West. Res. Law Review*, **17**, 529.
12. HOFFMEYER, H., NØRGAARD, M. and SKALTS, V. 1967. Abortion, sterilization and contraception. Experiences with the Mothers' Aid Centres in Denmark. *J. Sex Res.*, **3**, 1.
13. LEVY, D. 1955. A follow-up study of unmarried mothers. *Social Casework*, **36**, 27.
14. LEWIS, H. 1964. Unmarried mothers. *Corresp., Brit. med. J.*, **1**, 1636.
15. LEWIS, H. 1965. The psychiatric aspects of adoption. In *Modern perspectives in child psychiatry.* (J. G. Howells, ed.). Edinburgh: Oliver and Boyd.
16. MACDONALD, E. K. 1956. Follow-up of illegitimate children. *Med. Offr.*, **96**, 361.
17. MORRIS, F. S. 1956. What happens to illegitimate babies? *Child Care*, **10**, 4.
18. PARKES, J. 1951. Problems of early infancy. *J. Macy Foundation, 2nd Conference* New York.
19. SETON, G. 1882–4. On illegitimacy in Scotland. *Proc. roy. Soc. Edin.*, **12**, 18.
20. SKALTS, V. and NØRGAARD, M. 1965. *Mothers' aid in Denmark.* Copenhagen: Der Danske Selskab.
21. SWAINSON, M. 1961. *Student mental health.* London: World University Service Report.
22. VINCENT, C. E. 1961. *Unmarried mothers.* The Free Press of Glencoe.
23. WIMPERIS, V. 1960. *The unmarried mother and her child.* London: Allen & Unwin.
24. YOUNG, L. 1954. *Out of wedlock.* New York: McGraw-Hill.

XXIV

THE PSYCHOLOGICAL MANAGEMENT OF HANDICAPPED CHILDREN IN THE FIRST YEAR OF LIFE

DAVID MORRIS

F.R.C.P., D.C.H.

Paediatrician
London
England

1

Introduction

There are few conditions which call for such skill and sensitivity in immediate and long-term management as the family with the handicapped child. It is the management during the early phases that may determine the whole future attitudes of the parents, the siblings, and the child himself.

The desired aim is a family who can eventually accept the child's handicaps without remorse or guilt, and will treat him in a way which is neither over-protective nor too spartan. Acceptance usually implies a somewhat passive frame of mind, whereas in such a family it means an *active* process of achievement of "coming to terms" with the reality of the situation. There is the acute pain of disappointment, as in bereavement; but the grief need not impede an eventual positive attitude. If parents have affection for their child, they will be able to provide him with the essential requirements and the opportunity for him to function to the optimum of his ability. How the family and the child can be helped towards these ends will be the subject-matter of this chapter.

It is not inappropriate that in this series "handicapped" should be the adjective of choice. It was not all that long ago that terms like "crippled", "disabled", paralysed" or "defective" were in current use. "Handicapped" is not simply a contemporary semantic fashion: it indicates a basic change in attitude towards those who are "disadvantaged". It emphasizes, by implication, the ability of the individual, and at the same time recognizes the limitations imposed by the condition.

Recently the correspondence columns of the *Lancet*[16, 20] have carried strong arguments in favour of "handicapped" rather than "retarded". The very origin of the word, which dates back to the twelfth century, is not without interest. It originates from the phrase "hand-in-cap", a reference to the forfeit money being deposited in the cap held by the umpire by two parties competing in a game. It came to mean "a lottery to another, who offered something in exchange: an umpire being chosen to decree the respective values". By the eighteenth century it came to mean a match between two horses, in which the umpire decided the extra weight to be carried by the superior horse. It was then used for competitive racing, and finally the term "handicap" has been used to indicate that which holds one back, or limits one.

Whereas the ordinary well-adjusted person who is adequate learns to function within his limitations, hopeful and motivated by reward from his effort and endeavour, those who are handicapped may be imprisoned by the concentration upon their inabilities, and fail to utilize what abilities they possess.

There are, however, outstanding examples of mastery over handicap. One of these is Brown.[2] Only his left foot was spared in an otherwise totally incapacitating cerebral palsy, and although this was the only part of his body he could use for feeding and dressing himself, he eventually wrote a very worthwhile book, besides executing many interesting paintings. Carlson[4] vividly describes how his parents fought for his right to be educated, in spite of the forlorn total despair and lack of help they encountered from both doctors and educationalists. He is a living example of how an individual, with no apparent ability or use of his body, could become a pioneer and a leader in the struggle to provide for the disabled. Down's syndrome did not prevent Nigel Hunt[10] from writing his autobiography; and although an exceptional achievement, it does demonstrate that with opportunity, encouragement and belief individuals are capable of achievements never previously thought possible.

Guttman[7] has shown how those severely paralysed from spinal cord injury can be helped to overcome their disability, learn a way of life which is satisfying, and contribute to the community. Previously they were immobilized in plaster, and spent their hopeless lives on their backs, totally inactive and dying prematurely from preventable secondary infection. Children with limbs affected from Thalidomide taken by their mothers during pregnancy[15] have constituted a new challenge to parents, teachers, physicians and remedial medicine.

One such child, with all four limbs affected, was attending a school for physically handicapped children which was totally unsuitable intellectually for his particular needs. His father, with support from understanding doctors and teachers, found him a place in an ordinary preparatory school, where he has proved himself capable of leading the same sort of life as the rest of the boys in his class. Of particular interest has been the rigid and limiting attitude of those who have provided him with his prostheses. They could only envisage him moving when wearing them, which rendered him robot-like in his movements: once he was free of them, he moved around in his own way almost as quickly as the others. In competitive games he always won when the others had to race against him on their knees, as their handicap. Protective knee-caps and a lightweight low four-wheeled trolley have enabled him to overcome what were thought to be insuperable problems (Wigglesworth[25]).

A hallmark of civilized society is the way in which it regards and treats its less fortunate members, providing for them opportunities and facilities to enable them to function to their optimum abilities. In well developed countries, with the present relatively excellent state of health of the childhood population, there has been a gradual shift of emphasis from diagnostic and curative medicine to preventive medicine and health promotion. Visiting less developed countries exposes the circumstances and accompanying attitudes that existed in most countries at one time—physical disease which kills and maims significant proportions of the childhood population against a background of poor housing, sparse education and inadequate nutrition.

Preoccupation with survival determines the level of priorities; enuresis, sleep disorders, or food faddism are low in priority. The handicapped child is an added burden to an already heavily burdened family and society. The survival of ordinary mature normal infants is enough of a challenge: prematurity, "small-for-dates" infants, and those born malformed, fall by the wayside because of their relative unimportance. Society's attitude towards the child who is born with a handicap and the services which exist to help him and his family leave much to be desired. The struggle to help these children and their families has fortunately been considerably influenced by the interested groups of parents of the handicapped, who have formed themselves into "parent-bodies", such as the National Society for Mentally Handicapped Children, the Spastics Society, and the Spina Bifida Group in the United Kingdom. They have helped by revealing the scarcity of facilities available for these children's development, and have influenced both Government and society to change their attitude and provide for them, albeit in a limited way.

The prevailing apathy and the paucity of provision are understandable; for many of those who are handicapped—even given the very best of conditions—will never be sufficiently active and contributory to be regarded as useful citizens. There has, however, been a growth of humanism and an increase in tolerance towards the less fortunate members of society.

2

The Normal Development in the First Year

General

The natural development of the child during the first year of life follows a fairly consistent pattern. Sheridan[24] has provided us with the details of the normal "stepping stones" of development. By knowing how normal children grow and develop and what can be expected of them at different ages, we are enabled to detect the earliest deviations from the normal, so that they may be corrected or treated as early as possible.

Developmental assessment has become a part of the infant welfare service, and is already reaping rich rewards: the routine testing of children's hearing at four months of age has brought to light a number of children with auditory defects which might not have been detected till much later and after harm had been done. The "at risk register", which has now become widely accepted, pays special attention to those infants who have been at some perinatal disadvantage. Babies born "small-for-dates", those who required resuscitation or were in special care after birth, infants with neo-natal illness such as prolonged jaundice or respiratory distress syndrome, are but a few of those whose condition had put them at risk with possible effects on their development. The widespread practice of individual assessment during the first year has through experience improved the skill and efficiency of the Local Health Authority doctors in the preventive field.

Stages of Development

Each phase of development of a normal child acts as a stimulus to his mother to help him on to the next. It influences the way she handles the child and the way in which she carries out her daily routine care of him. Although, of course, he is totally dependent on her care to begin with, he does respond to his own needs, indicating in his own way when he is hungry or discontented, satisfied or sleepy. His growth and development reinforce all the loving endeavour with which the mother tends him and plays a big part in the rate of progress he makes. A mother with a handicapped child is deprived of such stimulation, and has to find other sources to enable her to cope.

One Month. At one month of age the child is beginning to show his awareness of the world around him, although most of his time is spent sleeping. He stops crying when he is picked up and spoken to; he is startled by a sudden or loud noise, and reacts to a soothing voice. Within a few weeks he will be smiling and beginning to watch his mother's face when she feeds him or talks to him. He will turn his head towards the light, and may follow a slowly moving toy. He has little control of his head at this age, but placed supine or prone his head will turn to one side. His hands are mostly closed with the thumbs turned in.

Three Months. By three months of age he will lie on his back with his head in the midline. He now moves his limbs more smoothly, and less randomly. His hands are now mostly open, and he can bring them into the midline over his chest when held in the sitting position. He can now control his head for several seconds before it flops forward. He is now visually alert and actively moves his head to look around him, either following moving objects or out of interest. He shows recognition of familiar objects like his bottle, to which he reacts with eagerness. He cannot yet fix his glance for more than a few seconds at a time. A sudden loud noise will still disturb him, and he responds increasingly to his mother's comforting voice. Familiar sounds, such as footsteps or doors opening, evoke excitement. He may react to sound by turning his head, but it is more likely that at this age he will move his head from side to side. He now looks at his mother as she feeds him and he reacts to familiar sights with smiles and excitement. If he is played with, talked to, or tickled, he will respond with utter pleasure. He may hold on to a rattle for a few seconds when it is placed in his hand.

Six Months. At six months of age he can raise his head from the pillow and lift his leg and grasp his foot. If supported, he can sit in his cot and move his head from side to side as he looks around him. He now uses his arms purposefully and holds them outstretched to be picked up. When his hands are held he will pull himself up and stand somewhat uncertainly bearing his weight on his feet. He can roll from front to back and may sit on his own momentarily. He will support himself on his arms extended in front of him when he is placed downwards on his face. He now moves his head in all directions non-stop, and he uses his eyes harmoniously and effectively in looking at small objects close to him, which he reaches out to grasp. He uses the whole of his hand for grasping; but when a toy falls from his hand, he soon forgets it and does not search for it.

When the six-months-old child hears his mother's voice, he turns immediatetly and vocalises freely, using single and double syllables. He laughs and chuckles, shows annoyance, and will scream if upset. He responds briskly when a noise occurs at one-and-a-half feet from him, by turning and visually localizing the sound. He uses his hands singly or together competently for reaching, grasping, and manipulating small objects; and he tends to put everything in his mouth. He begins to take part in his feeding by patting his bottle or attempting to support it. He uses a rattle purposefully as he watches it intently. With strangers he is still friendly, but he may show some shyness or anxiety, especially if his mother is not around.

Nine Months. By nine months of age any doubts about a child's development will have been confirmed or dispelled. Up to this time there is always the possibility that the child's delay in arriving at his milestones is due to a temporary slowness and not to inherent retardation. It is at this age that the handicapped child can be recognized with some certainty.

The normal child can now sit on his own for a variable time, and can at the same time turn to look sideways whilst he stretches out to grasp or pick something up. He starts to become mobile in an experimental way, attempting to crawl or shuffle. He attempts to stand by holding on, and when his hands are held he takes steps purposefully: the beginning of walking. He is alert, attentive, and observant. He reacts to an object of interest by reaching out and grasping it, first in one hand, and then using both, passing it from one hand to the other. The dexterity of his fingers enables him to use his index finger as a prodder and he can grasp small objects between finger and thumb in a pincer fashion. When he drops a toy he can direct his attention to the right place and follow it with his eyes.

The nine-months-old child watches with absorbed interest all that happens, and can concentrate on things for variable periods. He uses his voice to communicate, shouting to attract attention and waiting for a response. There is a musical intonation in his babbling, which is taking shape, and is recognizable. He understands, and says "Bye bye" and repeats "No, no". This is the stage of mimicry—both for actions and in speaking. He manipulates food and toys with skill and dexterity, demonstrating his hand-eye-mouth co-ordination. He tends to feed himself, for instance with a biscuit, attempts to hold the cup or bottle and tries to get hold of the spoon with which he is fed. When annoyed or unwilling, he uses his whole body and voice. Strangers are now recognized by him, and he relates to them with caution and uncertainty, immediately turning to those familiar if he is uncertain. This is the time when he can take part in games activity, like peek-a-boo, or looking for a toy which has been covered over.

One Year. When he is one year old, the child will sit on his own for most of the time and will be abe to get himself into the sitting position if he has been lying down. He crawls with great speed. He pulls himself up into the standing position, and is able to let himself down. He walks sideways, by holding on, occupying a lot of his activity, and he may be able to stand on his own momentarily. His manual skill enables him to pick up small objects with smooth accuracy, and he experiments with cause and effect as he watches what happens when he drops something, following its movement with an intent gaze. He indicates with his finger what he wants, using his own speech for it. His manipulative skill enables him to bang two objects together.

The one-year-old child responds to his name, vocalizes most of the time, and understands an increasing number of words, gestures and commands. He shows great glee and responsiveness when played with, and enjoys playing a game with a ball. He can drink out of a cup on his own, chews his food, but cannot quite use the spoon effectively to feed himself. He begins to participate in dressing, and understands a lot of what is involved. He puts less into his mouth, and skilfully places objects into a cup or box. Everything he comes in contact with absorbs his interest, and he reacts by looking, handling, and talking about it. He likes to have his mother within sight and sound most of the time.

Emotional Relationship

Up to three months of age the child is aware only of what he feels and experiences, he cannot distinguish between himself and the outside world. He is not aware of his mother's absence, and will react indiscriminately to anyone who looks after him. His range of experience is confined to hunger, feeding and satisfaction; and he is preoccupied with his mouth and its function. Experiences are transitory and he is susceptible only to what is happening at a given time, with little influence from what has been experienced before. His mother at this stage accepts his demands without reserve. It is during this stage that the infant learns by experience his reliance and confidence in those who look after him.

After six months of age the baby will be acutely aware of his mother's absence, and will react accordingly, at first by protest and then by passive submission. He has also learnt who is familiar and who is strange, and reacts accordingly. This is also the time when memory begins to operate. Levy[14] has shown how children can remember their inoculations, especially if the interval is short. A good example of a normal child's intellectual development towards the end of the first year of life is the realization that objects still exist when they cannot be seen (Piaget[17]). The baby's reactions will be determined by his social and emotional experience; a child who has had a good loving experience up to six months of age and then becomes ill will cope with the illness better than a child who has been deprived of good maternal care. Erikson[5] emphasises that childhood experience is not lost, but affects the psychological growth of the child for good or bad.

In every child's life there are stresses of different kinds which affect each individual child in a different way, depending on the severity and the duration of the stress and on the help the parents are able to give the child at the time and afterwards. If the stress is extreme, such as in a major surgical procedure, then the parents and those looking after the child will only minimally be able to reduce the pain and relieve anxiety by the most tender loving care. Children also suffer because of the lack of realization of the effect of such experience upon the child by parents and by doctors. Embargos on affection are imposed to avoid his being spoilt, toughening him up by infrequency of visits, and by limits on close physical contact. An infant with severe burns may have to be nursed in isolation and a bacteria-free environment, but if the infant's needs are recognized, then ways and means will be found for his mother to maintain contact with him, such as by telephone, or other visuo-auditory means. To cope with the infant's very deep distress, those who look after these children in hospital develop a type of "protective deafness and blindness" which helps them to carry out these painful but necessary procedures. In this process it often happens that the child and his needs are neither recognized nor met.

The Handicapped Child

Initially the handicapped child who has to undergo painful experiences starts life with some mistrust and uncertainty, due to the lack of fulfilment of his basic needs; these feelings can very seriously influence his subsequent development. His need for a continuance of loving, mothering care by the same person has been well demonstrated by Rheingold.[19] Babies receive more social and verbal stimulation when looked after by a single mother-figure than when cared for by a number of different nurses. A continuous one-to-one mothering relationship, which recognizes his deep needs, will form the basis of his long-lasting attitudes and images of people and relationships. In animal studies Harlow and Zimmerman[8] have shown how young infant monkeys react to mothers and mother-like objects which, if made of cloth, provide the infant with "contact comfort" that can prove more important than food. Some babies have been shown by Schaffer[22] to suffer less from a period of understimulation in hospital if they are both active and mobile, than those who are unable to be so active.

Much of what the child will eventually feel about himself will have been determined in the formative first year of life. His subsequent acceptance of himself will reflect his acceptance by his parents and the family. The appreciation of his aptitudes, and the recognition of his abilities will direct him away from his inherent tendency to be preoccupied by his own condition. This will encourage him to be outgoing and to relate to those around him, but it will call for a great deal of contact with him. Depending upon his particular disability, ingenious ways and means have to be found to stimulate him through different pathways: if his hands are disabled, visual, auditory and leg stimulation will need to be designed. Even if he is immobilized on his back, he can still be helped to play with interesting objects of different consistency. Sensory stimulation and what physical activity can be devised are all-important if he is to develop his aptitudes. Care must be taken not to overdo it; every child needs certain periods of inactivity.

There is an inherent tendency for the normal child to assert himself and to express wishes and dislikes. Whilst he enjoys the care he receives, he does at the same time start to demonstrate his own prowess as he masters each new skill and phase of development. He holds his rattle and bangs it incessantly. When he learns to reach out and can hold on to an object of interest, he will repeat the exercise and will learn to drop his toy over the side of his pram when his mother, or others, are present. When he finds his feet, having mastered crawling, there is no stopping his marathon-like walking activities. This is the basis of his individuality, personality, independence and character. The handicapped child may be deprived of many of these normal satisfactory achievements—aided and abetted by those who look after him. With the very best intentions in the world they find it easier, quicker, and "kinder" not to let him struggle with each of his daily tasks, thereby interfering with his normal growth of independence.

3

The Effects of Handicap on the Child

A child born with a condition which, like spina bifida for instance, requires surgical treatment, will have a great deal of adverse experience to contend with: restraint, pain, interference with his normal spontaneous activities and the lack of the ordinary reassurance and comfort he would normally receive at moments of need. We cannot realize what it means to a child to be tied down with a restrainer, to be always fed while lying on his back, to have contact with the world only through his eyes and ears, to be forcibly prevented from moving his body and establishing any physical contact with other people.

Sometimes there are *the effects of the condition itself*, as in the metabolic disorders, like galactosaemia and phenylketonuria; for without special diet both the intellect and physical growth will be grossly affected. Congenital heart disease may limit the child's activities, even in the first few months of life; if he develops heart failure this will render him an invalid. The pain and discomfort of congenital bladder-neck obstruction or intestinal obstruction, oral, facial, palatal, pharyngeal or oesophageal malformations will severely impede him, interfere with his feeding, and be accompanied by frequent vomiting. The effect of all this during the first year of life cannot be over-estimated.

At each phase of development the pain, the discomfort and the lack of satisfaction will preoccupy the infant's attention and mitigate against his moving on successfully to the next phase of his development. When a surgical procedure has to be repeated, the infant is subjected to further insult to his developing feelings and subsequent personality and character.

Certain conditions will be more harmful than others, involving especially *sensitive organs* like the mouth or the genitalia, which may seriously and adversely affect him for the rest of his life.

It is a common tendency to imagine that children with certain disabilities will all have the same type of personality and character. An image is created in the minds of parents that their child will be just like all the other handicapped children they have seen. It is almost as though there is no individuality about these children, and that they are all "very much of a muchness'. The disability appears to outweigh any particular individual characteristic. The child's likes and dislikes, the way in which he reacts to pleasure and to pain, his patience and impatience, are all seen as common to all; whereas each particular child has his own individual traits, reactions and behaviour patterns. This denial of individual personality is part of the denigrating effect that a handicapped child has on the parents, who cannot see any good in him at this stage.

However, parents of a child with, for instance, Down's syndrome learn to recognize that child's special characteristics, as they do with their other children. Emotionally handicapped children's reactions will be determined by their experience and what added burdens their particular disability causes; feeding an infant with cerebral palsy can make life very arduous for the child and his parents. In the child with spina bifida micturition and defacation entail a lot of effort and patience; the blind infant will suffer the physical discomfort of banging into things until he learns the particular technique of coping with the world. Another child, because of his immobility and dependence, may be deprived of natural contact with every-day objects and of normal interaction with others; he has to lie most of the day in his cot on his back, limited in his experience; this may make him passive, disinterested and withdrawn.

Infant and early childhood activity is continuously reinforced by varied outside stimuli of contact with people and things. It requires special effort by parents to provide the necessary compensation for the child's limiting disability; frustration, anger and disillusion are ways in which the child and his parents may react.

All children have the same basic needs for experiences of being loved and cared for; they build up their feelings from their day-to-day, minute-to-minute experience. Each of their wants should be recognized, and attempts made to provide for them. When the child is hungry he is fed, when thirsty he is given a drink, he is comforted when miserable, and given a cuddle for cuddle's sake. Mothers learn to recognize, understand and satisfy a normal child's wants. With a handicapped child it may not be so easy; for he may be persistently irritable, dissatisfied and difficult to settle. His failure to respond to her endeavours may be very wearing, and drain her resources, with increasing iritability and impatience on her part. The child will, of course, sense her disapproval, and this will add to her difficulties, especially when she is feeling guilty and tries to make up to him with excessive care and attention. This preoccupation with the child's needs will be influenced by his demands, which may leave little time and feeling for the mother to show her appreciation and approval of him and of what he does.

In the normal stages of development there is a close sequence of events as the child rapidly expands his activity, awareness and responsiveness, each evoking in his parents a rich feeling of satisfaction, which they express freely. But with the handicapped child the phases of development may be long drawn out, and hope may dwindle, until finally, when, for instance, he is able to chew something a little solid, the pleasure is very thin and there is little sense of reward for this attainment.

The actual physical contact between the child and his parents may be distorted by his condition. His paralysis may interfere with the normal holding and cuddling mothers practise with their infants. The healing of a large spinal wound may necessitate conscious avoidance of contact between mother and child. By nine months of age, the deaf infant is strangely apart from auditory contact with his parents and the world around him. The blind child is deprived of the visual, eye-to-eye smiling and head-shaking reactions of his mother; his only line of intake is from what he hears and by what he touches and feels.

If procedures have to be carried out, such as exercises for disabled limbs, as in cerebral palsy—an important newly recognized role of parents in the day-to-day management of active help for their children, (Finnie[6])—he may dislike them, or react to them with crying and upset which may cause estrangement between parent and child. The baby cannot understand that what they are doing is for his benefit; he only knows of the discomfort it causes, and becomes antagonistic and hostile. This does not, of course, make for easy relationships between child and parents; and even if they can overcome their reaction to his anger, it may still take a long time before they can see in him a response to the comfort they offer him.

Over-indulgence is very common with the handicapped child; for how else can the parents make up to him for all the disadvantages he has, and the normal pleasures denied him. The presence of a handicapped child in the family may have an important influence on the siblings—it can have corroding effects on their personalities, making them feel excluded and not all that important in the life of the family. Resentment and jealousy can affect their behaviour, rendering them assertive or aggressive, withdrawn or devious. Deprived of their normal love requirement, they may show disorders of sleep, feeding or behaviour, all of which add to the parents' problems. To find the right balance between sensitive and tender care without it becoming excessive, and acceptance of the reality of the child's disability without shame or remorse can be a most difficult task, even for the very best of parents!

4

The Effects of Handicap on the Mother

During the first year of the child's life the attitude of the parents and the way they have reacted to the situation will influence them in the way they handle the child, and may well have considerable bearing on his subsequent emotional and intellectual development. We know how normal children are influenced by maternal feelings and the handling they experience. The "growth of love" of a mother for her baby and of the baby for his mother depends upon a variety of factors: her wish to be pregnant, and the pregnancy itself, her relationship with her husband and children, the delivery, the sort of baby she produces, and her experiences in the lying-in period. Her own childhood and the parenting she received will determine many of her attitudes towards her marriage, her husband and her children. Compensation for her own poor background may motivate her to make doubly sure that her own child will get what she lacked; but if she over-compensates, it can be to the developmental detriment of her child. She may, however, like so many women, fulfil her own and her child's needs in a healthy way.

How much greater, then, is the disturbance of this natural process of mother-child interaction if she gives birth to a child with any recognizable deformity? What loving and cherishing feelings she might have had for her baby are totally disrupted by her anguish and despair, and it may take a long time before she can overcome her sadness, disappointment and anger at having produced such a baby. The effect of the impact will depend upon many factors; the severity of the condition, the psychological make-up of the parents, the nature of the family, how they learn the news, in what way it will finally affect the child, and how much independence he will eventually have.

It may take the mother a long time to establish a close bond with her baby and to feel confident that she can manage him without further harm. The deadening of her feelings at the impact of the "bad news" may be over-whelming and completely occupy her, leaving no thought or feeling for the baby. This ice-bound feeling may thaw if she can be helped and supported by her husband and by a skilled social worker; but the feeling may take the form of open and overt rejection, with adamant and emphatic refusal to see or handle her child. This is exceptional, but it does occur; and it creates a serious problem for the midwife, the general practitioner and the paedia-trician, who may have to place the child in residential care. It takes a long time before parents' mixed feelings settle. These feelings not only fluctuate between pessimism and optimism, between hope and despair, but also between loving and hating the child, and sometimes feeling both these emotions almost at the same time. This conflict of emotions may be intense and may interfere with the development of a comfortable relationship with the child. In a study reported in 1954[15] a number of parents of handicapped children admitted that they had experienced strong feelings of both resent-ment and irritation, mingled with their feeling of love. This leads some parents to push their children to excessive independence, while other parents cannot let the children develop any independence.

If a woman gives birth to a premature or an ill baby needing care in a special nursery, lack of contact with the baby may seriously interfere with her "growth of love" for him; thus it may be a long time after she gets home before she is able to identify with him and respond to his requirements. This enforced separation of mother and child at this stage can cause serious disturbances of the mother-child emotional relationship (Caplan[3]).

How much a mother does for her handicapped child will depend on her hopes and expectations. She may appreciate the "long-term investment" she is making, and the dividends she gets will influence her activities. Her reactions will be far from consistent, and may fluctuate between extremes of depressive despair and exalted over-optimism. What self-pity there is may be aggravated by the pity she receives from others.

The mother has to cope with the child's medical care as well as with his upbringing. She is involved in providing for his needs with affection, tender loving care, guidance and discipline, exactly as if he were a normal child. There is an understandable tendency for parents neither to apply the same control to nor to have the same expectations from a handicapped child, and to over-indulge and over-protect the child. The controls mothers normally apply will tend to be less, especially if he has required medical or surgical treatment, if he has difficulty with his feeding and sleeping, and if he is subject to discomfort or pain.

It is understandable that in these circumstances the mother should swing between an excessive zeal and a loss of hope; and this will impose a heavy emotional toll on her. She will succeed if she can find a balance between her extremes of hope and despair. The fact that so much can now be done for

children born handicapped will be a source of great comfort and encouragement to the parents. Medical and surgical techniques are steadily improving
and, even in such unalterable conditions as mental subnormality, social
acceptance and the services provided for these children will encourage the
parents to care for their child at home.

The ultimate aim of all child-rearing is to enable the child to function
with independence, to hold a job, to enjoy the company of others, and perhaps even to marry and raise a family. The handicapped person may be
denied some of these experiences in varying degrees; but parents can now
look forward to the help their child will receive to render him capable of
leading a life as normal and productive as possible. The earlier a child receives the necessary stimulation, correction of his deformity, and loving care
and attention both to his physical and emotional needs, the better chance he
will have to realize his potential.

5

The Effects of Handicap on the Parents

What happens between husband and wife when the child is born with a
congenital malformation may have far-reaching consequences. Whilst the
mother is much more directly involved with the child and emotionally
suffers very intensely, the father may also be seriously affected. At this time
they may find mutual support and comfort in each other, but on the other
hand they may drift apart. Sometimes parents can play at "make-believe",
conniving together to try and pretend that nothing is wrong and nothing is
amiss. This parental fantasy is well-illustrated in Albee's play *Who's afraid
of Virginia Woolf?* Such pretence can indeed become very real: they never
talk about the abnormality, as though by ignoring it they make it non-
existent. By so avoiding the reality, husband and wife become increasingly
estranged and the child too will be affected by this attitude that there is
"nothing the matter".

Parental reactions are individual and varied, from hostility and resentment
to sympathetic understanding and support, throughout this turbulent period.
The resentment may be directed towards the hospital where the child was
born, towards the obstetrician or the paediatrician, or, later, towards those
who treat the child and who fail to make him "normal". The loneliness felt
by couples in these particular circumstances is almost universal, and is
reinforced by their withdrawal from all other contacts. They may provide
each other with comfort by sharing their anxiety, but it can also become a
shrinking from reality. This self-imposed isolation may make it all the more
difficult for them to be realistic about their child's condition, to help him
to function to the best of his ability, and to accept him for what he is.

Part of the agony parents experience is related to their own feelings and
to the feelings they have toward their children as an extension of themselves;

so much of what we feel about ourselves determines our particular attitude towards our children. We strive to provide for them as a fulfilment of our own ambitions. We are motivated by our own "self-interest", vicariously finding satisfaction through our children and their achievements. Hence, when they are born handicapped the pain is all the greater if the parents have an inherent sense of inadequacy or a feeling of a personal lack of "worth-whileness". The whole subject of "self-blame" and guilt may be related to early childhood, when egocentric thoughts lead to believing that ill-happenings are due to our own naughtiness, or it may bring to light unsolved guilt over some past happening. The parents' self-esteem may suffer a severe set-back when a child is malformed at birth or is in any other way disabled.

Sensitivity is all the more affected by the attitude of near relations, friends and neighbours. Susceptibilities are highlighted when parents think the handicapped child has lowered them in the eyes of near relations. The child's appearance, his demeanour, the degree of obviousness of his particular deformity, and his unusual behaviour, will all add to the parents' sensitivity reaction to others. Indeed, it takes a long time and much work before they are able to withstand the way in which people look at their "unfortunate' child, the things they say and what they ask about him, as well as the advice so freely and frequently given—and of such little help to them. Sometimes, after they have made good progress, and feel particularly pleased and optimistic, a well-intentioned chance remark (often a reflection of the anxiety that handicap brings out in others), can bring back those earlier feelings of depression and hopelessness. At other times, when parents have got so used to their child's particular condition that it has become part of their every-day life, they may be very suddenly and rudely reminded of the handicap and its disadvantages all over again.

6

The Effects of Handicap on the Family

"It is no exaggeration to say that in the background of every individual handicapped child there is always a handicapped family", wrote Sheridan.[23]

Sometimes the involvement of coping with the handicapped child may indeed alter the whole way of life of the family. The interests and activities, outings and pastimes previously enjoyed by the family become a thing of the past. Parents often say to me: "I don't understand how I can still enjoy myself, when my child is going through so much suffering." They feel they ought not to be involved in any pleasurable activity which excludes their child; any pleasure they allow themselves seems to them to be at the child's expense. They can no longer have a life of their own, and this distortion may not, in fact, be helpful to the child.

If there are other children in the family, they can be very seriously affected, either by becoming part of the "unspoken and unfaced tragedy", with all the toll it will take of them, or by the interference with their normal upbringing. They may be helped to understand and cope with their handicapped sibling in a sensible way, thereby developing their sense of responsibility and generosity.

Public interest is reflected in an article which recently appeared in a Sunday newspaper:[11] "Without adequate help, the birth of a handicapped child can be the final straw that breaks a marriage apart. Often the other children in a family with a spastic child are in danger emotionally because the handicapped member of the family is given all the love and attention." Sometimes, to compensate for the failure of having a handicapped child, the other children will be expected to work harder and be more successful than others.

Invariably, the family of a handicapped child goes through feelings of guilt, resentment, confusion, despair, and overall isolation. Schaffer[21] found that if families do not break down they can become too cohesive, with the danger that the handicapped child may become over-dependent, because of the over-protectiveness of his parents. This over-protectiveness is intimately linked with having produced a handicapped child, and they feel differently towards him because he is handicapped; sometimes they think they are not doing as much as they feel they could or should. Their feelings may be in conflict between wanting to keep the child at home and having to consider sending him away because he causes the other children to be neglected.

7

Management

The way parents first learn about their child's handicap will depend on the attitude of the professional workers involved.

There is always an interval between the baby's birth and the moment when the mother is told of her child's handicap. The inevitable first question, "Is he all right?" is side-stepped or evaded with some non-committal answer. The grosser the deformity the more difficult the task of breaking the news. The situation is always intense and evokes considerable feelings of sympathy and solicitude, especially in the nursing staff who will do all they can to comfort the mother warmly and tenderly. While all are agreed that women are at this time in a highly susceptible frame of mind, this does not justify the withholding of the news and letting the mother believe she has a normal child. The emotional impact on the mother, however experienced and sensitive the staff, is always highly intense and varies from total numbness and depression to the extremes of hysterical and uncontrollable emotional reaction. At this initial interview there is little that can be imparted of a factual kind about the condition, why it occurred, what treatment is available, and how it will affect the child. But once having realised the situation, the parents are eager to learn as much as they can; and for this a senior doctor, preferably the consultant, should be available to talk to them, rather than a junior member of the staff. Perhaps the most meaningful service for the parents is the knowledge that the consultant will be readily available to see them in the coming months. One mother, whose first baby had died at four months from cerebral trauma, was referred by me to a consultant obstetrician for her second confinement; she later told me how she had been touched most of all by the fact that he had given her his private telephone number.

In those conditions which are present at birth and are easily recognizable there is, apart from Down's syndrome, no holding back of information, although there is often some delay before the news is broken and the mother is allowed to see her baby. There is added tension when, after having been told about her baby's condition, she is then shown the baby. Sometimes mothers are relieved, because they had imagined the condition to be much worse than it is. A mother may say that she cannot bear to see the child, but this is exceptional and, however reluctant she might be, every effort should be made to establish contact between her and the baby. The task is an onerous one, entailing much subjective emotion for the individual general practitioner, obstetrician, or paediatrician; but it is no different from breaking the news of a still-birth or a neonatal-death. Informants differ in their techniques. Sometimes the husband's advice is asked on how best to break the news to his wife, and not infrequently he will choose to tell her himself.

If a baby is born with Down's syndrome, the situation is often handled quite differently. Some parents recognize the condition and ask directly, "Is he a Mongol?" To this question there can only be a "yes" or "no" answer. But the majority of parents have no awareness that there is anything the matter with the baby. Paediatricians differ markedly as to when the parents should be told; some still say, "wait until the parents realize the child is slower than he should be in his development". The parent's suspicion that something is amiss is then confirmed by the paediatrician, who will then "break the news". This was common paediatric teaching and practice, rationalized by the belief that it was less of a shock and less traumatic if they came to the realisation gradually. But parents of Mongol children have made it clear that they feel cheated when they learn that the doctor knew all along and that they had been lulled into a false sense of security. From my experience, I am of the opinion that parents are entitled to know of their child's condition as soon as the doctor is sure of the diagnosis. I have not experienced a higher incidence of total rejection, which some contend is brought about by this method. Sometimes one cannot be absolutely sure of the diagnosis; then it is better to wait on confirmation or refutation by chromosome analysis.

In those conditions where the diagnosis of a handicap does not become clear till, say, three or six months, the parents are alerted and prepared by being told that their child might be "at-risk". The actual management of the parents and the nature of the initial and subsequent interviews are the same as in the first group.

The child born with a deformity, such as congenital dislocation of the hip, exomphalos, or spina bifida, necessitating immediate surgical treatment, creates its own havoc with the mother's feelings. There is first of all the anxiety about his survival, for understandably a newborn infant, so small and helpless, who has to undergo major surgery, is at considerable risk. So often, if not invariably, the mother is confined to bed in the maternity hospital or at home, far from the hospital where her child is being treated. She feels acutely the absence of her baby, who has with such suddenness been taken from her, and is uncertain whether her child will ever return. His survival is her main concern at this stage. Should he survive, she further wonders what sort of child he will be and how he will be affected by his condition and the operation. When the mother finally goes to visit him, she will be highly susceptible to how he looks and what she is told about him. It is during this time that she needs much help. The information she has so far received is likely to have been conveyed to her through her husband, who in turn may have imperfectly understood a young surgeon's or house physician's explanation. If the mother is in hospital, the ward sister will do what she can to bolster up her spirits; if she is at home, a devoted general practitioner may be able to give her some detailed information which he has gathered from the hospital. But the unavoidable uncertainty of the immediate and eventual outcome will be something that nobody can alter. Ideally, someone from the hospital, directly involved with the child, should visit the mother at home; this would be of very great help to her.

The help that can be given to the mother during this time is that of support, respect for her anxiety and concern, and care by someone professionally skilled, who can enable her to talk out her feelings. This therapeutic role can be carried out by a midwife, a health visitor, the general practitioner, or the paediatrician. It is a skill which can be taught and learnt. In essence, it entails the allocation of time, albeit as short as twenty minutes or as long as an hour: the ability to be able to listen to what the other person has to say, and perhaps the skill of helping her to express herself by such opening phrases as "Many mothers in these circumstances wonder what will happen", or "It must be difficult just to sit and wait for news about one's baby". The know-how of interpretation, proffered with such remarks as, "I have the impression that", or "I wonder what it must be like for the baby". There is a tendency for professional medical personnel to try to stop the mother from being upset by offering her "shallow reassurance" such as "Of course he'll be all right", when in fact this may be far from being the truth. What the mother needs in these circumstances is the opportunity to express her feelings and her anguish, and perhaps to be able to clarify her thoughts in so doing.

Whatever the condition, and whenever it occurs, the help provided should be more than just diagnosis and treatment; the understanding of the cause of the handicap appears to mean a lot to parents, rendering them in some instances more readily available for "coming to terms". By contrast, the insatiable hunger for an explanation of the "why and how" seems to haunt many parents. In a number of them, however, their personal emotional difficulty remains unaffected whether or not the cause of the disability is known. In those cases where the cause is unknown, there is a tendency for them to feel a greater sense of personal parental responsibility and guilt for the condition; whereas, when the cause is known, such as in a chromosome aberration, or a cerebral birth incident, they tend to dissociate themselves from it.

I would emphasize the actual technique of talking *with* the parents. Whereas the principle is applicable to all doctor-patient relationships, it is particularly relevant in this context. Balint[1] highlights the apostolic role of the doctor, and contemporary undergraduate medical training does little to change the image. The doctor who tells the parents may have little if any effect on them if he fails to empathise with their emotional states and particular needs. Korsch[12] in her work at the Children's Hospital, Los Angeles, has demonstrated how the doctor, explaining to parents about a child's illness, may be on a different "wave-length", even when he does what he thinks is right with great sincerity and effort. Objectively, on tape-recording, the explanation sounds excellent; but the mother, interviewed after the consultation, will express her dissatisfaction, and its failure to fulfil her expectation. This happens because at no point did the doctor allow himself to "tune-in" to her and so enable her to express her thoughts, fears and apprehensions about her child's illness. To take one example, an inflammation of her baby's ear, otitis media, a clear-cut medical entity, well-defined, and circumscribed, was linked by the mother with the deafness in other members of the family!

Except in dire circumstances, such as impending death or gross disease, time and its limitations are the commonest excuse for doctors imparting their information in passing, in a hurry, in a corridor. Why should it be so rare for doctors to talk with patients in privacy? Is it really that they are too busy, or could it be that they consider that their way of dealing with this situation is right? Their approach is rarely discussed, and what the recipient of the information they impart thinks and feels is not known by them.

In the psychological management of the handicapped child, the attitude and feeling of the parents is of the utmost importance; and it is incumbent upon us all to do whatever we can to help them. To achieve this end, both time and privacy are essential. It may even be time-saving for the doctor, who could otherwise (as so very often happens) be repeatedly approached for more information by the anxious parents. The professional satisfaction experienced by being positively helpful to the parents more than justifies the effort entailed.

Both parents (fathers are too often left out) need to talk of what they feel, although to do so may sometimes be both difficult and painful, especially at first. As with bereavement, there is a tendency to avoid facing the issue and talking about it, because of the revival of grief feelings. However, helping the parents to talk may provide comfort and understanding about the present situation and about the future; during the very susceptible period of the first year this understanding may indeed affect their attitude to the handicapped child, and the way in which they treat him.

The anguish, the forlorn despair, the sense of utter hopelessness parents experience are not easily overcome: and unfortunately they may be given little help to change these persistent and overwhelming feelings. It is no wonder that self-pity, so fruitless a state of mind, should be so common in the parents and in the near relations of a handicapped child. Part of the benefit that comes from such help is the way in which it affects parents in their day-to-day life, especially with strangers. Social changes in attitudes are reflected in the number of handicapped children now seen in public with their parents, who are no longer ashamed of them. Some parents may even use these social occasions therapeutically for themselves and their child: each time they can deal successfully with the embarrassment of being seen with the child and talking about him, they gain a little more strength and overcome part of their difficulty. Eventually they may even feel relatively comfortable whenever the child is discussed. However, there is a strong feeling all the time of wanting to hide the handicap, and so forget its existence—an attitude which will determine the child's own particular attitude towards his disability.

The individual's conscious realization of his handicap and all that it means does not of course apply during the first year of life; it is only the parents who are involved in this long-range and very real problem. The child's future will depend not only upon the degree of his ability and the degree of his disability, but also on the particular way in which he is helped to adjust and adapt to it, the compensations he can devise, and the sublimations he can achieve. The parents' attitude and the way in which they can handle him will to a great extent determine the nature of the outcome. The Danish National Institute of Social Research carried out an extensive study[13] on this subject and found that (a) when the physical disability is compensated for, the handicapped person has a relatively high degree of self-reliance while (b) social and working adjustments are negatively influenced by anxiety and depressive tendencies, even when the handicap is rather mild.

However, long before this time the parents will be concerned over how much their particular baby differs from his peers, and whether he will be able to lead a life approaching normality. The help parents receive during the first year may come from a variety of different sources—sometimes from too many, with consequent confusion. The general practitioner may indeed become the key person, depending upon the nature of his previous relationship with the family and personal reaction to these particular circumstances.

Quilliam[18] has pointed out that general practitioners may not possess the knowledge or have the personal experience required. I have known general practitioners who have become the most important element in holding the whole family together. It is not only his presence and his attitude, but also the practical help he can organize, that will enable the family to cope with the ordinary every-day events.

Such mundane practical details as getting the child to and from the hospital, obtaining financial help, finding someone to look after the other children, and somebody to prepare the meals, may make all the difference and save the family from being submerged. These problems can indeed be very demanding, and call for vigorous action to provide the necessary help to enable the family to cope. A "home-help" may be a salvation for a situation which looks disastrous, and a volunteer from one of the local parents' groups may be able to offer much help in an emergency. A period of relief from being with the child twenty-four hours a day may save the mother from giving up the struggle, and our realization and acceptance of this fact is most important in enabling her to accept such help.

The health visitor may be in the picture from the start when the child arrives home from the maternity hospital, or when the midwife leaves. She may be just right for that particular family, because of her personality and attitude and may be able to assist in many ways. For instance, she may introduce the mother to others with a similar problem, and, even if it will be some time before the parents are able to face such meetings, when they can become part of a group of parents with similarly handicapped children, such an introduction may prove of inestimable value. "You are not alone" is one of the dictums of the National Society for Mentally Handicapped Children; and if this feeling of loneliness can be overcome, the parents will then be in a better position and frame of mind to manage the situation.

The relationship between parents and the hospital specialists may also be helpful, especially when the latter have the ability to recognize the parents' needs. Medical social workers have indeed done much to influence hospital doctors in this particular direction. Medical social workers are often involved in assisting the parents of handicapped children; but, for a variety of reasons, their skills and resources are not used to the full. Hewett,[9] in her study of 180 spastic children cared for in their own homes, found that when parents were asked, "If you needed help or advice, who would you go to first?", none chose the hospital medical social worker!

Part of ongoing "counselling" is to forewarn and forearm parents for the many difficulties they will encounter. The quality of help that others, whoever they may be, can give, will depend upon their "sharing ability" emotionally and practically. "Supportive" is a common professional catchphrase, a convenient short-cut, which needs to be fully understood. It entails a sense of comfort and warmth, which comes from being with somebody who makes you feel that his mere presence is of help, and thus counteracts the abject sense of loneliness and isolation which is so common.

REFERENCES

1. BALINT, M. 1968. *The doctor, his patient, and the illness.* London: Pitman Paperbacks.
2. BROWN, C. 1954. *My left foot.* London: Secker and Warburg.
3. CAPLAN, G. 1964. *Principles of preventive psychiatry.* London: Tavistock Publications.
4. CARLSON, E. R. 1952. *Born that way.* Evesham: L. James.
5. ERIKSON, E. H. 1965. *Childhood and society.* London: Penguin Books.
6. FINNIE, N. R. 1968. *The handling of the young cerebral palsied child at home.* London: Heinemann.
7. GUTTMAN, L. 1956. *Victory over paraplegia.* (Sir Ian Fraser, ed.). New York: St. Martin's Press.
8. HARLOW, H. F. and ZIMMERMAN, R. R. 1959. Affectional responses in infant monkeys. *Science,* **130,** 421.
9. HEWETT, S. 1970. *The family and the handicapped child.* London: Allen & Unwin.
10. HUNT, N. 1967. *The world of Nigel Hunt: the diary of a mongoloid youth.* Beaconsfield: Darwen Finlayson.
11. KEENAN, M. 1968. Centre for spastics. *Sunday Times, 31st March.*
12. KORSCH, B. Personal communication.
13. KUHL, P. A. 1967. *The physically handicapped in Denmark,* Vol. 6: Psychological characteristics. Copenhagen: Teknisk Forlag.
14. LEVY, D. M. 1960. The infant's earliest memory of inoculation: a contribution to Public Health procedures. *J. genet. Psychol.,* **96,** 395.
15. New York City Board of Educational Research. 1954. The child with orthopaedic limitations. *Pub. No. 33, June.*
16. PAYNE, R. 1969. Deficiency. Correspondence in *Lancet,* ii, 1422.
17. PIAGET, J. 1970. *The psychology of the child.* London: Routledge & Kegan Paul.
18. QUILLIAM, T. A. 1965. Clinical communication—a contemporary problem. *Med. Biol. Illus.,* **15,** 66–68.
19. RHEINGOLD, H. L. 1956. The modification of social responsiveness in institutional babies. *Monogr. Soc. Res. Child Developm.,* **21,** No. 2.
20. ROBERTS, T. 1969. Deficiency. Correspondence in *Lancet,* ii, 1256.
21. SCHAFFER, H. R. 1964. The too-cohesive family. *Int. J. Soc. Psychiat.,* **10,** No. 4.
22. SCHAFFER, H. R. 1966. Activity levels as a constitutional determinant of infant reaction to deprivation. In *Child development* (p. 395). London: Tavistock Publications.
23. SHERIDAN, M. 1965. The handicapped child and his home. London: National Children's Home.
24. SHERIDAN, M. 1968. *The developmental progress of infants and young children.* London: H.M.S.O., No. 102.
25. WIGGLESWORTH, R. 1962. Thalidomide. Correspondence in *Lancet,* ii, 349.

AUTHOR INDEX

SUBJECT INDEX

This index covers volumes 1 to 5 of the Modern Perspectives in Psychiatry series, the figure in bold type denoting the volume of the entry.

Vol. 1

MODERN PERSPECTIVES IN CHILD PSYCHIATRY

CONTENTS

Vol. 2

MODERN PERSPECTIVES IN WORLD PSYCHIATRY

CONTENTS

Editor's Preface
Introduction   *Lord Adrian*, o.m.

PART ONE: SCIENTIFIC

PART TWO: CLINICAL

Vol. 3

MODERN PERSPECTIVES IN INTERNATIONAL CHILD PSYCHIATRY

CONTENTS

Vol. 4

MODERN PERSPECTIVES IN ADOLESCENT PSYCHIATRY

CONTENTS

Editor's Preface

PART ONE: SCIENTIFIC

PART TWO: CLINICAL